Spontaneous Hypertension

Its Pathogenesis and Complications

Edited by

KOZO OKAMOTO, M. D.

Professor, Department of Pathology, Faculty of Medicine
Kyoto Univresity, Kyoto, Japan

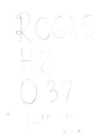

IGAKU SHOIN LTD. TOKYO
SPRINGER-VERLAG BERLIN · HEIDELBERG · NEW YORK

PUBLISHERS

© First edition, 1972 by IGAKU SHOIN LTD., 5-29-11 Hongo Bunkyo-ku, Tokyo.
Sole distribution rights for Europe (including the United Kingdom), U. S. A. and Canada granted to
SPRINGER-VERLAG, Berlin • Heidelberg • New York.
Library of Congress Catalog Card Number 72–86725

ISBN 3-540-05942-3 Springer-Verlag Berlin-Heidelberg-New York
ISBN 0-387-05942-3 Springer-Verlag New York-Heidelberg-Berlin

Printed and bound in Japan

PREFACE

The separation of a colony of the Spontaneously Hypertensive Rats (OKAMOTO and AOKI) (SHR) was reported in 1962 and 1963. At that time the following points regarding these rats were described: (1) The incidence of hypertension was 100 per cent in the rats over several months of age. (2) The blood pressure was markedly high. (3) These rats showed hypertensive cardiovascular diseases in high frequency at the advanced stage of hypertension. Therefore, it was emphasized that SHR was by far an excellent material for hypertension research in contrast with the other animals with spontaneous hypertension or with already known experimental hypertensions.

Since then 10 years have passed. Meanwhile, we established an inbred strain of SHR at the Department of Pathology, Faculty of Medicine, Kyoto University, in October, 1969. Various and numerous reports, more than 150 were published on SHR not only from our Department but also from some of more than 100 domestic and foreign laboratories and institutions to which these animals were donated. Finally, time was ripe for an international symposium on this SHR, which was held on Oct. 18–22, 1971 in Kyoto as U.S.-Japan Seminar on Spontaneously Hypertensive Rats (organizers; U.S.—S. UDENFRIEND, Ph. D., Japan—K. OKAMOTO, M. D.). In this seminar 25 members and 22 observers from the U.S., Japan and other countries participated. They presented 46 reports in 9 sessions, joined the lively discussions and obtained satisfactory results.

This book consists of the precious manuscripts which were donated by the participants in the seminar in memory of my retirement from Kyoto University. I would like to express my cordial thanks to the contributors for their kind donation.

I reported a review of the studies on SHR as of the end of 1968 [Spontaneously Hypertension in Rats, Int'l Review of Experimental Pathology, (G. W. RICHTER and M. A. EPSTEIN, eds.), Vol. 7, 227–270, Academic Press, New York and London]. The present book covers the tremendous progress in the studies on SHR which have been made all over the world during the past few years following the publication of the review. Consequently, this book will enable us to gain up-to-date knowledge on the pathogenesis of hypertension, the pathogenesis of the complications in SHR and the application of SHR for the screening of antihypertensive agents, and I believe that these studies on SHR compared to the studies in other experimental hypertensions will inform us of a different and more valuable data for the clarification of human hypertension, especially, essential hypertension. Moreover, the studies on SHR supply us with very important data in search for the methods of the prediction and prophylaxis of hypertension and its complications; this kind of study is obviously impossible in the other forms of experimental hypertension. Therefore, I hope that these studies will be evaluated as an opening of a completely new field, the future of hypertension research.

The aforementioned U.S.-Japan Seminar was supported by the National Science Foundation of the United States and the Japan Society for the Promotion of Science. I express my hearty gratitude for their support, and would like to express my appreciation to the precious collaboration of Drs. S. UDENFRIEND, S. SPECTOR, the members of the Council for SHR and the following corporative members of the Council; Takeda Chemical Industries, Ltd., Sankyo Co., Ltd., Kowa Co., Ltd., Fujisawa Chemical Industries, Ltd. and Nippon Merck-Banyu Co., Ltd. and others. My deepest thanks are also extended to Drs. F. HAZAMA, R. TABEI, S. NOSAKA and Y. YAMORI for their active cooperation in preparing this edition.

January 1, 1972

KOZO OKAMOTO, M.D.

Professor, Department of Pathology
Faculty of Medicine
Kyoto University, Kyoto, Japan

CONTENTS

Chapter I. DEVELOPMENT AND HEREDITY

Chapter II. CATECHOLAMINE METABOLISM

Chapter III. NEURAL FACTOR AND BEHAVIOR

Chapter IV. CARDIOVASCULAR DYNAMICS

Chapter VII. RENAL FACTORS AND ELECTROLYTES

Chapter VIII. ESSENTIAL HYPERTENSION AND SPONTANEOUS HYPERTENSION

LIST OF CONTRIBUTORS

Ivan ALBRECHT, M.U.Dr. — Staff, Institute of Physiology, Czechoslovac Academy of Sciences, Prague, Czechoslovakia. (121)

Shigeru AMANO, M.D. — Research Associate, Department of Pathology, Faculty of Medicine, Kyoto University, Kyoto, Japan. (129, 134)

Kyuzo AOKI, M.D. — Associate, Department of Internal Medicine, Nagoya City University Medical School, Nagoya, Japan. (23, 37, 173)

Yoshitomo ARAMAKI, Ph.D. — Head, Pharmacological Department, Biological Research Laboratories, Research and Developmental Division Takeda Chemical Industries, Ltd., Osaka, Japan. (149)

Leslie BAER, M.D. — Assistant Professor, Department of Medicine, Columbia University College of Physicians and Surgeons, New York, N.Y., U.S.A. (203)

Barry BERKOWITZ — Staff, Department of Pharmacology, Roche Institute of Molecular Biology, Nutley, New Jersey, U.S.A. (41)

F. Merlin BUMPUS, Ph.D. — Chairman, Research Division, Cleveland Clinic Foundation, Cleveland, Ohio, U.S.A. (227)

David W.J. CLARK, B.Sc. M. Pharm. — Staff, Wellcome Medical Research Institute, Department of Medicine, University of Otago Medical School, Dunedin, New Zealand. (18)

Lewis K. DAHL, M.D. — Senior Scientist and Chief of Staff, Hospital of the Medical Research Center, Brookhaven National Laboratory, Upton, New York, U.S.A. (218, 225)

Akio EBIHARA, M.D. — Associate, Department of Internal Medicine, Faculty of Medicine, University of Tokyo, Tokyo, Japan. (214)

Lionel FINCH, Ph.D. — Staff, Department of Experimental Medicine of F. Hoffmann-La Roche & Co., Ltd., Basle, Switzerland. (97)

Björn FOLKOW, M.D., Ph.D. — Professor, Department of Physiology, University of Göteborg, Göteborg, Sweden. (103)

Edward D. FREIS, M.D. — Senior Medical Investigator, Veterans Administration Hospital, Washington, D. C. and Professor of Medicine, Georgetown University, Washington, D.C., U.S.A. (231)

Motohatsu FUJIWARA, M.D. — Professor, Department of Pharmacology, Faculty of Medicine, Kyoto University, Kyoto, Japan. (119)

Marcel GEROLD, M.D. — Staff, Department of Experimental Medicine, F. Hoffmann-La Roche & Co., Ltd., Basle, Switzerland. (51)

Eftimija GLAVAŠ, M.D. — Staff, Department of Pharmacology, Medical Faculty, University of Skopje, Skopje, Yugoslavia. (46)

Christopher R. GRESSON, B. Sc. — Assistant Professor, Wellcome Medical Research Institute, Department of Medicine, University of Otago Medical School, Dunedin, New Zealand. (18)

Arthur GROLLMAN, M.D., Ph.D. — Professor of Experimental Medicine, Department of Pathology, University of Texas Southwestern Medical School, Dallas, Texas, U.S.A. (238)

Stojka GUDESKA

Research Fellow, Department of Pharmacology, Medical Faculty, University of Skopje, Skopje, Yugoslavia. (46)

Hideyuki HAEBARA, M.D.

Associate, Department of Pathology, Faculty of Medicine, Kyoto University, Kyoto, Japan. (1, 129, 134, 155)

Guenther HAEUSLER, Ph.D.

Staff, Department of Experimental Medicine, F. Hoffmann-La Roche & Co., Ltd., Basle, Switzerland. (97)

Margareta HALLBÄCK

Research Associate, Department of Physiology, University of Göteborg, Göteborg, Sweden. (103)

Carl T. HANSEN, Ph.D.

Chief, Genetics Unit, Animal Production Section, National Institutes of Health, Bethesda, Maryland, U.S.A. (13)

Fumitada HAZAMA, M.D.

Associate Professor, Department of Pathology, Faculty of of Medicine, Kyoto University, Kyoto, Japan. (1, 129, 134)

Martha HEINE, B.A.

Staff, Medical Department, Brookhaven National Laboratory, Upton, New York, U.S.A. (218)

George C. HOFFMAN, M.B., B. Chir., M.R.C. Path.

Staff, Division of Laboratory Medicine, Cleveland Clinic Foundation, Cleveland, Ohio, U.S.A. (227)

Ken HOTTA, Ph.D.

Professor, Department of Physiology, Nagoya City University Medical School, Nagoya, Japan. (37, 173)

Nobuko IKEDA

Research Associate, Department of Internal Medicine, Nagoya City University Medical School, Nagoya, Japan. (173)

Susumu IKEHARA

Graduate Student, Department of Pathology, Faculty of Medicine, Kyoto University, Kyoto, Japan. (155)

Kimiho IRINODA, M.D.

Professor, Department of Ophthalmology, Hirosaki University School of Medicine, Hirosaki, Japan. (243)

Junichi IWAI, M.D.

Associate Scientist, Medical Department, Brookhaven National Laboratory, Upton, New York, U.S.A. (218, 225)

David R. JONES, B.Sc. Dip. Sci.

Staff, Wellcome Medical Research Institute, Department of Medicine, University of Otago Medical School, Dunedin, New Zealand. (18)

Chujiro KASHII, M.D.

Associate Professor, Department of Internal Medicine, Osaka Medical College, Takatsuki, Osaka, Japan. (166)

Kioko KAWAI

Associate, Department of Pathology, Nagasaki University School of Medicine, Nagasaki, Japan. (177)

Hisanori KAWAJI, Ph.D.

Associate Researcher, Pathological Department, Biological Research Laboratories, Research and Development Division, Takeda Chemical Industries, Ltd., Osaka, Japan. (149)

Kenzo KIKUCHI, Ph.D.

Senior Scientist, Pharmacological Department, Biological Research Laboratories, Research and Development Division, Takeda Chemical Industries, Ltd., Osaka, Japan. (149)

Jun KIRA, M.D.

Research Associate, Department of Internal Medicine, Faculty of Medicine, Kyoto University, Kyoto, Japan. (210)

Abbie KNOWLTON, M.D.	Assistant Professor, Department of Medicine, Columbia University College of Physicians and Surgeons, New York, N.Y., U.S.A. (203)
Knud D. KNUDSEN, M.D.	Scientist, Medical Department, Brookhaven National Laboratory, Upton, New York, U.S.A. (218, 225)
Simon KOLETSKY, M.D.	Professor, Department of Pathology, Case Western Reserve University Medical School, Cleveland, Ohio, U.S.A. (194, 199)
J. KŘEČEK	Staff, Institute of Physiology, Czechoslovac Academy of Sciences, Prague, Czechoslovakia. (121)
Masahito KUCHII	Department of Pharmacology, School of Medicine, University of Hawaii, Honolulu, Hawaii, U.S.A. (119)
Yoshikiyo KUDO	Associate, Department of Pathology, Hirosaki University School of Medicine, Hirosaki, Japan. (142)
Michiko KUMADA, M.D.	Research Associate, Department of Pathology, Faculty of Medicine, Kyoto University, Kyoto, Japan. (185)
Kazuyoshi KURAHASHI	Research Associate, Department of Pharmacology, School of Medicine, University of Hawaii, Honolulu, Hawaii, U.S.A. (115)
Masahisa KYOGOKU, M.D.	Professor, Department of Pathology, Kobe University School of Medicine, Kobe, Japan. (1, 155)
John H. LARAGH, M.D.	Professor, Department of Medicine, Columbia University College of Physicians and Surgeons, New York, N.Y. U.S.A. (203)
Yen LUNDGREN	Research Associate, Department of Physiology, University of Göteborg, Göteborg, Sweden. (103)
Toshiro MARUYAMA, M.D.	Research Associate, Department of Pathology, Faculty of Medicine, Kyoto University, Kyoto, Japan. (185)
Masao MATSUMOTO, M.D.	Associate, Department of Pathology, Faculty of Medicine, Kyoto University, Kyoto, Japan. (1)
Masato MATSUNAGA, M.D.	Assistant Professor, Central Clinical Laboratories, Kyoto University Hospital, Kyoto, Japan. (210)
Takao MATSUO, Ph.D.	Associate Researcher, Biochemical Department, Biological Research Laboratories, Research and Development Division, Takeda Chemical Industries, Ltd., Osaka, Japan. (149)
Shuichi MATSUYAMA, M.D.	Assistant Professor, Department of Ophthalmology, Hirosaki University Medical School, Hirosaki, Japan. (243)
Meiki MATSUZAKI	Staff, Institute of Microbial Chemistry, Tokyo, Japan. (31)
Susumu MIZOGAMI	Associate, Department of Pharmacology, Toho University School of Medicine, Tokyo, Japan. (93)
Katsuyoshi MIZUNO, M.D.	Professor, Department of Ophthalmology, Tohoku University School of Medicine, Sendai, Japan. (23)
Kimiko MIZUTANI	Associate, Department of Biochemistry, School of Dentistry, Aichi-Gakuin University, Nagoya, Japan. (31)

Kazuo MORI, M.D.

Associate, Department of Internal Medicine, Kobe University School of Medicine, Kobe, Japan. (64)

Toshio MORI

Research Fellow, Institute of Cerebrovascular Diseases, Hirosaki University School of Medicine, Hirosaki, Japan. (142)

Akinobu NAGAOKA, B.S.

Staff, Pharmacological Department, Biological Research Laboratories, Research and Development Division, Takeda Chemical Industries, Ltd., Osaka, Japan. (86, 149)

Ikuko NAGATSU, M.D.

Professor, Department of Anatomy and Physiology, Aichi Prefectural College of Nursing, Nagoya, Japan. (31)

Toshiharu NAGATSU, M.D.

Professor, Department of Biochemistry, School of Dentistry, Aichi-Gakuin University, Nagoya, Japan. (31)

Keiji NAKAMURA

Senior Staff, Research Division, F. Hoffmann-La Roche Inc., Nutley, New Jersey, U.S.A. (51)

Branislav NIKODIJEVIĆ, M.D.

Professor, Department of Pharmacology, Medical Faculty, University of Skopje, Skopje, Yugoslavia. (46)

Shozo NISHIDA, M.D.

Assistant Professor, Department of Ophthalmology, Nagoya City University School of Medicine, Nagoya, Japan. (23)

Shoichiro NOSAKA, M.D.

Associate, Department of Pathology, Faculty of Medicine, Kyoto University, Kyoto, Japan. (67, 73, 79)

Koichi OGINO, M.D.

Assistant Professor, Department of Internal Medicine, Faculty of Medicine, Kyoto University, Kyoto, Japan. (210)

Tomio OHTA, M.D.

Associate Professor, Department of Neurosurgery, Osaka City University Medical School, Osaka, Japan. (67, 155)

Kozo OKAMOTO, M.D.

Professor, Department of Pathology, Faculty of Medicine, Kyoto University, Kyoto, Japan. (1, 9, 67, 73, 83, 89, 129, 134, 155, 185)

Tadashi OKUDA, M.D.

Head, Laboratory of Clinical Pathology, Kansai-Denryoku Hospital, Osaka, Japan. (1, 155)

Akira OOSHIMA, M.D.

Research Associate, Department of Pathology, Faculty of Medicine, Kyoto University, Kyoto, Japan. (1, 9, 73, 129, 134, 155)

Masayori OZAKI, M.D.

Associate Professor, Department of Pharmacology, Nagoya City University Medical School, Nagoya, Japan. (37)

Katsuko OZAWA

Associate, Department of Ophthalmology, Nagoya City University Medical School, Nagoya, Japan. (23)

Chonraku PARK, M.D.

Research Associate, Department of Pathology, Faculty of Medicine, Kyoto University, Kyoto, Japan. (1)

Edward L. PHELAN, B.Sc.

Staff, Department of Medicine, Wellcome Medical Research Institute, Medical School, University of Otago, Dunedine, New Zealand. (18)

Jose RIVERA-VELEZ M.D.

Research Associate, Department of Pathology, Case Western Reserve University Medical School, Cleveland, Ohio, U.S.A. (199)

Akira SASAKI, M.D.

Assistant Professor, Institute of Cerebrovascular Diseases, Hirosaki University School of Medicine, Hirosaki, Japan. (142)

Subha SEN, D.Sc.

Staff, Research Division, Cleveland Clinic Foundation, Cleveland, Ohio, U.S.A. (227)

Shoji SHIBATA, M.D., Ph.D.

Professor, Department of Pharmacology, School of Medicine, University of Hawaii, Honolulu, Hawaii, U.S.A. (115, 119)

Kiro SHIMAMOTO, M.D.

Director, Biological Research Laboratories, Research and Development Division, Takeda Chemical Industries, Ltd., Osaka, Japan. (86)

Patricia SHOOK

Research Associate, Department of Pathology, Case Western Reserve University Medical School, Cleveland, Ohio, U.S.A. (199)

Ramon SIVERTSSON, M.D., Ph.D.

Department of Clinical Physiology II, University of Göteborg, Görteborg, Sweden. (103)

Albert SJOERDSMA, M.D., Ph.D.

Vice President, Research Merrell International (Division of Richardson-Merrell, Inc.) and Director, Merrell International Research Center, Strasbourg, France. (27)

Robert R. SMEBY, Ph.D.

Staff, Research Division, Cleveland Clinic Foundation, Cleveland, Ohio, U.S.A. (227)

Sir Frederick Horace SMIRK, K.B.E., M.D., F.R.A.C.P. (Hon.), F.R.C.P., D.Sc. (Hon. Hahnemann)

Emeritus Professor, Wellcome Medical Research Institute, Department of Medicine, Medical School, University of Otago, Dunedin, New Zealand. (250)

Hirofumi SOKABE, M.D.

Associate Professor, Department of Pharmacology, Toho University School of Medicine, Tokyo, Japan. (93)

Sydney SPECTOR, Ph.D.

Section Chief, Department of Pharmacology, Roche Institute of Molecular Biology, Nutley, New Jersey, U.S.A. (41)

Nicholas T. STOWE, Ph.D.

Research Fellow, Research Division, Cleveland Clinic Foundation, Cleveland, Ohio, U.S.A. (227)

Hajime SUGIHARA, M.D.

Assistant Professor, Department of Pathology, Faculty of Medicine, Nagasaki University, Nagasaki, Japan. (177)

Milka ŠAKAROVA

Research Fellow, Pharmaceutical Industry ALKALOID, Skopje, Yugoslavia. (46)

Yoshio SUZUKI

Director, Central Research Laboratories, Sankyo Co., Ltd., Tokyo, Japan. (9)

Ryo TABEI, M.D.

Associate Professor, Department of Pathology, Faculty of Medicine, Kyoto University, Kyoto, Japan. (185)

Shigeki TAKAHASHI, M.D.

Assistant Professor, Department of Ophthalmology, Hirosaki University School of Medicine, Hirosaki, Japan. (160, 243)

Shuji TAKAORI, M.D.

Associate Professor, Department of Pharmacology, Faculty of Medicine, Kyoto University, Kyoto, Japan. (83, 89)

Tadasu TAKATSU, M.D.

Professor, Department of Internal Medicine, Osaka Medical College, Takatsuki, Osaka, Japan. (166)

Tomio TAKEUCHI — Associate Director, Institute of Microbial Chemistry, Tokyo, Japan. (31)

Chikako TANAKA, M.D. — Assistant Professor, Department of Pharmacology, Faculty of Medicine, Kyoto University, Kyoto, Japan. (62, 83, 89)

Toshinari TANAKA, M.D. — Research Associate, Department of Pathology, Faculty of Medicine, Kyoto University, Kyoto, Japan. (1, 129, 134)

Hisao TANASE, B.S. — Staff, Fukuroi Branch of the Central Research Laboratories, Sankyo Co., Ltd., Fukuroi, Shizuoka, Japan. (9)

James TARVER — Staff, Department of Pharmacology, Roche Institute of Molecular Biology, Nutley, New Jersey, U.S.A. (41)

Hans THOENEN, M.D. — Professor, Department of Pharmacology, Biocenter, University of Basle, Basle, Switzerland. (51)

Noboru TODA, M.D. — Associate, Department of Pharmacology, Faculty of Medicine, Kyoto University, Kyoto, Japan. (119)

Tatsuya TOMOMATSU, M.D. — Professor, Department of Internal Medicine, Kobe University School of Medicine, Kobe, Japan. (64)

Hideo TSUCHIYAMA, M.D. — Professor, Department of Pathology, Nagasaki University School of Medicine, Nagasaki, Japan. (177)

Sidney UDENFRIEND, Ph.D. — Director, Roche Institute of Molecular Biology, Nutley, New Jersey, U.S.A. (254)

Yasuyuki UEBA, M.D. — Assistant Professor, Department of Internal Medicine, Kobe University School of Medicine, Kobe, Japan. (64)

Yutaka UMEHARA, M.D. — Professor and Director, Institute of Cerebrovascular Diseases, Hirosaki University School of Medicine, Hirosaki, Japan. (142)

Hamao UMEZAWA, M.D. — Professor, Department of Microbiology, Faculty of Medicine, Tokyo University and Director, Institute of Microbial Chemistry, Tokyo, Japan. (31)

Domnika VETADŽOKOSKA, M.D. — Assistant Professor, Department of Pharmacology, Medical Faculty, University of Skopje, Skopje, Yugoslavia. (46)

M. VÍZEK — Staff, Institute of Physiology, Czechoslovac Academy of Sciences, Prague, Czechoslovakia. (121)

Shih-Chun WANG, M.D., Ph.D. — Professor, Department of Pharmacology College of Physicians and Surgeons, Columbia University, New York, N.Y., U.S.A. (79)

Lilian WEISS — Research Associate, Department of Physiology, University of Göteborg, Göteborg, Sweden. (103)

Yoshikazu YAMAZAKI M.D. — Research Associate, Department of Pathology, Faculty of Medicine, Kyoto University, Kyoto, Japan. (134)

Yukio YAMORI, M.D. — Associate, Department of Pathology, Faculty of Medicine, Kyoto University, Kyoto, Japan. (1, 9, 59, 67, 73, 155)

Chapter I

DEVELOPMENT AND HEREDITY

ESTABLISHMENT OF THE INBRED STRAIN OF THE SPONTANEOUSLY HYPERTENSIVE RAT AND GENETIC FACTORS INVOLVED IN HYPERTENSION

K. OKAMOTO*, Y. YAMORI*, A. OOSHIMA*, C. PARK*,
H. HAEBARA*, M. MATSUMOTO*, T. TANAKA*,
T. OKUDA*, F. HAZAMA* and M. KYOGOKU*

In 1962 and 1963, OKAMOTO [6], OKAMOTO and AOKI [9] reported that they had produced a colony of Spontaneously Hypertensive Rats (SHR hereafter) by selective inbreeding of Wistar rats from the Animal Center Laboratory, Kyoto University Faculty of Medicine (abbreviated hereafter as Wistar-Kyoto). At that time, SHR colony had reached the sixth generation.

Since then we have continued the brother-sister inbreeding of that colony up to the present. We obtained the twenty-first generation in October of 1969 [8, 10]. In other words, in October of the year before last, we succeeded in obtaining the inbred strain of SHR which was so-called 'pure' from the biological viewpoint.

Here, we would like to review briefly the blood pressure, pathological lesions and pathogenesis, mainly based on the recent works, at first, and then report the characteristics of 3 substrains of SHR which we have at present.

1. Blood pressure

The elevation of blood pressure in the recent generations occurs earlier than in their antecedents. They frequently reach the hypertensive level as early as 5 weeks after birth, develop hypertension without exception at the 7th week of life and maintain higher blood pressure than those of the previous generations [7, 9]. This might be mainly attributed to the fact that the recent SHR as an inbred strain possess most of the hypertensive factors.

2. Pathological lesions

Pathological findings in the SHR which died a natural death over 6 months old are shown in Table 1. It is noteworthy that the incidence of cerebral lesions is relatively low, and that the incidence of myocardial lesions, nephrosclerosis and malignant vascular lesions is remarkably high in SHR with severe hypertension.

3. Pathogenesis of hypertension

a) Genetic analysis of blood pressure in SHR. Since our SHR has already become the inbred strain, as mentioned above, we are now in the stage where we can make the genetical studies on this hypertension.

---

* Department of Pathology, Faculty of Medicine, Kyoto University, Kyoto, Japan

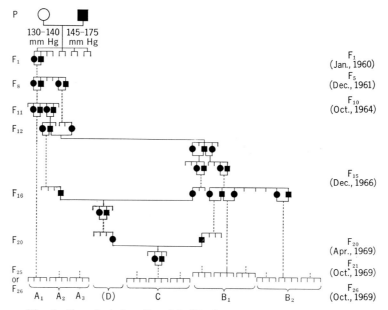

Fig. 1 Genealogical outline of A, B̄ and C substrains of SHR (1971).

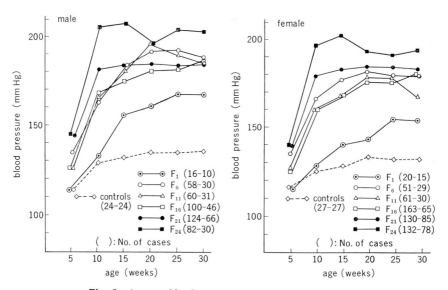

Fig. 2 Average blood pressure of SHR according to age.

We used inbred SHR (F_{21}) and Wistar-Mishima rats, an authentic inbred strain of Wistar (F_{58}), and mated them to produce hybrid F_1, and then they were intercrossed to produce F_2 segregates and backcrossed with SHR (BC_1) and Wistar-Mishima (BC_2).

We calculated the degree of genetic determination by the statistical analysis of the blood pressure in these cross-generations and tried to estimate the number of major genes according to Wright's formula. The former showed 0.86–0.96 and the latter 1.4–3.1 at the age of 15–30 weeks after birth [10]. So, the conclusion of our genetic analysis revealed the great importance of the genetic factors in the spontaneous hypertension, that

Table 1 Pathological findings in SHR after natural death.

Kind of lesions		Incidence (%)	
		SHR[7] (91* cases)	Severe SHR (111** cases)
Hypertensive cerebral lesions (hemorrhage, softening etc.)		8	12
Myocardial lesions (infarction, fibrosis)		19	72
Nephrosclerosis	Benign	5	22
	Malignant	12	18
Malignant vascular lesions	PN+	30	55
	PN−	7	2
Pneumonia		84	67
Miscellaneous (abscess etc.)		24	31

PN: periarteritis nodosa
* : ♂...51, ♀...40; **: ♂...57, ♀...54
Severe SHR: rats with blood pressure over 200 mm Hg.

is, the development of hypertension is mainly controlled by the genetic factors and the mode of the inheritance is not in accordance with the simple Mendelian law, but consistent with the additive mode of inheritance. Moreover, our results suggested that a relatively small number of major genes are involved in this hypertension.

Consequently, we can regard the hypertension of SHR as a disease due to some genetical disorders. Such concept led us to the speculation that there would exist some disorders in enzyme activity in the organs of our SHR.

b) Enzymes in SHR. Firstly, we detected that there existed abnormalities in the pattern of esterase isozyme in the kidney [15], liver [15], arteries and many other organs, except for a small number of organs, such as medulla of suprarenal gland, prostate, heart muscle, spleen and so on.

Secondly, we could detect an abnormality in the pattern of acid phosphatase only in the liver. In this organ, the intense isozyme band of the control Wistar-Kyoto, extended toward the cathode side, and there was also a pretty dense band near the top of the anode side. On the other hand, these bands in SHR showed the opposite pattern.

Moreover, we have obtained some other findings in this field [7, 8]: The activity of acid phosphatase is increased histochemically in the follicular cells of the thyroid, in the nerve cells of some definite nuclei of the hypothalamus, midbrain and medulla oblongata, and in the nerve cells of superior cervical sympathetic ganglia in SHR. The activity of G-6-P dehydrogenase or TPN diaphorase in the adrenal cortex, and that of ATPase or AMPase in the arterioles are also increased in SHR.

However, whether the majority of these biochemical findings are intimately related with the pathogenesis of hypertension or not is not yet determined.

Anyhow, the genetic factor is very important in the development of hypertension in SHR. It may induce the functional abnormality as a pathogenetic mechanism of hypertension in some organs through the biochemical abnormalities.

c) Significance of some characteristics in SHR. We have already clarified the various characteristics of SHR. In order to determine the relationship between some of these characteristics and hypertension, we made the cross-generations between inbred SHR and inbred Wistar-Mishima, as mentioned before, and examined the weights of the heart, pituitary, adrenal and thyroid and some enzyme activities in the F_2 segregate generations which showed the widest distribution of blood pressure from normotension to hypertension. Then we studied the coefficient of correlation between each characteristic and blood pressure, and the significance of the coefficient. Consequently, the significant positive correlations with blood pressure were proved in the heart weight, pituitary weight and adrenal weight. The total activity of ACPase in the thyroid also showed a slight positive correlation to blood pressure level, while the aromatic L-amino acid decarboxylase activity of the brainstem [13] had a slight inverse correlation to blood pressure, but the G-6-P dehydrogenase activity of adrenal no correlation. The esterase isozyme pattern of the kidney in the F_2 segregate generation was separated into 3 types, that is, SHR-, hybrid- and normal types, in the ratio of 1 to 2 to 1. And the distribution of blood pressure and the average of the blood pressure in each F_2 segregates, BC_1 and BC_2 with the different isozyme patterns indicated that the esterase isozyme patterns of the kidney were loosely correlated to blood pressure.

Therefore, this kind of genetic analyses also confirmed that the pituitary, adrenal and thyroid had a relationship to the development or maintenance of hypertension in SHR and it can be supposed that 3 enzymes cited here might also have a certain relationship to hypertension.

d) Mechanism of the development of hypertension. In the above-mentioned and the other studies [1–5, 7, 11, 12, 14], we have been working on the various organs of SHR to detect their morphological or functional abnormalities. As the summary of these studies, we confirmed the following findings.

(1) There are some slight but regular hyperfunctions in the hypothalamo-hypophyseo-adrenocortical system, (2) and also in the hypothalamo-hypophyseo-thyroidal system. (3) Hypersecretion of neurosecrets. In addition, (4) increased pressor activity at the periphery induced by hyperactivity of the pressor center of the medulla oblongata, which was probably produced by the dysregulation of the pressor and depressor mechanisms of the hypothalamus.

We suppose all these factors somehow contribute to the development and maintenance of hypertension. Of course, we need further detailed studies on this problem and it is our great hope to have many topics concerning this problem in the following chapters of this book.

4. Substrains of SHR

a) Separation of substrains. In the SHR with severe hypertension, it is generally difficult to produce successive generations only by their brother-sister breeding and in certain generations in the process of establishing an inbred strain, it is difficult to produce the offspring. We were faced with such difficulties several times. To avoid such difficulties in maintaining the strain, we used to produce the offspring by cross breeding as well as by brother-sister breeding.

In these circumstances, at present, we can regard our SHR strain as consisting of 3 substrains, and named them, A, B and C strains.

The A strain is the original one and it was obtained only by successive brother-sister breeding for 26 generations. The B strain was separated from the original strain at the F_{12} generation by non-brother-sister breeding and was kept by brother-sister breeding thereafter, and consists of 2 groups, *i.e.* B_1 and B_2 strains. Next, at the F_{16} generation, a male from A strain and a female from B strain were mated and their offspring were kept as D strain by brother-sister breeding. However, to our regret no more D rats of strain exist now. The C strain was obtained at the F_{20} generation by the mating between a female from D strain and a male from B strain, and this C strain has been kept by brother-sister breeding up to the present (Fig. 1).

There is no marked difference in the blood pressure elevation and external appearance among these three substrains. However, as shown in Table 2, there do exist some differences in alkaline phosphatase isozyme of the liver and serum, esterase isozyme of serum, and also in the appearance of serum post albumin. According to those characteristics, we can group 3 substrains into two: A and combined B and C, because we can not distinguish C from B only by these methods.

Table 2 Characteristics of A, B and C substrains in SHR, compared with Wistar-Kyoto.

		SHR			Wistar-Kyoto		
		A	B	C			
Zymogram	Alkaline phosphatase of liver	S.	D.	D.	−	+	B. (8.5)
	Alkaline phosphatase of serum	S.	D.	D.	−	+	H. (8.0)
	Esterase of serum*	D.	S.	S.	−	+	H. (8.0)
	Esterase of kidney,** liver, artery	D.	D.	D.	−	+	B. (8.5)
	Acid phosphatase of liver*	D.	D.	D.	−	+	B. (8.5)
	Acid phosphatase of thyroid gl.	D.	D.	D.	−	+	B. (8.5)
Serum post albumin		++ − +++	± − ++	± − ++	− − ±		

S.: same, D.: different, B.: borate buffer, H.: histidine buffer, ( ): pH.
*: zymogram is different in Wistar-Mishima.

However, when we experimentally loaded young male SHR, 45–60 days after birth, with a high fat-cholesterol diet (tempura oil: 20%, cholesterol: 5%, bile powder [crude sodium cholate]: 2%, stock chow: 73%) with 1% of salt in the drinking water, we observed a difference in the serum cholesterol level in these experimental groups. As shown in Fig. 3, A strain showed a rapid increase in the initial period and the level was always higher than that of B_2 strain. C and B_1 strains showed almost the intermediate level between A and B_2 strains. This difference in the serum cholesterol level among these substrains was already clear one week after the loading of special diet (A, B_2, C, B_1 and Wistar-Kyoto showed 190 ± 30.3 (M$\pm$SD), 123 ± 19.2, 159 ± 26.1, 164 ± 33.1 and 109 ± 8.6 mg/dl, respectively).

b) Cardiovascular lesions in substrains under loading with special diet. The experiment of feeding these A, B_2, C strains of SHR and Wistar-Kyoto at the age of 45–120 days on such

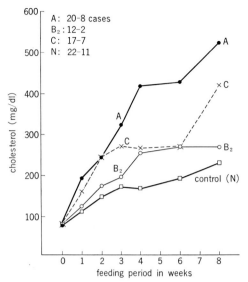

Fig. 3   Serum cholesterol of male A, B and C substrains in SHR and control rats, fed on fat-cholesterol-salt diet (cholesterol determination by ZURKOWSKI's method).

Table 3   Incidence of cerebral lesions in SHR substrains and control Wistar-Kyoto, loaded with 1% NaCl in the drinking water with or without fat-cholesterol diet.

Diet	Fat-cholesterol-salt				Salt		
Kind of rats	A	B_2	C	Control (Wistar-Kyoto)	A	B_2	Control (Wistar-Kyoto)
Loading period in days (died or sacrificed)	57 ± 20.7	64 ± 41.0	56 ± 12.0	66 ± 36.6	56 ± 18.9	101 ± 67.0	142 ± 98.6
Total No. of rats	67	29	24	30	28	17	20
Incidence of cerebral lesions — No. of rats	43 (+10)	4 (+6)	12 (+2)	0 (+0)	19 (+3)	2 (+4)	0 (+0)
Incidence of cerebral lesions — %	64 (79)	14 (34)	50 (58)	0 (0)	68 (79)	12 (33)	0 (0)

(+):   rats with histological cerebral lesions.
( ):   incidence of rats with histological and macroscopical lesions.
Rats, 45–120 days after birth, were used.
Fat-cholesterol Diet: tempura oil 20%, cholesterol 5%, bile powder 2% and stock chow diet (Japan CLEA-CE 2) 73%.

high fat-cholesterol-salt diet showed a difference in the incidence of the cardiovascular lesions, especially cerebral lesions, that is, cerebral hemorrhage and or softening among these 3 substrains. The incidence of them was 79% in A, while 34% in B_2. Moreover, the cerebral lesions in A was larger in size in comparison with that in B_2, and most of them were noted macroscopically. The incidence of the cerebral lesions in C was 58%, and it ranged intermediately between A and B_2 strains. None of the cerebral lesions were observed in Wistar-Kyoto, and also in non-treated SHR before 6 months of age. The fatty deposition in arteries as well as arterioles (Arcus aortae, Aorta abdominalis, A. carotis communis, A. renalis, heart arterioles) was observed in a higher degree in A strain, in a lower degree in B_2 strain, but in the Wistar-Kyoto, there was no change.

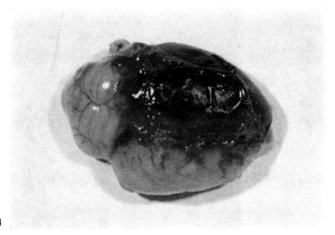

Fig. 4

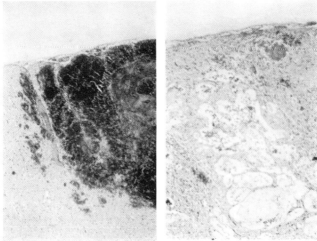

Fig. 5   Fig. 6

Fig. 4   The brain of a male 100-day-old SHR, died after loading with 1% of salt in the drinking
water for 55 days. A large hemorrhage in the left temporal lobe is shown.
Fig. 5   Microscopical appearance of cerebral hemorrhage in the above-mentioned case. (H.E., ×40)
Fig. 6   The brain of a male 95-day-old SHR, died after loading with 1% of salt in the drinking
water for 60 days. Microscopical appearance of softening in the cerebral cortex is shown.
(H.E., ×40)

Next, SHR, 45–120 days after birth, were fed on the ordinary stock chow diet with
1% of salt in the drinking water. Although they were not loaded with fat and cholesterol,
the incidence of cerebral lesions (Figs. 4, 5, 6) was 79% in the A strain, only 33% in
the B_2 strain, but there was no incidence in Wistar-Kyoto and non-loaded SHR before 6
months of age. These results were almost coincident with the previous experiment of high
fat-cholesterol-salt loadings. In this experiment, there was no marked increase in the serum
cholesterol, and no marked difference in it was noted between A and B_2 strains. Consequently, we can conclude that the increase in serum cholesterol is not necessary for high
incidence of cerebral lesions. The details of the cerebral lesions and other cardiovascular
lesions in these experiments and the results in the similar researches, will be presented
in two papers in Chapter V.

In short, (1) SHR is susceptible to cerebral vascular lesions under the condition of
high fat-cholesterol diet with salt or simply with salt loading. (2) The incidence of these
lesions was different among the substrains. (3) It seems that there is a parallelism between

the vulnerability to the vascular, especially cerebral lesions and the elevation of serum cholesterol level by the loading of high fat and cholesterol diet with 1% of salt in the drinking water.

ACKNOWLEDGEMENT

This investigation was supported by a grant (HE 10762) from the National Heart Institute of the National Institutes of Health (U.S.A.), by a grant-in-aid for scientific research from the Japanese Ministry of Education.

The authors would like to express their deep gratitude to Drs. M. FUKUSHIMA, K. ICHIJIMA, M. KUMADA, T. MARUYAMA, T. MORISAWA, T. MOTOYOSHI, S. NOSAKA, Y. SUZUKI, R. TABEI, T. TAKEDA and H. YAMABE in the Department of Pathology, Kyoto University Faculty of Medicine for their collaboration.

REFERENCES

1. HAEBARA, H., ICHIJIMA, K., MOTOYOSHI, T. and OKAMOTO, K. (1968): Jap Circ J, 32, 1391.
2. ICHIJIMA, K. (1969): Jap Circ J, 33, 785.
3. MARUYAMA, T. (1969): Jap Circ J, 33, 1271.
4. MATSUMOTO, M. (1966, 1967, 1969): Jap Circ J, 30, 743; 31, 1187; 33, 37 and 411.
5. NOSAKA, S., and OKAMOTO, K. (1970): Jap Circ J, 34, 685.
6. OKAMOTO, K. (1962): Nippon Naibunpi Gakkai Zasshi, 38, 782.
7. OKAMOTO, K (1969): International Review of Experimental Pathology (G.W. RICHTER and M.A. EPSTEIN, eds.), Vol 7, p 227, Academic Press, New York and London.
8. OKAMOTO, K. (1971): Jap J Nephrol, 13, 23.
9. OKAMOTO, K. and AOKI, K. (1963): Jap Circ J, 27, 282.
10. TANASE, H., SUZUKI, Y., OOSHIMA, A., YAMORI, Y. and OKAMOTO, K. (1970): Jap Circ J, 34, 1197.
11. THANT, M., YAMORI, Y. and OKAMOTO, K. (1969): Jap Circ J, 33, 501.
12. YAMABE, H. (1970): Jap Circ J, 34, 233 and 245.
13. YAMORI, Y., LOVENBERG, W. and SJOERDSMA, A. (1970): Science, 170, 544.
14. YAMORI, Y. and OKAMOTO, K. (1969): Jap Circ J, 33, 509.
15. YAMORI, Y. and OKAMOTO, K. (1970): Lab Invest, 22, 206.
(Most of references cited in OKAMOTO's review of SHR (1969) [7] are omitted in this paper.)

FURTHER GENETIC ANALYSIS OF BLOOD PRESSURE IN SPONTANEOUSLY HYPERTENSIVE RATS

H. TANASE*, Y. SUZUKI*, A. OOSHIMA**,
Y. YAMORI** and K. OKAMOTO**

In the previous experiments, it was shown that the blood pressure level in SHR strain was genetically determined to a considerable degree [4], and that the mode of inheritance was additive with some dominance [5]. Furthermore, these experiments suggested that the number of genes involved in this hypertension might be relatively small, and we could not eliminate even the possibility of the existence of a single major gene in the etiology of this hypertension. The purpose of the present study is to confirm the genetic mechanism, especially the number of genetic factors involved in the blood pressure level of SHR strain. In the first presentation of this session Prof. OKAMOTO brieffly reviewed the genetic studies performed independently in his laboratory using the inbred SHR and normotensive controls consisting of Wistar-Kyoto or inbred Wistar-Mishima. TANASE and SUZUKI [4, 5] coincidentally obtained almost the same data. Therefore, to avoid overlaping of the results, we will present mainly the data obtained in Sankyo laboratory.

Systolic blood pressure was measured on the caudal artery of unanaesthetized animals using a tail-water plethysmographic method when they were at the fifteenth week of age. This age was determined from the result of the previous experiment [5]. The average of three readings was recorded as the blood pressure for each rat. The SHR strain, originally from Kyoto University, was introduced through Toho University into Sankyo laboratory in 1966, and it has been maintained by full sib-matings. The rats used here were in the fourteenth generation of inbreeding. Blood pressures were measured in six strains: Wistar-Imamichi, Donryu, Jaundice, Sprague-Dawley, Holtzman and SHR strains. The mean blood pressure of SHR strain was distinctly higher than those of the other five strains, and the difference was significant. Consequently, the latter strains of rats were considered to be normotensive strains. However, some differences were observed among these normotensive strains. Wistar-Imamichi rats were selected as a normotensive strain in the study of genetic analysis for the following reasons. First, both SHR and Wistar-Imamichi rats derived from the same ancester. Second, their blood pressures were relatively stable. Third, they had good reproductive ability.

For the study of segregate generations, reciprocal crosses were made between SHR and Wistar-Imamichi rats. These hybrids, derived from a cross between male SHR and female Wistar-Imamichi rats, were intercrossed and backcrossed to the parental strains. Blood pressures in these non-segregate and segregate generations were measured. The average blood pressures in the hybrids obtained by the reciprocal crosses were intermediate between those in the parental strains, and they did not significantly differ from the mid-parent value. The variance of blood pressure in F_1 hybrids derived from a cross between male Wistar-Imamichi and female SHR was significantly greater than that in the hybrids, from the reciprocal cross. Therefore, maternal and/or paternal influences might exist. The variance in F_1 hybrids did not differ from that in Wistar-Imamichi rats,

* Central Research Laboratories, Sankyo Co., Ltd., Tokyo, Japan
** Department of Pathology, Faculty of Medicine, Kyoto University, Kyoto, Japan

but the variance in SHR strain was significantly greater than in the Wistar-Imamichi and F_1 hybrids. This inhomogeneity of variances indicates the presence of genotype-environment interaction. F_2 mean was also intermediate between the means of parental strains. Backcross means were intermediate between those of F_1 and respective parent strains. However, the means of F_2 and backcross generations were some what lower than the values expected from the assumption of completely additive inheritance. There was no evidence for pronounced bimodality in backcross generations nor was there seen the expected 1:2:1 ratio in the F_2 generation. The distribution of blood pressures tended to be positively skewed, especially in the F_2 generation.

From the result of cross analysis, the blood pressure level in the SHR strain seems to be regulated by so-called polygenic mechanism. However, when we consider that almost 100 per cent occurrence of spontaneous hypertension was observed even at the third generation of selection [2] and that this trait could be readily fixed in comparison with the New Zealand strain of genetic hypertension [3], we have to presume that the number of genes involved should be relatively small.

From this assumption, upward selection was made for elevated blood pressure from the F_2 generation. Selection in subsequent generations was practiced in both sexes. Full sib-mating system was used in each generation. The mean proportion selected per generation was 14.9 per cent in females and 14.4 per cent in males. Assuming a normal distribution, selection intensity depends on the proportion of population included in the selection and it can be read from a graph prepared by FALCONER [1]. As a result, mean selection intensity was about 1.58 in both sexes. The blood pressure level became approximately equal to that of the SHR strain at the third generation of selection. After that, selection response was decreased in both sexes. This result was similar to the original report by Prof. OKAMOTO and Dr. AOKI [2] that almost 100 per cent occurrence of spontaneous hypertension was observed at the third generation of selective inbreeding. Next, to estimate the realized heritability of blood pressure during five generations of upward selection, the selection differential and response were calculated. Selection differential is calculated as the difference between the mean of the animals selected as parents and the mean of the generation they belonged to. Selection response is the difference in the mean phenotypic value between the offspring of selected parents and the entire parental generation before selection. The selection differential and response values are then cumulated over generations. The least square technique yields a linear regression line fitted to these values. This regression line is equal to the realized heritability [1] with the standard error of the former regression line corresponding to the standard error of the latter. The realized heritability of blood pressure was 73.6 ± 8.6 per cent in females and 82.3 ± 6.3 per cent in males. Both values were very significant. Consequently, this trait is regulated to a large extent by the additive effect of genes.

The result of the selection experiment suggested a relatively small number of genes involved in this genetic hypertension. We cannot exclude the possibility of the existence of a single major genetic factor in the etiology of this hypertension through a specific physiological pathway. If the high blood pressure in the SHR strain is regulated by a single major gene, it would be possible to introduce the gene into the genetic background of a normotensive strain by successive backcrosses, and to breed a congenic strain for the major gene.

Then, successive backcrosses were carried out from this assumption. They have reached the fourth generation up to the present. The distribution of the blood pressure in these generations seemed to become bimodal. However, segregate ratio was not 1:1 exactly as expected under a single major gene. Subsequently, males and females with the highest blood pressure at the third generation of successive backcross were intercrossed. Although, the distribution did not show 1:2:1 segregating ratio as expected under the assumption of a single major gene, there was a small peak in the upper end of the distribution. Therefore, it can be considered that the high blood pressure in the SHR strain would be regulated by a relatively small number of major genes. But the number of major genes involved could not be determined exactly by this experiment.

The results of the selection experiment and the successive backcrosses would support the hypothesis in the previous experiment that the blood pressure level in the SHR strain appeared to be regulated by a relatively small number of major genes acting additively. However, the high blood pressure in the SHR strain could not be explained by these major genes only. The average blood pressure in the F_2 and backcross generations were lower than the values expected from assumption of completely additive inheritance, and the distribution of blood pressures in segregate generations tended to be positively skewed. Therefore, complex genic interaction might exist among genes. In addition, the influence of environmental factors was already reported, and the presence of genotype-environment interaction was presumed from the inhomogeneity of the variances among the non-segregating generations. Maternal and/or paternal influences might exist as shown in the difference of the variances in the F_1 hybrids from reciprocal crosses. Furthermore, as shown in the strain comparison, strain difference existed in normotensive strains. So, several or more genes with minor effect, which cause the strain difference, would be involved in the heredity of this high blood pressure. Consequently, this character would be regulated by a relatively small number of major genes and many genes with minor effect, and complex interaction might exist between gene and environment and among genes.

According to these results, a congenic strain with a characteristic related to the pathogenesis of hypertension could be separated by successive backcrosses to a normotensive strain. Since the major gene is not only one, different kinds of congenic strains might be established. By using these congenic strains, we could analyze genic interaction among these genes, and solve the etiology of hypertension in the SHR strain. These studies seem to contribute to the elucidation of the pathogenesis and to the establishment of the prescience or prevention in human essential hypertension.

Finaly, the SHR strain was supplied to various laboratories at the early stage during the development of the inbred strain. In Sankyo laboratory, the SHR strain was introduced twice. When the blood pressure levels of these two lines and the fifth generation of upward selection in the present study were compared with each other, a significant difference was observed in blood pressure levels. This result would be a matter of course if we take the genetic mechanism of this character into consideration. Moreover, it is supposed that genetical subdivision not only in relation to blood pressure level but also in relation to various other traits might occur in SHR lines separated from the SHR-Kyoto strain at the early stage of inbreeding. Therefore, it is necessary to take this point into consideration when comparing the results of similar experiments carried out by different workers using different SHR lines.

REFERENCES

1. FALCONER, D. S. (1960): "Introduction to Quantitative Genetics." Ronald Press, New York.
2. OKAMOTO, K. and AOKI, K. (1963): Jap Circ J, **27**, 282.
3. PHELAN, E. L. (1968): N Z Med J, **67**, 334.
4. TANASE, H. and SUZUKI, Y. (1971): Exp Anim, **20**, 1.
5. TANASE, H., SUZUKI, Y., OOSHIMA, A., YAMORI, Y. and OKAMOTO, K. (1970): Jap Circ J, **34**, 1197.

A GENETIC ANALYSIS OF HYPERTENSION IN THE RAT

C. T. HANSEN*

INTRODUCTION

Animal models for the study of hypertension have been developed by selective breeding by SMIRK and HALL [11], DAHL, et al. [6], and OKAMOTO and AOKI [9]. While these models have been useful for the study of many aspects of hypertension, they all suffer from the limitation of representing a narrow genetic base which limits their value for the study of cause and effect relationships. An understanding of such relationships are necessary to determine the basic factors involved in the regulation of blood pressure. Thus, additional models are needed which will complement those models already available.

The techniques involved in developing these complementary models depends upon the genetic nature of the characteristic studied. If the characteristic is determined by a simple genetic system, the development of these models is relatively simple. However, the evidence presented by ALEXANDER, et al. [1] in rabbits, STURKIE, et al. [12], in chickens, McKUSICK [8], in man, SCHLAGER and WEIBUST [10], in mice, and TANASE, et al. [13] and TANASE and SUZUKI [14], in rats all show that blood pressure regulation is polygenically determined. Thus, the procedures used in developing the complementary models are of necessity those used for the study of polygenic inheritance. The material presented in this chapter is based on the preliminary results of experiments designed to further analyze the genetic basis of blood pressure regulation in the rat with the goal of developing additional models.

MATERIALS AND METHODS

The data presented here are the results of two experiments. The first consisted of measuring the blood pressures in 17 inbred strains of rats to determine if strain differences were present. In this experiment, 12 males were measured in each strain. The number and sex were limited by the time available. The second experiment consisted of determining the blood pressures of F_1 male progeny produced from mating of males of the SHR/N strain of rats with females from five of the inbred strains used in the first experiment.

The blood pressures were measured in the unanesthetized animal using the indirect tail plethysomograph described by WILLIAMS, et al [15]. The average of three readings was the record of blood pressure for each animal. Recordings were made at 4, 6, 8 and 10 weeks of age. The 10 week age was chosen as the final recording on the assumption that if strain differences were present, they would have been evident at this age. The recordings at 4, 6 and 8 weeks of age were made for the purpose of determining if strain differences in blood pressures were evident at these ages.

The strains were perpetuated by brother-sister matings and were produced in a modified SPF barrier type facility. The animals were fed a commercially available autoclavable diet.

* Laboratory Aids Branch, Division of Research Services, National Institutes of Health, Bethesda, Maryland, U.S.A.

RESULTS

The average blood pressures at 4, 6, 8 and 10 weeks of age for the males of 17 inbred strains are presented in Table 1. Significant differences ($P<.01$) were found between the strains for the 10 week blood pressures despite the limited number of animals measured. The blood pressures ranged from 182 mm Hg for the SHR/N strain, which had been selectively bred for high blood pressures (Okamoto and Aoki [9]) to 116 for the ACI/N

Table 1 Mean (SD) Blood Pressures [a] at 4, 6, 8, and 10 weeks of age and standard deviations of blood pressure at 10 weeks of age for males of 17 inbred rat strains and the analysis of variance of strain differences for blood pressure at 10 weeks of age.

| Strain | blood pressures | | | | |
	4 wk	6 wk	8 wk	10 wk	SD
SHR/N	121	143	166	182	5
OM/N	110	136	153	160	6
RHA/N	114	139	151	158	11
SD/N	102	141	150	156	5
ALB/N	100	143	145	143	14
F344/N	106	120	131	140	4
RLA/N	103	130	135	137	7
LA/N	102	124	133	136	6
CAS/N	103	120	131	136	6
MR/N	97	118	126	132	7
CAR/N	96	125	128	131	7
MNR/N	101	121	125	129	7
BUF/N	102	110	126	129	10
PETH/N	101	122	126	128	7
W/N	105	121	126	128	6
M520/N	104	110	128	124	9
ACI/N	101	110	118	116	6
	104	125	135	139	7

Source	df	Mean Square
Total	203	
Between Strains	16	3188**
Within Strains	187	60

**   ($P<.01$)

[a]   N=12

strain. The distribution of the blood pressures of the unselected strains, that is, excluding the SHR/N, appeared to be continuous. This might be considered as additional evidence for the multifactorial inheritance of blood pressure. The distinction between a hypertensive and normotensive strain is an arbitrary one. On the basis of these results, those strains which fell within the 125–135 range were defined as normotensive and those outside this range either hyper- or hypotensive. Using these ranges as a working definition for the normal state, five of the strains (OM/N, RHA/N, SD/N, ALB/N, and F344/N) could be considered as hypertensive in addition to the SHR/N and one as hypotensive (ACI/N). Although, if more strains were measured, this definition might have to be changed.

The strain variation tended to be distributed at random. There was almost a three-fold range in the standard deviations among the strains, but there did not seem to be any relationship between the means and variances. These data are too limited to determine if these strains characterized by the larger standard deviations are still segregating for blood pressures despite long inbreeding, or if these are the consequence of a limited sample size. However, the sample size must be increased to obtain a better measure of the strain variation.

The strains also differed with respect to their blood pressures at 4, 6, and 8 weeks of age. At 4 weeks of age, the blood pressure of the SHR/N strain was higher when compared to the remainder of the strains and remained so until 10 weeks of age. The blood pressures of the remainder of the strains reached their peak levels at either 6 or 8 weeks of age. However, again these data were too limited to draw any conclusion with respect to strain differences. The change of blood pressure with age is an important consideration when making a choice of animal models.

Table 2   Average 10 weeks blood pressure and the standard errors of F_1 males from crosses of females of five inbred strains with SHR/N males.

Female parent	Male parent	F_1 progeny
W/N	SHR/N	174 ± 2.1 (19)[a]
SD/N	SHR/N	167 ± 2.0 (17)
RHA/N	SHR/N	161 ± 2.2 (9)
ACI/N	SHR/N	139 ± 1.9 (25)
PETH/N	SHR/N	136 ± 2.0 (8)

[a] Number of Animals Tested

Table 2 presents the average blood pressures of the F_1 male progeny from mating females of five inbred strains with males of the SHR/N strain. As in the case of the strain comparisons, considerable variation was found in the progeny from these five combinations. The blood pressures ranged from 174 mm Hg for the progeny from the W/N × SHR/N to 136 mm Hg for the progeny from the PETH/N × SHR/N matings despite the fact that W/N and PETH/N strains were characterized by identical blood pressures. This would suggest a more complex form of inheritance than indicated from the selection studies. The blood pressures of the progeny from the SD/N and RHA/N strains mated with the SHR/N strain were in a similar range as that of the W/N × SHR/N progeny, whereas, that for the ACI/N × SHR/N progeny were near that of the PETH/N × SHR/N mating. Again, additional data are needed to confirm these results, but further analysis of these hybrids may be of interest.

DISCUSSION

The results obtained from this study, while preliminary, suggest that additional models are available which might complement those already developed by selective breeding. As far as the distributions of blood pressure are concerned, they appear to be similar in rats as in mice [10]. Since these rat strains have been developed for a variety of purposes ranging from cancer studies to behavioral differences, the study of cause and effect relationships are possible utlizing these different strains in different hybrids among themselves as well as with the selectively bred strains such as the SHR/N.

An example is the relationship of behavior to elevated blood pressures. Four of the strains included in this experiment were selected for behavioral differences. Two of the strains, MNR/N and MR/N, were selectively bred for low and high emotionality respectively, on the basis of an open field test [5]. There was essentially no difference in the blood pressures between these two strains. This might lead to a conclusion that emotional differences are not important in affecting blood pressure. However, a different situation occurred when comparing the RHA/N and RLA/N strains. The RHA/N strain was selectively bred for a high avoidance to an electric shock, whereas, the RLA/N strain was bred for a low avoidance to an electric shock [3]. The blood pressure of the RHA/N strain was significantly higher than that of the RLA/N strain suggesting that the genetic factors involved in this particular behavioral pattern are also related to elevated blood pressures.

The results of this survey can be considered from another view. A number of the strains, while representing different genetic backgrounds were characterized by nearly identical blood pressures. For example, the blood pressures of the OM/N, RHA/N, and SD/N strains were all in similar range, but elevated. The question is whether the factors which contributed to these elevated but similar blood pressures are the same or different. This is also true for those strains with lower but similar blood pressures.

The data obtained from the crosses of the W/N and PETH/N strains which were characterized by identical blood pressures with the SHR/N suggests that different regulatory systems were present in these two strains since the blood pressures of the W/N×SHR/N progeny were much higher than that of the PETH/N×SHR/N cross. A detailed physiological study of the progeny of these two hybrids might provide an insight into some of the factors involved in the regulation of blood pressure. More such unique combinations may exist, but can be only determined by further testing. The PETH/N strain was originally derived from a stock of rats exhibiting retinal dystrophy [4].

The importance of extending the testing to additional strains is demonstrated by the above results. The data obtained from the W/N×SHR/N hybrids agree with those reported by TANASE, et al. [13], which confirms their results and conclusions. However, the strains that they used for their study were similar to the W/N strain. The generality of the conclusions with respect to the genetic nature of blood pressure regulation depends upon the results from extending similar studies to more strains.

The ACI/N strain may also provide important information with respect to the role of the kidney in regulating blood pressure. This strain is characterized by a frequency of about 20% of unilaterally missing or abnormal kidneys [7]. Thus, comparisons of this strain with rats in which kidney function has been artificially impaired may provide further insight to the role of the kidney in regulating blood pressure. Also, by back crossing this strain with the SHR/N, there is a chance that the characteristic frequency of unilaterally missing kidneys can be introduced in the SHR/N strain.

Many possible combinations of this kind exist. Clearly, it would be an enormous task to examine all of the possible mating combinations among the 17 strains used in this study. However, further studies are planned to study the blood pressures of the progeny from all possible matings of the strains characterized by extreme measurements, both high and low.

The next logical step beyond the F_1 crosses is to carry these out to the F_2 followed by the development of new inbred strains from the F_2 segregants. The purpose of extending these studies beyond the F_1 is that genetic segregation occurs in the F_2 and if enough new strains were formed from the F_1 population, the new strains would be characterized by the same genes as the initial inbred populations but in different combinations. These new strains would then provide the opportunity to study cause and effect relationships. BAILEY [2] has proposed a similar technique for finding linkages and functions for histocompatibility genes in mice. While this technique is slow and time consuming, it probably represents the best possibility for studying cause and effect relationships involved in the regulation of blood pressure.

The development of these complementary models for the analysis of the factors involved in the regulation of blood pressure represents a challenge, both to the geneticist as well as the investigator. The challenge for the geneticist lies in the fact that he can utilize the tools developed for the analysis of complex genetic traits to further study the underlying genetic nature of blood pressure regulation and to provide the investigator with a series of results and models which are relevant for human medicine.

REFERENCES

1. ALEXANDER, N., HINSHAW, L. B. and DRURY, D. R. (1954): Proc Exp Biol Med, **86**, 855.
2. BAILEY, D. W. (1971): Transplantation, **11**, 325.
3. BIGNAMI, G. (1965): Anim Behav, **13**, 221.
4. BOURNE, M. C. and GRUENBERG, H. (1939): J Hered, **30**, 131.
5. BROADHURST, P. L. (1960): *In* "Experiments in Personality, Vol. 1, Pyschogenetics and Pysochopharmacology," (H. J. EYSENCK, ed.), p. 1, Routledge and Kegan Paul, London.
6. DAHL, L. K., HEINE, M. and TASSINARI, L. (1962): Nature, **194**, 482.
7. DERINGER, M. K., and HESTON, W. E., (1956): Proc Exp Biol Med, **91**, 312.
8. McKUSICK, V. A. (1960): Circulation, **22**, 857.
9. OKAMOTO, K. and AOKI, K. (1963): Jap Circ J, **27**, 282.
10. SCHLAGER, G. and WEIBUST, R. S. (1967): Genetics, **55**, 497.
11. SMIRK, F. H. and HALL, W. H. (1958): Nature, **182**, 727.
12. STURKIE, P. D., WEISS, H. S., RINGER, R. K. and SHEAHAN, M. M. (1959): Poult Science, **38**, 333.
13. TANASE, H., SUZUKI, V. D., OOSHIMA, R., YAMORI, Y. and OKAMOTO, K. (1970): Jap Circ J, **34**, 1197.
14. TANASE, H. and SUZUKI, V. D. (1971): Exp Anim, **20**, 1.
15. WILLIAMS, J. R., HARRISON, T. R. and GROLLMAN, A. (1939): J Clin Invest, **18**, 373.

THE DEVELOPMENT AND INHERITANCE OF THE HIGH BLOOD PRESSURE IN THE NEW ZEALAND STRAIN OF RATS WITH GENETIC HYPERTENSION

E. L. PHELAN*, D. W. J. CLARK*, C. R. GRESSON*,
and D. R. JONES*

The elucidation of the mechanisms responsible for the initiation and maintenance of high blood pressure in rats with hereditary forms of hypertension [8, 11] is of value in understanding the pathogenesis of human essential hypertension. In most forms of experimental hypertension the rise of blood pressure is the consequence of a specific procedure which may be precisely defined as to its nature and time of occurrence. In rats bred to develop hypertension there has been no intervention to precipitate the hypertension, and the factors responsible for the rise in blood pressure are of natural occurence. As in human essential hypertension there is no obvious derangement of physiological systems which may be said to initiate the high blood pressure. The hereditary nature of the hypertension in rats is a further analogy with much human hypertension which it is not possible to duplicate in other experimental models.

The origin of the New Zealand strain of rats with genetic hypertension (GH rats) has been described previously [9]. The rats of this strain are descended from a mating in 1955 between a pair of rats with over average blood pressures from the Otago stock colony of albino rats. This stock colony, the progenitors of which were brought to New Zealand from England in 1930, is ultimately of Wistar origin. The mean systolic blood pressure of the Otago stock colony for both males and females is approximately 110–120 mm Hg when measured under light ether anaesthesia by a tail cuff method, and has remained constant over the last 15 years; pressures exceeding 140 mm Hg are rare.

The descendants of this single mating have now been propagated by brother-sister matings between rats with the highest blood pressures in each generation for over 30 generations. Over this period of 15 years the blood pressure of rats of the hypertensive strain has risen at a mean rate of just less than 2 mm Hg per generaion, [10], until in males of the 30th generation it averages 178 mm Hg. This slow and steady rise in blood pressure over several generations of inbreeding is in strong contrast to the situation in the Japanese colony of rats with spontaneous hypertension (SHR) in which very high levels of blood pressure were achieved after only three generations of selection [8]. In the New Zealand colony the increase in blood pressure is not easily explicable by environmental changes nor by the presence of a few genes which strongly influence the blood pressure but is compatible with multifactorial genetic control of the blood pressure.

It is important to quantify the inheritance of the hypertension in GH rats and to define the relative roles of genetic and environmental factors in determining the level of the blood pressure. In this paper are reported the results of an experiment which further indicates that the blood pressure of the New Zealand GH rats is inherited in a graded fashion presumably through the action of many genes of relatively small individual effect.

A random selection of pure line hypertensive rats of the 25th generation of GH rats (21 male and 37 female) and of the 39th generation of a pure line of normotensive (BS) rats [9] (30 male and 30 female) comprising rats born in the same month, were recipro-

* Wellcome Medical Research Institute, Department of Medicine, University of Otago Medical School, Dunedin, New Zealand.

cally mated to produce an F_1 generation. When these F_1 rats were 12 weeks old a selection was randomly mated to produce the F_2 generation. Concurrently a further F_1 generation was produced by remating the parent strains and the backcross matings ($F_1 \times GH$ and $F_1 \times BS$) were also made at the same time. Thus it was possible to reduce environmental and seasonal variation by measuring the blood pressures of the second F_1, the F_2 and two backcross generations in rats reared at the same time and under similar conditions. These rats were aged between 11 and 13 weeks when their pressures were measured. The blood pressures of the rats from the parent GH and BS strains were determined at the ages of 11 and 28 weeks and the means and variances did not change significantly during this time. Values reported are systolic blood pressures measured under light ether anaesthesia by a tail cuff method [4] and are the means of three replicates. All measurements were made between 9 a.m. and 12 noon. The results are shown in Figs. 1 and 2.

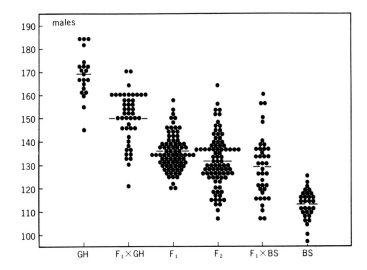

Fig. 1 Distribution of blood pressure in males of the GH (hypertensive) and BS (normotensive) strains, the F_1 and F_2 generations and the backcrosses from the F_1 to the parent strains. The mean blood pressure, the variance and the number of rat in each generation were:

GH (168 mm Hg, 93.2, 21);
$F_1 \times GH$ (150 mm Hg, 113.7, 46);
F_1 (136 mm Hg, 57.7, 79);
F_2 (131 mm Hg, 125.9, 85);
$F_1 \times BS$ (129 mm Hg, 173.2, 39);
BS (113 mm Hg, 38.2, 30).

Inspection of these figures shows that the mean blood pressure of the F_1 generation in both males and females is close to the mid-parent means and that the F_2 means are also close to these values. The means of the backcrosses are also intermediate between the means of the F_1 generation and appropriate parental mean. This indicates that the level of the blood pressure is an inherited characteristic and that dominance effects, if present, are largely balanced. In males there is some suggestion of segregation of phenotypes in the $F_1 \times BS$ generation.

The phenotypic variance in the F_1 generations is due theoretically to environmental causes only, whilst the F_2 variance may be partitioned into environmental and genetic

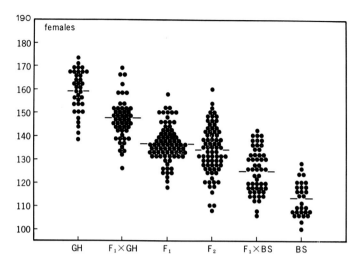

Fig. 2 Distribution of blood pressures in females of the GH and BS strains, the F_1 and F_2 generations and the backcrosses from the F_1 to the parent strains. The mean blood pressure, the variance and number of rats in each generation were:

GH (159 mm Hg, 75.8, 37);
$F_1 \times$ GH (148 mm Hg, 75.3, 51);
F_1 (137 mm Hg, 58.7, 79);
F_2 (134 mm Hg, 112.6, 75);
$F_1 \times$ BS (125 mm Hg, 87.2, 53);
BS (113 mm Hg, 48.1, 30).

components. The genetic determination of the blood pressure was calculated as the difference of these two variances divided by the F_2 variance and for males equals 0.54 ± 0.102 and for females 0.48 ± 0.120. These values are lower than, but not significantly different from, those obtained in SHR [12].

The results were analysed by standard biometrical techniques [1]. There was no evidence for significant interaction between genotype and environment in the non-segregating GH, BS and F_1 generations in either sex when the variances were tested for inhomogeneity by the Hartley and Pearson M-test. When the generation means were used to derive the genetic parameters representing additive effects (d) and deviations from additive effects (h) at any one locus, and also the three first order interactions (i, j, l) between loci, it was found that in females only the additive genetic component was significant whilst in males the four non-additive components were also significant (Table 1).

No meaningful results were obtained from an analysis of the generation variances into environmental and additive and dominance genetic components. Variances must always be positive quantities but in males a negative additive variance and in females a negative dominance variance were obtained. In females the failure of the analysis was surprising, as the generally accepted criteria had been met; however several other similarly discrepant results have been reported in the literature [1, 7].

The number of independently-segregating genetic determinants of the blood pressure was estimated by the formula derived by WRIGHT [13] and was greater than five for both sexes. While the validity of this formula has yet to be fully established for physiological variables, the result implies that a considerable number of genes are involved in the inheritance of the blood pressure level in GH rats.

Table 1

Genetic Parameters Derived from Generation Means
All values $\pm$ SEM

	Male mm Hg	Female mm Hg
d (additive effects)	21 $\pm$ 2.6*	22 $\pm$ 1.8*
h (dominance deviations)	29 $\pm$ 7.3*	11 $\pm$ 6.3
Non-allelic interactions		
i (d $\times$ d)	34 $\pm$ 7.2*	10 $\pm$ 6.0
j (d $\times$ h)	-14 ± 5.8*	-1 ± 4.0
l (h $\times$ h)	-39 ± 12.0*	10 $\pm$ 9.0

* Significant values P<0.05

In rats of the New Zealand strain with genetic hypertension aged about 12 weeks, we may conclude that there is strong genetic determination of the blood pressure but that environmental influences are of importance in determining its final level within the hypertensive range. The inheritance is multifactorial and probably additive polygenic in females, but in males dominance deviations and non-allelic interactions are significance.

These genetic findings suggest that the aetiology of hereditary hypertension in rats is complex and the search for a single fundamental defect is futile. Whatever the genetic differences between normotensive and GH rats may be which cause the latter to become hypertensive, it is obvious that these manifest themselves early in the rat's life. It has been shown that at the age of two days GH rats exhibit blood pressures significantly higher than those of normotensive rats [5]. Pressures higher than those ever encountered in mature normotensive rats occur in GH rats aged only four weeks, and by six weeks of age blood pressures of 160 mm Hg are common.

Many of the differences between relatively mature GH rats and normotensive rats appear to be the consequence of this early elevation of the blood pressure and thus yield information on the secondary processes contributing to or modulating genetic hypertension. Renin levels are normal in the kidney and plasma of GH rats aged 9 weeks or less and in older rats they may be depressed by 20% or more [6]. Cardiac hypertrophy occurs only in rats with considerable hypertension aged 6 weeks or more. Enhanced vascular reactivity of perfused mesenteric blood vessels to noradrenaline and serotonin first occurs in GH rats at the same age (JONES, unpublished).

While the sympathetic nervous system plays an important role in maintaining the level of the blood pressure in GH rats there is no clear demonstration that it plays a primary role in its elevation to hypertensive levels. In mature GH rats peripheral sympathetic nervous activity as assessed by the rate of disappearance of administered ³HNA is normal or reduced [10]. This reduction in sympathetic activity appears to be a homeostatic response to the high blood pressure, for in GH rats aged $5^{1}/_{2}$ weeks the rate constant for the decline of cardiac ³HNA following intravenous administration is 0.079 $\pm$ 0.0096 hr^{-1} which is identical to the value in similarly aged normotensive rats (0.078 $\pm$ 0.012 hr^{-1}). Administration of either anti-nerve growth factor or 6-hydroxydopamine to neonatal rats produces a widespread sympathectomy which appears to be life-long: GH rats so treated have intra-arterial blood pressures higher than those of untreated normotensive rats [2, 3] and thus genetic hypertension is not wholly dependent on an intact sympathetic nervous system.

It is of interest to note that these treatments which almost completely destroy the sympathetic innervation of the heart do not reduce the elevated heart rate of GH rats to control levels [2]. This elevated heart rate, like the high blood pressure, persists under anaesthesia. The heart rate of GH rats aged 10 days is $386 \pm$ S.E. 6.2 beats/min, compared with the normotensive rats' rate of 354 ± 9.0 beats/min, $P < 0.005$, (JONES, unpublished), and may be a contributing factor to the development of the hypertension. We have also found that one of the determinants of blood viscosity, and hence of vascular resistance, the packed cell volume is significantly greater in GH rats by the age of three weeks (GRESSON, unpublished).

The pathogenesis of genetic hypertension in SHR and GH rats is complex, but the differences between the two strains are such that both offer unique opportunities to study in the young animals those abnormalities of cardiovascular regulation which eventually lead to frank hypertension.

ACKNOWLEDGEMENTS

This work was supported by grants from the Medical Research Council of New Zealand and from the National Heart and Lung Institute, U. S. Public Health Service (Grant HE-10942). The authors wish to thank Associate Professor F. O. SIMPSON for his guidance of these studies and Emeritus Professor Sir HORACE SMIRK for helpful discussions. Thanks are also due to those technicians responsible for the care of rats of the hypertensive strain, and in particular Mrs. B. M. LYON, Mrs. D. C. FARMER and Mrs. E. E. HIGGINS.

REFERENCES

1. BROADHURST, P. L. and JINKS, J. L. (1961): Psychol Bull, **58**, 337.
2. CLARK, D. W. J. (1971): Circ Res, **28**, 330.
3. CLARK, D. W. J., LAVERTY, R. and PHELAN, E. L. (1972): Br J Pharmacol, **44**, 233.
4. DOWD, D. A. and JONES, D. R. (1968): J Appl Physiol, **25**, 772.
5. JONES, D. R. and DOWD, D. A. (1970): Life Sci, **9**, 247.
6. McKENZIE, J. K. and PHELAN, E. L. (1969): Proc Univ Otago Med Sch, **47**, 23.
7. NEWELL, T. G. (1970): J Comp Physiol Psychology, **70**, 37.
8. OKAMOTO, K. and AOKI, K. (1963): Jap Circ J, **27**, 282.
9. PHELAN, E. L. (1968): N Z Med J, **67**, 334.
10. PHELAN, E. L. (1970): Circ Res, **27**, Suppl. II, 65.
11. SMIRK, F. H. and HALL, W. H. (1958): Nature, **182**, 727.
12. TANASE, H. and SUZUKI, Y. (1971): Exp Anim, **20**, 1.
13. WRIGHT, S. (1968): *In* "Evolution and Genetics of Populations", Vol. 1, p 383. University of Chicago Press, Chicago.

HEREDITARY RETINAL DYSTROPHIC RATS IN STRAIN OF SPONTANEOUSLY HYPERTENSIVE RAT

K. MIZUNO*, K. OZAWA**, S. NISHIDA** and K. AOKI***

Retinal dystrophy in the rat, found by BURNE [1], involves progressive loss of photo-receptor cells, with onset during or soon after the developmental period. Several investigators had intensely studied this rat in order to clarify the pathogenesis of human retinitis pigmentosa. Functional, chemical and morphological data, however, obtained in the case of the rat indicated some differences from those of human retinitis pigmentosa. Accordingly we have long been looking for animals which spontaneously develop retinal dystrophy similar to human retinitis pigmentosa.

About two years ago Dr. AOKI told us that some old SHRs looked as if they were blind. We didn't believe him because he was not an ophthalmologist. One day after that I unexpectedly found a loss of visual cells in one of the pathological specimens obtained from SHR. Since that time, our attention was wholly taken up with the occurrence of retinal dystrophy and cataracts in a colony of SHR.

Since retinal dystrophy and cataracts were not the result of injury or intoxication, and the affected stock appeared in the ratio of about two to one in the colony of SHR, we concluded that a hereditary factor might be involved.

First we received from Dr. AOKI 19 SHRs, which were 12 to 14 months old, and examined them electroretinographically and morphologically. By gross inspection cataractous change was found in 6 animals. Electrical responses of SHR could be divided into two groups. The a-waves are divided into two groups bounded by 150 μV. The b-waves are also divided into two bounded by 450 μV (Fig. 1). No electrical activity was detected in 7 of the eyes in the group which showed low electrical activities. The ERG is an easy, convenient and reliable method for measuring the visual response of an animal. Low voltage response or extinction of the ERG, therefore, indicates dysfunction of the photoreceptors, especially some morphological changes in the photoreceptors. Both eyes of each animal which showed either subnormal electric response or extinct response to intense light stimuli were examined by light-and electron microscopy.

Animals of the subnormal ERG group showed a normal retinal architecture under light microscopic observations, while several early changes could be detected by electron microscopy. Primary disorganization of the outer segment was already present in the visual cell layer. The pigment epithelial process and cytoplasm appeared normal. Noteworthy, however, was an early change in the distal part of the pigment epithelium and Bruck's membrane. More or less deterioration could be seen on the basal infolding (Fig. 2). MIZUNO and NISHIDA [5] already mentioned, a few years ago, that the invasion of homogenous material into the cleft of the basal infolding and the partial loss of the basal infolding are characteristics of human retinitis pigmentosa. The same morphological changes as described in the human disease have already appeared in subnormal ERG group. The appearance of a fibroblast-like cell in the Bruck's membrane was also noticeable; the same change was found in human retinitis pigmentosa, too.

  * Department of Ophthalmology, Tohoku University School of Medicine, Sendai, Japan
 ** Department of Ophthalmology, Nagoya City University Medical School, Nagoya, Japan
*** Department of Internal Medicine, Nagoya City University Medical School, Nagoya, Japan

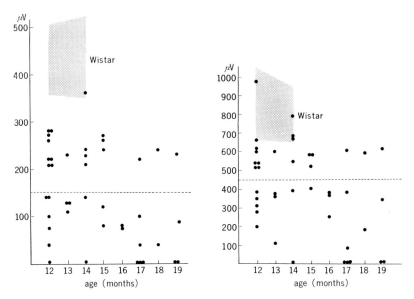

Fig. 1 Electroretinograms recorded from normal rats (Wistar) and SHRs. The a wave (left) and
b-wave (right) can be divided into two groups by the dotted line. Some animals are blind.

In the eyes of the extinct ERG group, light microscopy showed a retina in which the
photoreceptor outer segment layer was lost and rod cell nuclei decreased in number to
only about 2–3 rows of nuclei. Electron microscopy showed abundant disorganized outer
and inner segment materials. Membranes of the outer segment appeared to be arranged
in elongated bundles or sheets parallel to and closely opposed to the elongated pigment
epithelial processes. Cellular organelles of the pigment epithelium began to disorganize.
Its basal infolding was almost lost and flattened in part. Numerous fibloblast-like cells
appeared in Bruck's membrane (Fig. 3). In the choriocapillaris its basal lamina increased
in thickness, and the fenestration structure which is usually visible in the retinal side
endothelium of the normal choriocapillaris disappeared and was transformed into the
same structure as its scleral side. Thus, the retinal and choroidal lesion of this animal
bears a striking resemblance to the histologic appearances described in certain cases of
human retinitis pigmentosa.

Next an attempt was made to follow up electrical changes of SHR. Forty young SHRs
and 20 young Wistar rats were purchased from the Japan Rat Co., and their ERGs were
recorded every two months beginning 2 months after birth. Although the electrical
activity of control Wistar rats somewhat decreased with aging, the ERG change with
aging in SHR was much more significant. The ERG pattern of these SHR could be
divided into two groups as in the SHR given by Dr. Aoki. The ERG response continued
to attenuate by 4 to 6 months after birth. In several animals among them the response
became only a traceable one by 12 months.

Experiments like the above yielded an especially adequate comparison between the
ERG and the pathology of affected and unaffected animals because both groups of
animals were raised under the same conditions.

The electrophysiological and pathological conditions which we have described are a
hereditary progressive degeneration of the retina beginning with the death of the outer
segments. When we make a list of the characteristics which appeared in Burne's dystrophic rat (BDR), our spontaneously dystrophic rat (SDR) and human retinitis pigmentosa

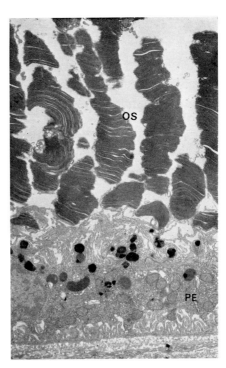

Fig. 2 Electron micrograph of affected animals which show subnormal ERG. Disorganized outer segment lamellae (OS), an early deterioration of basal infolding of the pigment epithelium (PE) and fibloblast-like cell in Bruck's membrane are seen.

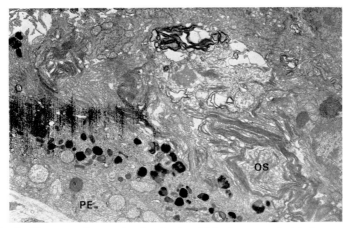

Fig. 3 Electron micrograph of animals which show no electrical response. Pieces of lamellar material of the outer segment (OS) have dislocated between the disorganized inner segment and the pigment epithelium (PE).

(HRP), we get a clear information of the differences among them (Table 1). In HRP, pathology has been studied only in mild or severe cases, and functional studies have so far in general served to define the early features of the disorder. Our clinical experiences, however, indicate that a few cases of HRP have apparently occurred in middle or old age. Therefore, SDR might be a model of senile HRP. Excessive production of rhodopsin and an associated abnormal lamellae tissue component before progressive loss of photoreceptors cells, confirmed in BDR by DOWLING and SIDMAN [2], definitely differ from HRP.

We are impressed by the striking resemblance with the fine structural features in the distal part of the pigment epithelium, Bruch's membrane and choriocapillaris seen in

Table 1   Discriminative significances of Burne's dystrophic rat (BDR) spontaneously dystrophic rat (SDR) and human retinitis pigmentosa (HRP).

	BDR	SDR	HRP
Onset	18–20 days	4–6 months*	Early age, or prime of life,* sometimes
Cataract	Absent	Present*	Present*
ERG	Normal to extinct	Normal to extinct	Subnormal to extinct
Abnormal lamellae	Present	Absent*	Absent*
Changes in pigment epithelium & Bruch's membrane	Absent	Present*	Present*

* represent something similar to each other

SDR bear to the electron microscopic appearance described in certain cases of HRP.

As far as we are aware, there has been no precise description of this lesion occuring in rats, nor of the exact mode of any progressive hereditary retinal lesion closely similar to the human disease.

It is very interesting to note in MIZUNO's paper [3,4] that increased catecholamine contents in the retina produced experimental retinitis pigmentosa in a rabbit. It is also interesting to refer to the paper of Dr. TABEI and his coworkers [7], concerning the increase of noradrenaline fluorescence in the peripheral vascular system of SHR, and to that of Dr. OZAKI and his coworkers [6] concerning increased adrenal noradrenaline contents in SHR.

The study of the retinal disease seen in SDR as a model of the inherited degenerative disorders is promising since more information will be available on the function, chemistry and structure of HRP than in studies using other experimental animals.

REFERENCES

1. BURNE, M.C., CAMPELL, D.A. and TANSLEY, K. (1938): Br J Ophthalmol, **22**, 613.
2. DOWLING, J.E. and SIDMAN, R.L. (1962):   J Cell Biol, **14**, 73.
3. MIZUNO, K. (1959): Acta Soc Ophthalmol Jap, **63**, 406.
4. MIZUNO, K. (1960): Acta Soc Ophthalmol Jap, **64**, 2186.
5. MIZUNO, K. and NISHIDA, S. (1967):   Am J Ophthalmol, **63**, 791.
6. OZAKI, M., SUZUKI, Y., YAMORI, Y. and OKAMOTO, K. (1968): Jap Circ J, **32**, 1367.
7. TABEI, R. MORISAWA, T. MARUYAMA, T. and SUZUKI, Y. (1967): Jap Circ J, **30**, 153.

Chapter II

CATECHOLAMINE METABOLISM

CATECHOLAMINE METABOLISM IN THE SPONTANEOUSLY HYPERTENSIVE RAT

A. SJOERDSMA*

I accept as a truism of research findings in human essential hypertension, that, whereas no convincing chemical evidence can be obtained to implicate excess activity of vasoconstrictor systems (such as the sympatho-adrenal system) in pathogenesis or maintenance of the hypertension, most of the effective antihypertensive drugs act by lessening vasoconstrictor activity, especially that mediated by the sympathetic nervous system. Furthermore, biochemical effects of such drugs are easily demonstrated, even in man [2]. Also, we have surmised that anti-adrenergic drugs with predominantly peripheral actions diminish markedly the availability of norepinephrine to vascular receptors and that only a small percentage of tissue noradrenaline is sufficient to maintain an existing hypertension [6].

Because of inherent limitations in research on human subjects, we welcomed the opportunity presented to us in 1966 to study the spontaneously hypertensive rat (SHR). It was at that time that Dr. TABEI, at the instigation of Professor OKAMOTO and Dr. UDENFRIEND, brought several F_{13} breeding pairs to the National Institutes of Health. The cooperation of Dr. HANSEN assured us an adequate supply of SHR's and normotensive Wistar/NIH animals and facilitated establishment of numerous other colonies of the SHR both in the USA and abroad.

A recurring problem in our work, as well as that of others, is the question of strain differences among normotensive animals used as controls. Numerous "apparent" abnormalities have been observed which may be related to this problem. In the case of catecholamines, such "abnormalities" in SHR range from alterations in levels of catecholamine enzyme activities to organ catecholamine contents. For example, elsewhere in this symposium OZAKI et al. and NAGATSU et al. report increased adrenal catecholamine content and synthesis rates, along with higher than "normal" levels of adrenal tyrosine hydroxylase and dopamine β-oxidase in SHR. On the other hand, we find little difference between SHR's and Wistar/NIH animals as regards adrenal catecholamine content but a markedly diminished synthesis rate (from ^{14}C-tyrosine and ^{3}H-dopa) along with a 50% decrease in dopamine β-oxidase activity in SHR's versus control animals. Recently, we have been studying also normotensive Kyoto-Wistar animals and some of our own most impressive "abnormalities" (*e.g.* decreased brain decarboxylase as reported by YAMORI et al. [8]) become less significant if we compare the SHR to Kyoto-Wistar. Perhaps this is not so critical since we might view the Kyoto-Wistar as possessing hypertensive traits. To re-emphasize, however, lack of a proper control animal

---

* Experimental Therapeutics Branch, National Heart & Lung Institute, Bethesda, Md., U.S.A.

is a continuing deterrent to studies on the pathogenesis of hypertension in the SHR and represents a challenge in animal genetics.

We have generally studied SHR's and matched controls at the time that blood pressure is rising rapidly in the SHR, *i.e.* from 8–15 weeks. Except for studies by Louis et al. [4, 5] in earlier generations, observations to be cited here were mainly in F_{20} to F_{26} animals. Recent generations of SHR/NIH exhibit a systolic blood pressure over 150 mm Hg as early as 8 weeks and usually greater than 200 mm Hg at 15 weeks of age [9].

The focus of our early studies [4, 5] was to ascertain whether there might be an overall or organ specific increase in norepinephrine synthesis and turnover rate which would reflect increased peripheral sympathetic nerve activity and thereby account for the hypertension. The answer as judged from studies on the heart was negative and indeed a somewhat decreased rate of turnover and release of norepinephrine suggested a secondary, compensatory state of sympathetic nerve activity, rather than an etiologically primary, overactivity. Similar conclusions could be drawn from the fact that plasma free fatty acid levels were "normal" and the total excretion of catecholamine metabolites in the urine was similar in SHR and Wistar/NIH. SPECTOR et al., reporting in this volume, also find evidence of a compensatory rather than primary mechanism in catecholamine studies on blood vessels.

Table 1 Organ weights in rats.

Animal	Age (weeks)	Heart mg/100 g	Adrenal (mg)	Thymus (mg)
Wistar	8	298 ± 7	26 ± 1	333 ± 10
SHR	8	309 ± 9	36 ± 1	$417 \pm 31*$
Wistar	12	265 ± 4	33 ± 2	258 ± 19
SHR	12	$313 \pm 11*$	$40 \pm 2*$	$320 \pm 24*$

Means $\pm$ SE =, n = 14 – 18, * p < 0.05. Also, see text.

Table 2 Tissue norepinephrine content in 9–11 week-old rats.

Animal	Norepinephrine (ng/g)				
	Brainstem	Spleen	Heart	Kidney	Submaxillary gland
Wistar	761 ± 14 (23)	1499 ± 60 (27)	663 ± 42 (6)	184 ± 9 (6)	806 ± 73 (6)
SHR	$594 \pm 11**$ (24)	$388 \pm 20**$ (28)	710 ± 66 (6)	$141 \pm 6**$ (6)	962 ± 92 (6)

Values are means ($\pm$ SEM); number of determinations in parenthesis; * = significant difference from Wistar controls (**p < 0.01).

Recently we have made a more extensive organ by organ comparison of male SHR's and Wistar/NIH animals regarding a number of parameters ranging from organ weights to norepinephrine synthetic rates. Although the body weights of age-matched animals were similar, significant differences in organ weights were noted as shown in Table 1 and were independent of sex. A significantly greater weight of heart (at 12 weeks), adrenals and thymus was observed in SHR. Minor differences were also noted in the weights of spleen and kidney (15% greater in SHR at various ages) but not in testes, liver and lung. These rather gross indices indicate the difficulties of attributing etiologic significance to differences between SHR and control animals.

Norepinephrine content of several organs is summarized in Table 2. Significantly lower values were found in brainstem, kidney and spleen, the low content of the latter in

SHR being particularly striking. Current observations on Kyoto-Wistar animals reveal average kidney norepinephrine values to be identical to that of SHR's, with intermediate levels in brainstem and spleen. Followup studies on norepinephrine synthetic rates in spleen and brainstem show an 80 and 30% decrease (compared to Wistar/NIH) respectively using the synthesis inhibition technique (injection of α-methyl tyrosine), and confirmatory values employing ^{14}C-tyrosine conversion to norepinephrine. The differences in spleen are probably related to a low endowment of sympathetic nerves since synthesis of norepinephrine from ^{3}H-Dopa is similarly affected, whereas the defect in brain is at the tyrosine hydroxylase step with incorporation of tritium into norepinephrine being similar in SHR's and control animals. Details of these studies will be published later.

One is left with similar conclusions to those presented earlier in this paper for the state of catecholamines and sympathetic nerve activity peripherally, with intriguing possibilities regarding a role of norepinephrine centrally. Studies by us [9] employing 6-hydroxydopamine to induce peripheral norepinephrine depletion support the contention that only a fraction of the normal norepinephrine content is sufficient to maintain hypertension in the SHR; probably a highly effective immunosympathectomy would inhibit development of hypertension, as reported by CLARK [1] for the New Zealand strain.

A detailed discussion of the possible role of norepinephrine in brain in the pathogenesis of hypertension in SHR and in the action of certain antihypertensive drugs is beyond the scope of this presentation. From available evidence [3, 7] there seems no doubt that hypotensive drug effects may be mediated by a central noradrenergic depressor system; we have previously speculated on the possible role of brain norepinephrine in blood pressure modulation [8], and still find the hypothesis of a central catecholamine deficiency in SHR an appealing possibility. I recall apparently successful induction of hypertension by YAMORI in preliminary studies on rats given 6-hydroxydopamine intraventricularly, but subsequently neither he nor de JONG could confirm the finding [9]. Further research on central noradrenergic mechanisms possibly in interaction with other stimuli, should be revealing. A reciprocal relationship between brain norepinephrine and serotonin with respect to blood pressure control also warrants consideration.

CONCLUSION

While it is premature to assume that the SHR is a reliable model of hypertension in man, clearly it is an excellent preparation in which to study hypertensive mechanisms and the effects of antihypertensive drugs. Strain differences among normotensive control animals may account for some of the "apparent" abnormalities in catecholamine metabolism in SHR's. Nonetheless, the weight of biochemical evidence favors normal or decreased sympathetic activity peripherally, suggesting a secondary rather than a primary state. To this writer, the future in this field appears to lie in more detailed studies on norepinephrine in brain.

ACKNOWLEDGEMENT

I recognize with pleasure the contributions to our research by three Visiting Scientists from Professor OKAMOTO's department, Drs. Ryo TABEI, Yukio YAMORI and Hirohiko YAMABE. Studies over the past $1^1/_2$ years represent primarily the efforts of Dr. YAMABE and Dr. Wybren DE JONG of Utrecht in collaboration with Dr. Walter LOVENBERG, head of our Section on Biochemical Pharmacology.

REFERENCES

1. CLARK, D. W. J. (1971): Circ Res, **28**, 330.
2. DEQUATTRO, V. and SJOERDSMA, A. (1968): J Clin Invest, **47**, 2359.
3. HENNING, M. and RUBENSON, A. (1971): J Pham Pharmacol, **23**, 407.
4. LOUIS, W. J., KRAUSS, K. R., KOPIN, I. J. and SJOERDSMA, A. (1970): Circ Res, **27**, 589.
5. LOUIS, W. J., SPECTOR, S., TABEI, R. and SJOERDSMA, A. (1969): Circ Res, **24**, 85.
6. SJOERDSMA, A. (1967): Circ Res, **20** and **21**, Suppl. III, 119.
7. YAMORI, Y., de JONG, W., YAMABE, Y., LOVENBERG, W. and SJOERDSMA, A. (1972): J Pharm Pharmacol, in press.
8. YAMORI, Y., LOVENBERG, W. and SJOERDSMA, A. (1970): Science, **170**, 544.
9. YAMORI, Y., YAMABE, H., de JONG, W., LOVENBERG, W. and SJOERDSMA, A. (1972): Eur J Pharmacol, **17**, 135.

ENZYMES OF CATECHOLAMINE BIOSYNTHESIS AND METABOLISM IN SPONTANEOUSLY HYPERTENSIVE RATS AND HYPOTENSIVE EFFECTS OF THE SPECIFIC INHIBITORS FROM MICROBIAL ORIGIN

T. NAGATSU*, K. MIZUTANI*, I. NAGATSU**,
H. UMEZAWA***, M. MATSUZAKI*** and T. TAKEUCHI***

We wish to report on (1) a pronounced hypotensive effect of the inhibitors of catecholamine biosynthesis in spontaneously hypertensive (SH) rats; and (2) the changes in the enzyme activities of catecholamine biosynthesis and metabolism in various organs of SH rats.

1. Hypotensive effects of the new inhibitors from microbial origin of tyrosine hydroxylase and dopamine β-hydroxylase on SH rats

Biosynthesis of epinephrine from tyrosine requires 4 enzymes; namely, tyrosine hydroxylase, DOPA decarboxylase, dopamine β-hydroxylase and phenylethanolamine N-methyltransferase. Tyrosine hydroxylase is the rate-limiting step in the catecholamine biosynthesis. Catecholamines are metabolized by 2 enzymes; namely, monoamine oxidase and catechol O-methyltransferase.

Several new inhibitors of tyrosine hydroxylase and dopamine β-hydroxylase from microbial origin have been discovered recently. Some of these microbial inhibitors, oudenone [11] and fusaric acid [1], were found to inhibit the catecholamine biosynthesis *in vivo* and to decrease the endogenous levels of catecholamines [5, 2]. These new inhibitors decreased blood pressure in various mammals including normal Wistar rats, but they had a more pronounced hypotensive action on SH rats [3].

Oudenone ((S)-2-[4,5-dihydro-5-propyl-2(3H)-furylidene]-1,3-cyclopentanedione) is a new microbial inhibitor of tyrosine hydroxylase discovered by UMEZAWA et al [11]. The chemical structure [6] is shown in Figure 1. This compound inhibited tyrosine hydroxylase both *in vitro* and *in vivo* and decreased the endogenous level of catecholamines [1].

Oudenone reduced the blood pressure of both normal Wistar rats and SH rats (Fig. 1, 2). Oudenone, at three different dosages, 50 mg/kg, 12.5 mg/kg, and 3.1 mg/kg, was administered orally to the rats three times every 24 hours. After the administration of oudenone, the blood pressure decreased slowly. The lowest level of blood pressure was maintained between 24 to 72 hours after the 3rd administration, and then the blood pressure returned to its original level. SH rats were significantly more sensitive to the enzyme inhibitors than normal Wistar rats, and more pronounced hypotensive effects of oudenone were observed (Fig. 2). OZAKI [7] also reported that α-methyl-p-tyrosine, a tyrosine hydroxylase inhibitor, has a marked hypotensive effect in SH rats.

SH rats under 30 weeks after birth were highly sensitive to the tyrosine hydroxylase inhibitor oudenone. SH rats over 30 weeks of age became less sensitive to oudenone.

Fusaric acid (5-butyl-picolinic acid) (Fig. 1) is an antibiotic produced by a fungus and discovered to be a new inhibitor of dopamine β-hydroxylase by HIDAKA et al [1]. This

* Department of Biochemistry, School of Dentistry, Aichi-Gakuin University, Nagoya, Japan
** Department of Anatomy and Physiology, Aichi Prefectural College of Nursing, Nagoya, Japan
*** Institute of Microbial Chemistry, Tokyo, Japan

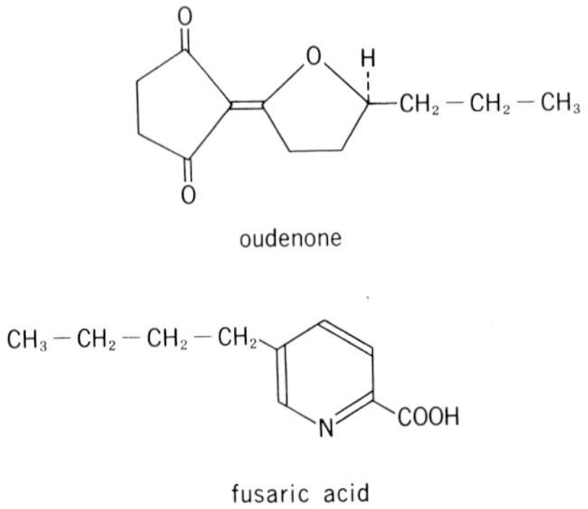

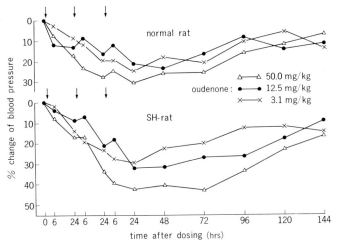

Fig. 1   Structures of oudenone and fusaric acid.

Fig. 2   Effect of oudenone (per os) on blood pressure of normal Wistar rats and SH rats.

compound inhibited dopamine β-hydroxylase *in vitro* and *in vivo*, and reduced the endogenous level of tissue catecholamines [2].

Fusaric acid reduced the blood pressure of both normal Wistar rats and SH rats (Fig. 3). Fusaric acid, at three different dosages, 50 mg/kg, 12.5 mg/kg, and 3.1 mg/kg, was administered orally three times every 24 hours. Blood pressure decreased rather rapidly within 6 hours and then recovered slowly. As shown in Figure 3, the SH rats were significantly more sensitive than normal Wistar rats to fusaric acid.

A relationship between hypotensive effect and dopamine β-hydroxylase inhibitor activity was observed with 5-alkyl-picolinic acid [9]. By increasing carbon numbers in 5-alkyl group of 5-alkyl-picolinic acid, the activity of dopamine β-hydroxylase inhibition and the hypotensive effect were increased simultaneously. 5-alkyl-picolinic acids with carbon numbers 4 and 5; that is, 5-butyl-picolinic acid (fusaric acid) and 5-pentyl-picolinic acid, both had the strongest hypotensive action and also the strongest inhibitor activity.

SH rats at any age from 8 to 46 weeks were highly sensitive to the dopamine β-hydroxylase inhibitor fusaric acid in contrast to the hypotensive action of the tyrosine hydroxylase

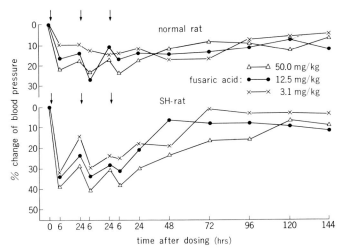

Fig. 3 Effect of fusaric acid (per os) on blood pressure of normal Wistar rats and SH rats.

inhibitor oudenone. As described above, SH rats under 30 weeks of age were sensitive to oudenone.

Another new microbial inhibitor of dopamine β-hydroxylase has been discovered. This compound, which has been named "dopastin," also had a pronounced hypotensive action on SH rats. The hypotensive effect of dopastin is similar to that of fusaric acid, and SH rats of any age from 8 to 46 weeks were highly sensitive to it. The chemical structure of dopastin is now under investigation.

A question is whether the hypotensive effect of these enzyme inhibitors is mainly due to the inhibition of the catecholamine biosynthesis and the resultant decrease in the endogenous levels of catecholamines. Since these inhibitors can reduce endogenous catecholamines, at least a part of the hypotensive effects appears to be due to the inhibition of the enzymes *in vivo*. However, the possibility of the hypotensive effect of the enzyme inhibitors due to some other mechanisms is also under investigation.

2. Enzymes of catecholamine biosynthesis and metabolism in SH rats

To investigate the high susceptibility of SH rats to the inhibitors tyrosine hydroxylase and dopamine β-hydroxylase, the activities of the enzymes involved in the catecholamine biosynthesis and metabolism in the organs of SH rats were examined [3,4]. Since we have found differences in relation to age in the hypotensive effects of the enzyme inhibitors on SH rats, the enzyme activities of SH rats at various ages were examined.

Normal male Wistar rats of the same age raised in the same conditions were used as controls. The rats were 4 to 26 weeks old. For the assay of enzyme activities, the rats were decapitated, and brains, hearts, adrenals, and spleens were quickly removed, frozen on dry ice, and stored.

Tyrosine hydroxylase was partially purified from soluble fraction of tissues by ammonium sulfate fractionation. Dopamine β-hydroxylase was solubilized from the particulate fraction of adrenals by using a detergent Cutscum and then fractionated with ammonium sulfate. These purification procedures of tyrosine hydroxylase and dopamine β-hydroxylase permit the determination of the enzyme activities which are proportional to the amount of the enzymes. Tyrosine hydroxylase activity was measured by radioassay

based on the formation of DOPA-^{14}C from L-tyrosine-^{14}C as substrate. DOPA decarboxylase activity was measured fluorometrically by the formation of dopamine from L-
DOPA as substrate. Dopamine β-hydroxylase was measured spectrophotometrically by
the formation of octopamine from tyramine as substrate. Phenylethanolamine N-methyltransferase activity was measured by radioassay of the formation of metanephrine-^{14}C
from normetanephrine and S-adenosyl-methionine-[methyl-^{14}C] as substrates. Catechol
O-methyltransferase activity was measured by radioassay of the formation of metane-
phrine-^{14}C from epinephrine and S-adenosyl-methionine-[methyl-^{14}C] as substrates.
Monoamine oxidase activity was measured fluorometrically by the formation of 4-
hydroxyquinoline from kynuramine.

The blood pressure of the SH rats was slightly higher than that of the normal Wistar
rats already 4 weeks after birth. The blood pressure of both the SH rats and the normal
Wistar rats increased up to about 12 weeks after birth. The blood pressure of the normal
Wistar rats remained at about 120 and 130 mm Hg, that of the SH rats at about 190 mm
Hg.

Wet weights of the adrenals of the normal Wistar rats and the SH rats were similar
at 4 weeks of age. The adrenal weights of both groups of rats increased gradually up to
about 16 weeks. The adrenal weights of SH rats increased slightly more rapidly than
those of the normal Wistar rats, but the adrenal weights of the normal Wistar rats and
the SH rats were not significantly different at 16 weeks of age.

The activity of tyrosine hydroxylase in the adrenals during the development of the
normal Wistar rats and the SH rats was examined. Tyrosine hydroxylase activity in
adrenals of the SH rats, expressed as units per adrenal glands, was higher than that of
the normal Wistar rats at 4 weeks after birth. The enzyme activity in the adrenals of the
normal Wistar rats increased gradually up to 16 weeks of age, while that of the SH rats
increased more markedly up to 16 weeks and remained at a level about two times higher
than that of the normal Wistar rats. Similar results were obtained when tyrosine hydroxylase activity was expressed on a per mg protein basis. The increase in the activity of
tyrosine hydroxylase may be attributed to the increase of the enzyme protein. The
results are consistent with the report of OZAKI [7] that the concentration of catecholamines
in the adrenal glands of SH rats doubles 4–5 months after birth. OZAKI [8] also found a
slight increase in tyrosine hydroxylase activity in the adrenal homogenates of SH rats.

The changes in the activity of DOPA decarboxylase in adrenal glands during the
development of normal Wistar rats and SH rats have been examined. The enzyme activity
of both the normal Wistar rats and the SH rats increased up to 8 weeks after birth and
then gradually decreased. The enzyme activity of the SH rats was about 1.3-fold higher
than that of the normal Wistar rats after 12 weeks of age.

Dopamine β-hydroxylase activity in the adrenals of SH rats was similar to that of
normal Wistar rats 4 weeks after birth. The enzyme activity in the adrenals of normal
Wistar rats increased slowly up to 16 weeks. The enzyme activity in the adrenals of SH
rats increased rapidly from 6 to 16 weeks, and then remained about 2-fold higher than
that of normal Wistar rats. Similar results were obtained when dopamine β-hydroxylase
activity was expressed on a per mg protein basis.

Phenylethanolamine N-methyltransferase activity in the adrenals of normal rats and
SH rats increased up to 12 weeks after birth and then gradually decreased. The enzyme
activity in adrenals of SH rats after 12 weeks of age was about 1.3-fold higher than that
of normal Wistar rats.

Monoamine oxidase activity in the adrenals of the SH rats was significantly higher
than that of the normal Wistar rats only during the period from 4 to 12 weeks after birth.

The enzyme activity in the adrenals of the SH rats increased more markedly up to 12 weeks and then decreased until 16 weeks to a level similar to that of the normal Wistar rats.

When the enzyme activities of catecholamine biosynthesis and metabolism in the adrenals of the SH rats and the normal Wistar rats at 16 weeks after birth were compared, all the activities of biosynthetic enzymes expressed as units per adrenal glands were higher in the SH rats [4]. However, the increase in the activities of tyrosine hydroxylase and dopamine β-hydroxylase was specifically pronounced and about 2-fold [3]. Similarly, the increase in the activities of tyrosine hydroxylase and dopamine β-hydroxylase was specific when the enzyme activities were expressed on a per mg protein basis.

Tyrosine hydroxylase activities in the brain stem, heart and spleen of 16 week-old SH rats and normal Wistar rats were compared. Tyrosine hydroxylase activities in the brain stem, heart, and spleen of SH rats were similar to those of normal Wistar rats.

TARVER, BERKOWITZ and SPECTOR [10] has recently reported a significant decrease in tyrosine hydroxylase activities in the mesenteric artery of SH rats. YAMORI, LOVENBERG and SJOERDSMA [12] reported lower DOPA decarboxylase activity in the brain stem of SH rats. These two findings were also reconfirmed in our laboratories. Therefore, characteristics of the activities of enzymes involved in catecholamine biosynthesis in SH rats are: 1) higher tyrosine hydroxylase and dopamine β-hydroxylase activities in the adrenals; 2) normal tyrosine hydroxylase activity in the brain, heart, and spleen; 3) lower DOPA decarboxylase activity in the brain stem as reported by YAMORI, LOVENBERG and SJOERDSMA [12]; and 4) lower tyrosine hydroxylase activity in the mesenteric artery as reported by TARVER, BERKOWITZ and SPECTOR [10].

We also found that tyrosine hydroxylase activity in the mesenteric artery was lower than that of normal Wistar rats, as reported by TARVER, BERKOWITZ and SPECTOR [10]. Two days after an adrenalectomy of the SH rats, tyrosine hydroxylase activity in the mesenteric artery was increased to the level of the normal Wistar rats. In contrast, the enzyme activity in the mesenteric artery of the normal Wistar rats slightly decreased after adrenalectomy. This result suggests that the increased biosynthesis of catecholamines in the adrenal glands may have some modulative effects on tyrosine hydroxylase in other tissues such as the mesenteric artery. However, the possibility that changes in adrenal cortical steroids may affect the tyrosine hydroxylase in mesenteric artery should also be considered.

The question is, which is the primary change for the development of hypertension in SH rats. However, it is clear from these results from different laboratories that some changes in the enzymes of catecholamine biosynthesis and metabolism do exist, and that the marked hypotensive effect of the inhibitors of tyrosine hydroxylase and dopamine β-hydroxylase in SH rats may be related to the changes of these enzymes in various organs of SH rats.

The relationship between the marked hypotensive effect of the inhibitors of tyrosine hydroxylase and dopamine β-hydroxylase and the changes of these enzymes in various organs of SH rats remains for further investigation.

REFERENCES

1. HIDAKA, H., NAGATSU, T., TAKEYA, K., TAKEUCHI, T., SUDA, H., KOJIRI, K., MATSUZAKI, M. and UMEZAWA, H. (1969): J Antibiot, **22**, 228.
2. NAGATSU, T., HIDAKA, H., KUZUYA, H., TAKEYA, K., UMEZAWA, H., TAKEUCHI, T. and SUDA, H. (1970): Biochem Pharmacol, **19**, 35.
3. NAGATSU, I., NAGATSU, T., MIZUTANI, K., UMEZAWA, H., MATSUZAKI, M. and TAKEUCHI, T. (1971): Nature, **230**, 381.
4. NAGATSU, I., NAGATSU, T., MIZUTANI, K., UMEZAWA, H., MATSUZAKI, M. and TAKEUCHI, T. (1971): Experientia, **27**, 1013.
5. NAGATSU, T., NAGATSU, I., UMEZAWA, H. and TAKEUCHI, T. (1971): Biochem Pharmacol, **20**, 2505.
6. OHNO, M., OKAMOTO, M., KAWABE, N., UMEZAWA, H., TAKEUCHI, T., IINUMA, H. and TAKAHASHI, S. (1971): J Am Chem Soc, **93**, 1285.
7. OZAKI, M. (1967): Jap J Constit Med, **30**, 155.
8. OZAKI, M. (1969): Proc Fourth Int Congr Pharmacol, 312.
9. SUDA, H., TAKEUCHI, T., NAGATSU, T., MATSUZAKI, M., MATSUMOTO, I. and UMEZAWA, H. (1969): Chem Pharm Bull, **17**, 2377.
10. TARVER, J.J., BERKOWITZ, B. and SPECTOR, S. (1971): Nature, **231**, 252.
11. UMEZAWA, H., TAKEUCHI, T., IINUMA, H., SUZUKI, K., ITO, M., MATSUZAKI, M., NAGATSU, T. and TANABE, T. (1970): J Antibiot, **23**, 514.
12. YAMORI, Y., LOVENBERG, W. and SJOERDSMA, A. (1970): Science, **170**, 544.

CATECHOLAMINE CONTENT AND METABOLISM IN THE BRAINSTEM AND ADRENAL GLAND IN THE SPONTANEOUSLY HYPERTENSIVE RAT

M. OZAKI*, K. HOTTA** and K. AOKI***

It has been demonstrated that norepinephrine (NE) and serotonin (5HT) are important transmitters of the nervous system. In addition, catecholamine and sympathetic stimulation produce vasoconstriction and high blood pressure (BP), and most of the anti-hypertensive agents are aimed at reducing sympathetic activity or inhibiting catecholamine metabolic pathway in synthesis, store or release. For these reasons many speculations and works have been done on the metabolism of catecholamine and 5HT in experimental hypertension.

OKAMOTO and AOKI [1] succeeded in the separation of a spontaneously hypertensive rat (SHR) colony through selective sib-breedings from the Wistar strain.

SHR [2] developed hypertension at about two months of age without any treatment and these particular rats seem to resemble human essential hypertension because of their spontaneous development of hypertension accompanied by cardiovascular lesions, degeneration of the kidney and other pathological changes.

The purpose of these studies is to ascertain whether the monoamines are consistently associated with the pathogenesis of hypertension or not. The studies are primarily concerned with a comparison between normotensive Wistar strain rats (NR) and SHR.

In 1965 [3], the author reported that in SHR the levels of 5HT in blood and heart were elevated by 25% over the levels of the NR at the age of 4 months. When 5-hydroxytryptophan was injected, 5HT levels in blood and heart of SHR were 20 to 30% higher than those of NR as determined after 60, 80 and 100 minutes.

Among the activities of aromatic amino acid decarboxylase, monoamine oxidase (MAO) and catechol-O-methyl transferase in the brain, heart, kidney and liver, only liver MAO activity showed a decrease in the SHR at the age of 6 to 8 months and over.

Tissue catecholamine levels were measured fluorometrically, in various tissues at the age of 2 to 3 months, 4 to 6 months and over 6 months, and only catecholamine levels of the adrenal gland in SHR were higher than that of NR. That is, the adrenal NE content in male SHR was almost twice as much as that in the control rats at 4 months of ages and over.

Next studies [4] were carried out to clarify whether any quantitative differences between SHR and NR were found in the releasable catecholamine contents of the adrenal gland.

For this purpose, the author performed a particular operation and under these conditions, it was possible to collect a blood sample of the left adrenal vein through the canula.

When the tyramine was injected intravenously, the catecholamine content of the sample from the SHR was markedly higher about 70% than that of the NR. In addition, the releasable NE content in the SHR heart after tyramine injection was also increased by about 20% over that of the NR.

* Department of Pharmacology, Nagoya City University Medical School, Nagoya, Japan
** Department of Physiology, Nagoya City University Medical School, Nagoya, Japan
*** Department of Internal Medicine, Nagoya City University Medical School, Nagoya, Japan

Using the homogenate of heart in SHR and NR, the activity of NE degradation was examined and it was found that SHR heart degradated NE in a little larger amount than that of NR during the incubation.

The rate limiting step in the biosynthesis of catecholamines is the hydroxylation of tyrosine. Therefore, the author examined tyrosine hydroxylase activity of the adrenal gland in SHR, because, as was mentioned above the NE content in the adrenal gland of SHR showed a great difference when compared with NR at 4 months of age and over. The tyrosine hydroxylase activity of the SHR was almost twice as much as that of the control rats. In addition to this, when one of the specific inhibitors of this enzyme, α-methyl-p-tyrosine (80 mg/kg. I.P.), was given to the rats, it was observed [4] that when the catecholamine levels were lowered in the brain, heart and adrenal gland, and also the BP simultaneously fell markedly in SHR during at least 2 to 6 hours after the injection.

The next studies [5] were carried out to determine the catecholamine contents quantitatively in the adrenal gland in relation to the development of hypertension in SHR. We measured the BP, NE and epinephrine (EN) levels in the adrenals in male SHR at various ages during the development of hypertension and thereafter, and compared the results with those in the age-mached male NR. Adrenal NE contents per adrenal, per animal and per gram of adrenal weight in SHR were almost twice as high as those in the NR at 4 months and over.

Nerve growth factor (NGF) antiserum was used for immunosympathectomy [6], that is, the antiserum was injected daily in new-born SHR (0.05 ml/1.5 g B.W. 16–20 days of age) and BP was measured of 7 weeks of age. At 7 weeks the rats which were given the antiserum showed rather lower BP than the nontreated animals. However, at the age of 11 weeks in the group given antiserum, the BP became over 180 mm Hg and no differences were observed when compared with the control rats.

The purpose of next experiments is to determine quantitatively the catecholamine contents in the brain-stem, heart and adrenal gland in relation to the development of hypertension in both sexes. Therefore, we measured the BP, NE and EN levels in these tissues in SHR at various ages during the development of hypertension, and compared them with the levels in NR. The average BP, mean body weight and catecholamine contents in tissues are shown in Table 1.

In the first stage (40–50 days of age) the BP of male SHR was a little higher than the control rats, and had already reached 150 mm Hg. In the second stage (110–140 days of age) the difference in BP between SHR and NR became much greater than in the first stage in both sexes. In body weight, however, SHR was lower than that of the control rats. The content of catecholamine in various tissues did not show noticeable differences at the first stage. Differences were obtained from the second stage (114–141 days of age) in both sexes of SHR.

The next studies were on the interrelationship between the central nervous system and the catecholamine content in the adrenal gland; that is how they influence the BP, and about their correlation with each other. For this purpose, we tried 1. hypophysectomy 2. splanchnicotomy at 40–60 days of age on the SHR and NR and then waited 3–4 weeks. During that period we measured BP once a week and finally measured the catecholamine content in the adrenal gland. The results are shown in Table 2. Hypophysectomized rats were shown to have lower BP in both SHR and NR when compared with the control rats. In the case of SHR, hypertension did not develop even 3–4 months thereafter. There was less increase of catecholamine in the adrenal gland and less body weight increase after the operation as compared with the control group.

Similar results were obtained after the splanchnicotomy as shown in Table 3.

Table 1 Blood pressure and tissue catecholamine content.

Experimental group		No. of animal	Age (days)	Body weight (g)	Blood pressure (mmHg)	Brain-stem NE (μg/g)	Heart NE (μg/g)	Kidney NE (μg/g)	Adrenal gland EN+NE	EN (mg/g)	NE
♂	NR	8	41	150	120± 7	0.83	0.79	0.38	0.386	0.340	0.046
	W/WK	2	50	120	120± 8	0.56	0.73	0.39			
	SHR	12	42	96	155± 5	0.81	0.90	0.40	0.474	0.422	0.052
♂	NR	5	137	419	135±13	0.70	0.78	0.32	0.856	0.700	0.156
	W/WK	5	119	268	134±12	0.71	0.88	0.32	0.622	0.552	0.170
	SHR	7	145	292	195± 7	0.72	0.61	0.33	1.168	0.864	0.304
♂	NR	3	335	461	136±10	0.94	0.96	0.53	0.835	0.675	0.160
	SHR	8	350	325	220± 5	0.98	0.78	0.48	1.246	0.952	0.294
♀	NR	6	145	288	125±10	0.80	0.83	0.39	0.671	0.611	0.060
	W/WK	4	119	212	130± 9	0.76	0.93	0.46	0.455	0.413	0.042
	SHR	7	120	210	175±13	0.77	0.81	0.41	0.720	0.607	0.113

NE: Norepinephrine.　　EN: Epinephrine.　　Each value is the mean (±SD in blood pressure)
NR: Normotensive Wistar rat.　　W/WK: Wistar rat from Kyoto Univ.

Table 2 Blood pressure and tissue catecholamine content after hypophysectomy.

Experimental group	No. of animal	Body weight (g)	Blood pressure (mmHg)	Brain-stem weight (g)	NE (μg/g)	Heart weight (g)	NE (μg/g)	Adrenal gland weight (g)	EN+NE	EN (mg/g)	NE
NR control	5	346	135± 8	0.65	0.74	1.03	0.71	0.62	0.82	0.73	0.08
NR operated	7	228	110±15	0.66	0.92	0.59	0.96	0.29	0.90	0.84	0.06
SHR control	5	265	178±22	0.59	0.71	1.33	0.88	0.49	1.16	0.97	0.19
SHR operated	7	150	135± 7	0.63	0.74	0.64	0.62	0.25	0.99	0.94	0.04

Table 3 Blood pressure and tissue catecholamine content after splanchnicotomy.

Experimental group	No. of animal	Body weight (g)	Blood pressure (mmHg)	Brain-stem weight (g)	NE (μg/g)	Heart weight (g)	NE (μg/g)	Kidney weight (g)	NE (μg/g)	Adrenal gland weight (g)	EN+NE	EN (mg/g)	NE
NR control	5	365	136±7	0.73	0.78	1.26	1.22	1.21	0.64	0.53	0.90	0.73	0.07
NR operated	7	410	125±5	0.66	0.85	1.20	0.93	1.32	0.56	0.43	0.74	0.69	0.05
SHR control	5	265	178±20	0.76	0.72	1.39	0.88	1.06	0.33	0.49	1.26	1.15	0.15
SHR operated	7	270	154±10	0.64	0.79	1.19	0.43	1.14	0.29	0.40	0.82	0.76	0.06

As previously reported the tyrosine hydroxylase activity of the adrenal gland of SHR was higher than that of NR after 4 months of age. When ^{3}H-tyrosine was given [7] to the rats, newly synthesized ^{3}H-catecholamine from the tyrosine during the infusion was almost twice as much in the adrenal gland of SHR as in that of NR.

In the present study, we tried ^{3}H-tyrosine infusion (5μCi/20 ml/1 hr) under urethane anaesthesia, on rats at 40–50 days of age, a rather younger stage than in the previous experiment. When we compared SHR and NR for determining the accumulation of ^{3}H-catecholamine right after the 30 minutes, 1 hour and 4 hour tyrosine infusion. There were no noticeable differences in the heart and adrenal gland in this younger stage.

When we considered chemical transmitters in the brain, we have to mention not only catecholamine but also other substances too. Table 4 shows the content of these substances and the comparison between the SHR and NR. They showed no differences except in the γ amino butyric acid (GABA) and glutamic acid content in the brain-stem which showed a little higher value in the SHR than in the NR.

Table 4   Monoamine and amino acid content in brain-stem (40–60 days of age ♂).

Experimental group	No. of animal	5HT (μg/g)	NE (μg/g)	Dopamine (μg/g)	GABA (mg/100g)	Glutamic acid (mg/100g)
NR	5	0.44	0.73	0.74	19.5	90.6
SHR	8	0.49	0.71	0.68	22.0	100.6

The next experiment was as follows; rats were anaesthetized with urethane, and we tried the injection of catecholamine and other substances into the lateral ventricle directly by stereotaxic method. The BP was recorded oscillographically. NE, EN, dopamine and aceylcholine in small doses caused an increase in BP, and GABA and 5HT showed a decrease in the BP. In the case of responses induced by dopamine (5–10 μg/0.02 ml) SHR was rather sensitive than NR.

SUMMARY

1. Development of hypertension in SHR followed upon increase of catecholamine content in the adrenal gland of both sexes.
2. Hypophysectomy or splanchnicotomy lowered BP and catecholamine content in adrenal gland greater in SHR than in NR.
3. Following intra-ventricle injection the brain of SHR was rather more sensitive to dopamine than that of NR.

REFERENCES

1. OKAMOTO, K. and AOKI, K. (1963): Jap Circ J, **27**, 282.
2. OKAMOTO, K. (1969): In "International Review of Experimental Pathology" (G.W. RICHTER and M. A. EPSTEIN, eds.), Vol 7, p 227, Academic Press, New York.
3. OZAKI, M. (1965): Japan-United States Neurochemistry Conference.
4. OZAKI, M. (1967): In "Proceeding of the 17th General Meeting of Japan Medical Association IV," p 509.
5. OZAKI, M., SUZUKI, Y., YAMORI, Y. and OKAMOTO, K. (1968): Jap Circ J, **32**, 1367.
6. OZAKI, M. (1968): Jap J Const Med, **31**, 225.
7. OZAKI, M. (1971): Jap J Const Med, **34**, 33.

CATECHOLAMINE BIOSYNTHESIS AND METABOLISM IN THE VASCULATURE OF NORMOTENSIVE AND HYPERTENSIVE RATS

S. SPECTOR*, J. TARVER* and B. BERKOWITZ*

The past few years has witnessed a considerable literature develop in regard to the regulation of catecholamine biosynthesis and metabolism. However, most studies have used heart, brain, adrenals and spleen and then extrapolated their findings to other adrenergically innervated tissues.

I should initially like to point out as others have also done, that the vasculature has an appreciable quantity of norepinephrine present, and in fact if one were to compare it with the heart tissue of various species it achieves a concentration that is much greater (Table 1).

Table 1 Concentration of norepinephrine in the aorta, mesenteric artery, vena cava and heart of the rat, guinea pig and rabbit.

Specie	Tissue Norepinephrine $\mu g/g$*			
	Aorta**	Mesenteric Artery**	Vena Cava**	Heart**
Rat***	0.52+0.10 (10)	2.75+0.48 (9)	2.97+0.0 (1)	1.02+0.07 (34)
Guinea Pig***	1.42+0.19 (12)	3.20+0.45 (10)	1.74+0.0 (1)	1.52+0.07 (43)
Rabbit***	2.26+0.75 (11)	2.70+0.21 (8)	3.33+0.64 (3)	1.14+0.1 (12)

Results are ± standard error of the mean and corrected for recovery loss and parenthesis indicates number of determinations.

Vessels were pooled for each determination. Rat, 5–7 aortas; 3–5 mesenteric arteries; 5 vena cavas. Guinea pig, 3–5 aortas; 3–5 mesenteric arteries; 1–3 vena cavas. Hearts were analyzed individually.

Rats were 200 g, females; guinea pigs were 200–300 g, males; and rabbits were 2 kg, males.

Table 2 Tyrosine hydroxylase activity in cardiovascular tissue.

Tissue	Rat		Guinea pig cpm/mg protein		Rabbit	
Heart	155+22	(8)*	511+71	(8)*	194+2	(2)*
Mesenteric Artery	18,434+3,436	(8)*	135,000+15,863	(8)*	22,140+13.962	(2)*
Aorta	333+50	(8)*	612+80	(6)*	437+115	(2)*

* Number of determinations

Figures represent mean ± standard deviation

Table 3 Monoamine oxidase activity in cardiovascular tissue.

Tissue	Rat	Guinea Pig mμ moles 5 HIAA/mg protein/25 min.	Rabbit
Heart	4.91± .46 (8)*	3.74± .47 (8)*	0.10± .02 (2)*
Mesenteric Artery	3.31± .51 (6)*	12.7±2.3 (8)*	0.72± .07 (2)*
Aorta	1.87± .56 (6)*	2.59± .23 (6)*	0.21± .07 (2)*

* Number of determinations

Figures represent mean ± standard deviation

---

* Roche Institute of Molecular Biology, Nutley, New Jersey, U.S.A.

Many tissues possess and active uptake mechanism for the catecholamines and so the question can be asked whether the norepinephrine present in the blood vessels is synthesized there. Table 2 and 3 shows the activity of an anabolic enzyme involved in norepinephrine biosynthesis namely tyrosine hydroxylase and a catabolic one, namely monoamine oxidase. Although I shall not present any data on catechol-o-methyl transferase, it too, is extremely active in the vascular system. I should like to point out that the blood vessels have a greater activity than seen in heart, and that the tyrosine hydroxylase activity in the mesenteric artery is comparable to the adrenal.

Using various techniques, such as rate of elevation of norepinephrine following blockade of monoamine oxidase or measuring rate of decline of the biogenic amine after the synthesis blocker alpha methyl para tyrosine or else labeling the tissue with H^3-norepinephrine and then measuring the rate of decline of the labeled material in order to obtain an indication of the turnover rate of norepinephrine in blood vessels, we came out with the following information. The half life of norepinephrine in heart, mesenteric artery and mesenteric vein is about 4.5 to 5.5 hours. The rate of synthesis of norepinephrine in these tissues is about four times that of the heart (Table 4). As a consequence, we propose that the vasculature may contribute a major fraction of the excreted catecholamines.

Table 4   Turnover of norepinephrine in rabbit blood vessels and heart.

Tissue	Half-Life (Hour)	KNE	Synthesis Rate (μg/g/hour)
Heart	5.7	.124	0.17
Mesenteric Artery	4.4	.169	0.64
Mesenteric Vein	4.5	.134	0.69

Many drugs which modify hypertension elicit their effects by interfering with the function of the sympathetic nervous system. Two drugs which drastically interfere with the activity of the sympathetic nervous system are 6-hydroxydopamine and nerve growth factor antiserum. A number of workers [2, 3, 4, 5, 7, 11] have reported that these two agents have a partial effect in antagonizing experimental hypertension. If one analyzed heart and spleen content after the administration of these agents, there is a marked depletion of norepinephrine. It has been postulated that the resistance of the adrenal catecholamines to these substances supports the elevated blood pressure. However, FINCH and LEACH [3, 4, 5], showed that 6-hydroxydopamine even after adrenal demedullation didn't have a profound effect on blood pressure. Rats and guinea pigs receiving two doses of 6-hydroxydopamine, using the same regimen as recommended by THOENEN and TRANZER(8), caused a smaller loss of norepinephrine from blood vessels when compared to heart or spleen. The adrenal norepinephrine content was not depleted (Table 5).

Table 6 shows that there was no significant change in the activities of monoamine oxidase in heart of rats treated with 6-hydroxydopamine, 50 mg/kg twice a day on day 1 and 100 mg/kg twice a day on day 7 and killed on day 15. The tyrosine hydroxylase declined about 30%. The mesenteric artery and aorta failed to show any change. MUELLER, THOENEN and AXELROD [10] showed an increase in tyrosine hydroxylase in the adrenal gland 2 days following a large dose of 6-hydroxydopamine. We didn't find any change in the adrenals 15 days after the first 2 doses, thus the increase in tyrosine hydroxylase may not be sustained. Rats treated with antiserum to nerve growth factor had their norepinephrine content of heart depleted to a larger extent than that of the aorta, mesenteric artery or mesenteric vein. The only tissue in which the vasculature has been reported to be depleted by immunosympathectomy have been in skeletal muscle and iris, while the adrenergic terminals in the intestines were resistant to immunosympathectomy [6], and

Table 5 Effect of 6-hydroxydopamine (6OH-D) on the concentration of catecholamine in the rat and guinea pig.

Species and Tissue	Noradrenaline μg/g*		% Decrease after 6OH-D
	Control	6OH-D	
Rat			
Heart	1.13+0.13	0.15+0.02**	87
Aorta	0.41+0.23	0.16+0.02	61
Mesenteric artery	3.39+0.75	2.43+0.43	28
Mesenteric vein	2.30−2.50	0.50−0.70	75
Spleen	0.30+0.04	0.05+0.01**	83
Adrenal glands	22.60+0.74	24.90+0.79	0
Guinea Pig			
Heart	1.59+0.13	0.07+0.03**	96
Aorta	2.50+0.64	1.08+0.58	57
Mesenteric artery	2.27+0.09	1.12+0.15**	51
Mesenteric vein	0.79−1.00	0.13−0.33	84

* The results are the mean of 5–6 determinations ± S.E.M. for heart, spleen and adrenal catecholamines. Vessels were pooled: 4 aortas, 3 mesenteric arteries and 5 mesenteric vein where the range of two determinations is given. 6OH-D was administered to 140 g rats i.v. twice within 24 hours on day 1, 50 mg/kg twice on day 7, 100 mg/kg and killed on day 15. 6OH-D was injected i.p., 50 mg/kg, to guinea pigs and sacrificed 24 hours later. Adrenal noradrenaline is as μg/per pair of adrenal glands.

** The difference between controls and treated animals statistically significant $p < .05$.

Table 6 Effect of 6-hydroxydopamine on tyrosine hydroxylase and monoamine oxidase activity in the heart, brain, adrenal and cardiovascular systems of the rat.

Tissue*	Tyrosine Hydroxylase**		Monoamine Oxidase**	
	Control	6OH-D	Control	6-HDM
Heart	0.12+0.04	0.08+0.04	8.80+2.6	7.2+2.1
Mesenteric artery	1.52+0.28	1.64+0.44	6.16+1.0	8.07+2.4
Aorta	—	—	5.5+0.5	4.6+0.8
Brain stem	—	—	19.1+2.0	16.6+1.8
Adrenals	4.72+0.32	5.24+0.32	—	—

* Heart, adrenal gland pairs, and brainstem were analyzed individually. The results of 3–4 tissues were averaged ± the standard deviation. For tyrosine hydroxylase 2 blood vessels were pooled and the results of 3–4 groups averaged. For monoamine oxidase, vessels were analyzed individually. 6OH-D was administered i.v. twice within 24 hours to 130 g male rats on day 1 of the experiment (50 mg/kg) and on day 7 (100 mg/kg) and rats were killed on day 15.

Tyrosine hydroxylase and monoamine oxidase were assayed as described in methods and results are expressed as mμ moles dopa/hr/mg protein and mμ moles indole acetic acid/20

** min/mg protein respectively.

FINCH and LEACH [3, 4, 5] also showed that rats are not hypotensive following immuno-sympathectomy. Also CAPRI and OLIVERO [1], showed that urinary catecholamines levels are not altered by immunosympathectomy and adrenal demedullation.

Another agent which effects the catecholamine content of the sympathetic nervous system, is reserpine. This compound casused a marked decrease in both levels of nor-epinephrine in various tissues as well as a reduction of blood pressure. THOENEN et al. [9, 10], showed that reserpine induces adrenal tyrosine hydroxylase and we investigated whether this drug influences catecholamine metabolic enzymes in the vasculature. Rats given 1.5 mg/kg 1 or 2 days show no change in either tyrosine hydroxylase or mono-amine oxidase activity in the heart. In contrast the tyrosine hydroxylase activity of the mesenteric artery is increased 75% after 2 days of treatment whereas the monoamine oxidase activity is significantly reduced after both time periods. Similar results are seen in the aorta. These changes may be a compensatory response caused by the hypotensive action of reserpine.

A comparison of the tyrosine hydroxylase activity in the untreated SHR compared with either normotensive or backcrossed indicated that the enzyme was significantly lower (50–68%) in the SHR (Table 7). It seems unlikely that these changes are due to hypertrophy or changes in the media-adventitia ratio as these are 15 week-old rats and no such changes have been observed in these animals at that time.

Table 7

	Blood Pressure (mm Hg)	Tyrosine Hydroxylase Activity Heart	Mesenteric Artery
Wistar	115	.092 ± .01 (6)	7.24 ± 1.12 (6)
Wistar × SHR**	135	.115 ± .03 (6)	4.84 ± .32 (6)
SHR	150–160	.110 ± .03 (6)	3.40 ± .08* (6)
SHR	180–190	.114 ± .03 (6)	2.84 ± .44* (6)

* mμ M Dopa/hr/mg protein
Figures represent mean ± standard deviation
( ) number of determinations
* Significantly different from backcrossed SHR p<.01
** Backcrossed SHR

Table 8 Histamine content in brainstem of normotensive and hypertensive rats.

Genotype	Blood Pressure (mm Hg)	Histamine (μg/g) Brainstem
Wistar (7)	110–120	42.6 ± 3.9
Male		40.0 ± 6.3 (4)
Female		46.1 ± 3.8 (3)
Wistar × SHR	130–150	56.3 ± 7.4 (7)
Male		57.6 ± 6.4 (4)
Female		54.7 ± 8.7 (3)
SHR	160–180	76.4 ± 6.3 (9)*
Male		72.5 ± 8.3 (5)
Female		81.3 ± 8.7 (4)

* p<0.001

It is known that histamine has a physiologic effect opposite to norepinephrine and many have speculated that endogenous histamine may act as an antagonist to norepinephrine. We have initiated some studies to ascertain firstly the endogenous content of the SHR and here we see that in the brain stem the histamine content of the SHR is elevated and that the backcross is intermediate between the normotensive and hypertensive animals (Table 8). We have no idea at the moment of the kinetics of the histamine in the SHR. However, it has been reported that in normotensive Sprague-Dawley rats it has a very rapid turnover rate. Although the focus has been on the relationship of catecholamine and hypertension, we feel that attention has to be given to the other biogenic amines to be found in the body.

REFERENCES

1. CARPI, A. and OLIVERIO, A. (1964): Int J Neuropharmacol, 3, 427.
2. CLARK, D. W. J. (1971): Circ Res, 28, 330.
3. FINCH, L. and LEACH, G. D. H. (1970 a): Br J Pharmacol, 39, 317.

4. FINCH, L. and LEACH, G. D. H. (1970 b): Eur J Pharmacol, **11**, 388.
5. FINCH, L. and LEACH, G. D. H. (1970 c): J Pharm Pharmacol, **22**, 354.
6. HAMBERGER, B., LEVI-MONTALCINI, R., NORBERG, K. A. and SJÖQVIST, F. (1965): Int J Neuropharmacol, **4**, 91.
7. MUELLER, R. A. and THOENEN, H. (1970): Fed Proc, **29**, 546.
8. THOENEN, H. and TRANZER, J. P. (1968): Naunyn-Schmiedeberg's Arch Exp Path Pharmak, **261**, 271.
9. THOENEN, H., MUELLER, R. A. and AXELROD, J. (1969 a): J Pharmacol Exp Ther, **169**, 249.
10. MUELLER, R. A., THOENEN, H. and AXELROD, J. (1969): Science, **163**, 468.
11. VARMA, D. R. (1967): J Pharm Pharmacol, **19**, 61.

ENDOGENOUS LEVEL OF NOREPINEPHRINE AND THE SENSITIVITY OF ADRENERGIC RECEPTORS IN SPONTANEOUSLY HYPERTENSIVE RATS

D. VETADŽOKOSKA*, S. GUDESKA*, E. GLAVAŠ*, M.SUKAROVA*
and B. NIKODIJEVIĆ*,

The role of catecholamines (CA) and the activity of the adrenergic nervous system take a very important part in the investigation of the pathogenesis both of essential human and experimental hypertension. Even in the renal hypertension of rats an important role of CA and of sympathetic tone has been stressed by several authors [1, 5, 10].

Spontaneously hypertensive rats (SHR, OKAMOTO and AOKI [11]) exhibit many features similar to human essential hypertension and present an excellent model for histopathological, biochemical and pharmacological studies.

The following aspects of the role of CA and of the adrenergic system in the pathogenesis of spontaneous hypertension will be considered in this report: concentration of norepinephrine (NE) in brain, heart and spleen, turnover of NE, relation between pool A and pool B of NE in the heart adrenergic nerve endings and the sensitivity of adrenergic receptors.

CONCENTRATION OF ENDOGENOUS NE

LOUIS et al. [6, 7] found a normal level of heart NE in SHR using male rats weighing 140–200 g, and 11–14 weeks old.

Table 1 Concentration of norepinephrine in SHR and in normotensive Wistar rat (M±SE).

Age (Months)	Rats	Systolic B.P. mm Hg	Norepinephrine μg/g		
			Brain	Heart	Spleen
3	Control	112±5.2	0.39±0.018	0.72±0.039	0.43±0.02
	SHR	143±5.1	0.30±0.015	0.59±0.021	0.39±0.018
9	Control	126±4.6	0.34±0.01	0.63±0.031	0.36±0.011
	SHR	185±6.3	0.31±0.018	0.36±0.014	0.38±0.018
15	Control	125±5.8	0.32±0.014	0.58±0.03	0.35±0.014
	SHR	190±6.8	0.31±0.011	0.31±0.012	0.36±0.019

We have determined the concentration of NE in whole brain, heart and spleen of SHR, of different ages, and the results are shown in Table 1.

There was no significant difference in the concentration of brain and spleen NE between control normotensive Wistar rats and SHR. However, a highly significant decrease in the heart NE level of SHR compared with the normotensive Wistar rats can be seen, especially at 9 ($p<0.005$) and 15 ($p<0.001$) moths of age.

It could be of interest to mention that MELVILLE et al. [8] found a similar fall in the heart NE level in a New Zealand strain of genetic hypertensive rats. DE CHAMPLAIN et al. [1] found such a decrease of heart NE level in DOCA hypertensive rats.

---

* Department of Pharmacology, Medical Faculty, University of Skopje, Skopje, Yugoslavia.

TURNOVER OF NE

Louis et al. [6, 7] indicated that both the rate of NE synthesis and its release were reduced in SHR, producing a diminished turnover rate of ^{3}H-NE. The authors proposed that the release of physiologically active NE from nerve endings would be less in hypertensive than in normal animals.

In a series of experiments we administered disulfiram, Ro4-4602 or alfa-methyl-5-hydroxytryptophan (AM-5-HTP), 200 mg/kg i.p., to SHR and to control normotensive Wistar rats, in order to inhibit NE biosynthesis at different levels. The animals were sacrificed 24 hours after the injection, and brain, heart and spleen used for determination of NE (Figs. 1, 2, 3):

All of the administered inhibitors provoked smaller decrease of NE concentration in brain, heart and spleen in SHR, than in control normotensive animals. These results

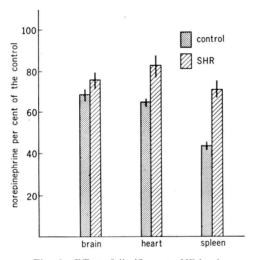

Fig. 1   Effect of disulfiram on NE-level.

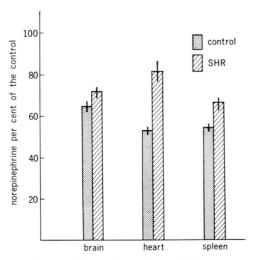

Fig. 2   Effect of Ro4-4602 on NE-level.

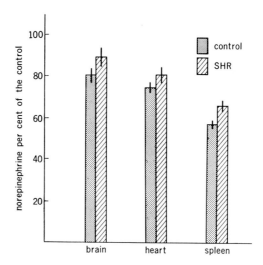

Fig. 3   Effect of AM-5-HTP on NE-level.

support the findings of Louis et al. [7], indicating a decreased turnover rate of NE in SHR.

On the other hand, an increased turnover rate of NE has been found in certain types of experimental hypertension: perinephritic hypertension [15], neurogenic hypertension [13], DOCA hypertension [2].

POOL "A" AND POOL "B" OF NE

TRENDELENBURG [14] proposed two pools of NE in the adrenergic nerve endings: a smaller one, pool A, available NE, that can be easily liberated by nerve impulses, and a larger one, pool. B, -bound NE. NE from pool A can also be liberated by tyramine, and NE from pool B by reserpine.

It has been emphasized many times that pool A is of high functional importance because NE liberated from it comes to the adrenergic receptors, and that it is quite possible that pool A is selectively enlarged in hypertension [9].

In a series of experiments carried out in this Department, we administered reserpine 1 mg/kg i.p., both to SHR and to normotensive control Wistar rats. The animals were sacrificed 24 hours after the injection, and NE determined in brain, heart and spleen.

In another series of experiments, tyramine 20 mg/kg i.p. was administered both to SHR and to normotensive control Wistar rats. The animals were sacrificed 3 hours after the injection, and NE also determined in brain, heart and spleen.

Results showed a more pronounced effect of reserpine on control normotensive rats than on SHR. However, tyramine provoked a more intense effect on SHR than on normotensive control rats. In control rats, there was a reduction of the heart NE level from 0.63 to 0.49 μg/g provoked by tyramine. The released amount of 0.14 μg/g of NE was probably pool A. Reserpine reduced the heart NE level from 0.62 to 0.17 μg/g in normotensive control Wistar rats. The released amount of 0.45 μg/g of NE was probably predominantly pool B. Thus, pool A in the heart of control Wistar rats contains 0.14–0.17 μg/g of NE, and pool B 0.45–0.49 μg/g, or 23–27 per cent for pool A, and 73–77 per cent for pool B (Fig. 4).

When we applied the same method of estimation for heart NE in SHR, we got the

Table 2 Heart norepinephrine level in SHR and in normotensive Wistar rats $(M \pm SE)$.

Rats	Pool—A	Pool—B	Total
Control	0.155	0.47	0.625
	(0.14–0.17)	(0.45–0.49)	(0.59–0.66)
SHR	0.18	0.21	0.39
	(0.17–0.19)	(0.18–0.24)	(0.35–0.43)

CONTROL RAT HEART
adrenergic nerve end.

0.49	0.14	Tyramine: 0.63→0.49
B	A	
0.45	0.17	Reserpine: 0.62→0.17

SHR HEART
adrenergic nerve end.

0.18	0.19	Tyramine: 0.37→0.18
B	A	
0.24	0.17	Reserpine: 0.41→0.17

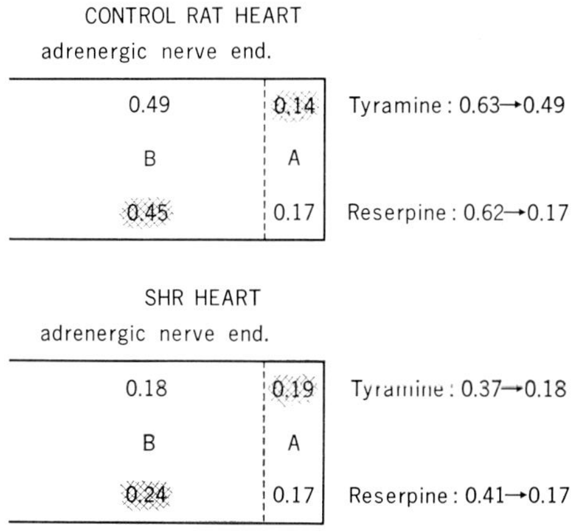

Fig. 4

following values: pool A contains 0.17–0.19 μg/g, and pool B 0.18–0.24 μg/g of NE, or 42–51 per cent for pool A, and 49–58 per cent for pool B (Table 2).

Consequently, it could be postulated that the reduction of the total concentration of heart NE in SHR was due to the reduction of pool B. Pool A, however, was not diminished, but rather was even absolutely enlarged for about 16 per cent, compared with the control normotensive Wistar rats.

SENSITIVITY OF ADRENERGIC RECEPTORS

OKAMOTO et al. [12] have shown an increased pressor response of SHR to administered NE, reduced to epinephrine (E), as well as an increased depressor response to acetylcholine. CLINESCHMIDT et al. [3] working on the isolated aortic strip failed to observe any alteration in the sensitivity of adrenergic receptors to NE. However, on the isolated perfused mesenteric artery, HAEUSLER and HAEFELY [4] have shown hypersensitivity of adrenergic receptors to NE.

We were studying vascular reactivity to certain adrenergic and cholinergic agonists on the whole animals, using SHR and MHR (metacorticoid hypertensive rats, produced by unilateral nephrectomy and administration of DOCA.).

Results showed a significant vascular hyperreactivity both in SHR and in MHR. The highest hyperreactivity in SHR was observed with NE and dopamine (in 70 per cent of the tested animals), and relatively less hyperreactivity to E (28 per cent), or to angiotensin (23.5 per cent). In MHR, however, the most striking hyperreactivity was observed with angiotensin and dopamine (73.3 per cent of the tested animals), and relatively less hyperreactivity to NE (60 per cent), or to E (26.6 per cent). It should be mentioned that vascular reactivity to isoproterenol or to acetylcholin was without change both in SHR and in MHR.

CONCLUSIONS

1.   A slightly increased pool A of heart NE in SHR was found, although total concentration of the transmitter was even reduced.

2.   A decreased turnover of NE in SHR was also found.

3.   An increased reactivity of alpha-adrenergic receptors in SHR was observed without alterations in the reactivity of beta-adrenergic or cholinergic receptors.

REFERENCES

1.   DE CHAMPLAIN, J., KRAKOFF, R. L. and AXELROD, J. (1967):   Circ Res, **20**, 136.
2.   DE CHAMPLAIN, J., MULLER, A. R. and AXELROD, J. (1969):   Circ Res., **25**, 285.
3.   CLINESCHMIDT, V. B., GELLER, G. R., GOVIER, C. W. and SJOERDSMA, A. (1970):   Eur J Pharmacol, **10**, 45.
4.   HAEUSLER, G. and HAEFELY, W. (1971):   Naunyn-Schmiedebergs Arch Pharmakol, **266**, 18.
5.   HENNING, M. (1969):   J Pharm Pharmacol, **21**, 61.
6.   LOUIS, J. W., SPECTOR, S., TABEI, R. and SJOERDSMA, A. (1968):   Lancet, **1**, 1013.
7.   LOUIS, J. W., SPECTOR, S., TABEI, R. and SJOERDSMA, A. (1969):   Circ Res, **24**, 85.
8.   MELVILLE, A., HODGE, J. V. and SMIRK, F. H. (1966):   Proc Univ Otago Med Sch, **44**, 17.
9.   MENDLOWITZ, M., WOLF, L. R. and GITLOW, E. S. (1970):   Am Heart J, **79**, 401.
10.   NIKODIJEVIĆ, B., TRAJKOV, T., CLAVAŠ, E., GUDESKA, S. and VETADŽOKOSKA, D. (1971): Naunyn-Schmiedebergs Arch Pharmakol, **268**, 185.
11.   OKAMOTO, K., AOKI, K. (1963):   Jap Circ J, **27**, 282.
12.   OKAMOTO, K., HAZAMA, F., TAKEDA, T., TABEI, R., NOSAKA, S., FUKUSHIMA, M., YAMORI, Y., Y., MATSUMOTO, M., HAEBARA, H., ICHIJIMA, K. and SUZUKI, Y. (1966):   Jap Circ J, **30**, 987.
13.   DE QUATTRO, V., NAGATSU, T., MARONDE, R. and ALEKSANDER, A. (1969):   Circ Res, **24**, 545.
14.   TRENDELENBURG, U. (1961):   J Pharm Exp Ther, **134**, 8.
15.   VOLICER, L., SCHEEN, E., HILSE, H. and WISWESWARAM, D. (1963):   Life Sci, **7**, 525.

DOCA-SALT AND SPONTANEOUSLY HYPERTENSIVE RATS: COMPARATIVE STUDIES ON NOREPINEPHRINE TURNOVER IN CENTRAL AND PERIPHERAL ADRENERGIC NEURONS

K. NAKAMURA*, M. GEROLD and H. THOENEN**

The role of the sympathetic nervous system in the pathogenesis of essential human hypertension is far from being clear. In spite of this, most of the drugs currently used in the therapy of essential hypertension act by modifying the disposition of norepinephrine (NE) in peripheral or central adrenergic neurons.

Although a representative model for essential human hypertension is not yet available, the analysis of the factors determining the development or maintenance of various forms of experimental hypertension in animals may provide new aspects for the pathogenesis and therapy of essential hypertension.

In previous experiments with DOCA-salt hypertensive rats, it has been shown that the NE turnover of the peripheral sympathetic nervous system increases in proportion to the rise in systolic blood pressure [5, 7, 17]. The increased cardiac NE turnover seems to result from an increased activity of the sympathetic nervous system, since it could be normalized by administration of ganglionic blocking agents [17].

However, in spontaneously hypertensive rats (SHR), the cardiac NE turnover has been found to be decreased in proportion to the elevation of the systolic blood pressure [15, 18].

In the present study, we wish to present the possible relationship between cerebral and peripheral NE turnover in both prehypertensive and hypertensive stages of two different types of hypertension in the rat.

METHODS

Hypertensive Animals. SHR, derived from a hypertensive mutant of a Wistar strain in Japan [19] was expanded (F-20–22 generations) by brother-sister imbreeding in our animal farm at Füllinsdorf. Male animals were used for the experiments when they had reached an age of 3 to 14 weeks. Age-matched male rats of a closed randomized colony of Wistar descent served as controls. For preparation of DOCA-salt hypertensive rats, male rats from a closed randomized colony of Wistar descent, initially weighing 100–120g, were made hypertensive by encapsulation of the left kidney by a plastic bag and by the subcutaneous implantation of a pellet of 25 mg DOCA. The animals were supplied with 1% saline instead of drinking water. Unoperated controls were kept under identical conditions in the same room but were supplied with tap water. The systolic blood pressure was measured in the unanesthetized animals by the method previously described in detail [10].

Norepinephrine Turnover. NE turnover was determined according to steady state kinetics [3, 8] either by measuring the decline in endogenous NE after inhibition of synthesis or by measuring the decline in the specific activity of NE after injecting ^{3}H-NE intravenously or into the right lateral ventricle of the brain. For blocking the NE synthesis [20], α-methyl-p-tyrosine methylester was given intraperitoneally in doses of 300 mg/

Laboratory of Experimental Medicine, F. Hoffmann-La Roche & Co. Basle, Switzerland
* On leave from Nippon Roche Research Center, Kamakura, Japan.
** Present address: Department of Pharmacology, Biocenter, University of Basle, Switzerland.

kg every 3 hours and the animals were killed 3, 6 or 9 hours after the first dose. For measuring the decline in the specific activity of ³H-NE in the peripheral organs [16] the animals were injected intravenously with 40μCi of dl-NE:7-³H hydrochloride (specific activity 7.47 Ci/mM) and killed 1, 3, 6 or 18 hours later. ³H-NE was purified before use by adsorption on alumina at pH 8.6 [2] and eluted with 0.2 N acetic acid. For the intraventricular injection of ³H-NE ,a permanent cannula was implanted into the right lateral ventricle [13]. 5 μCi of ³H-NE were dissolved in 10μl of Merlis solution and injected through the cannula. The animals were killed 1, 2, 4 or 6 hours after injection. The decline in the specific activity of ³H-NE was estimated in hypothalamus, medulla oblongata and the residual parts of brain, studied as a whole. Hypothalamus and medulla oblongata were dissected according to IVERSEN and GLOWINSKI [11]. To eliminate a possible influence of diurnal changes in NE turnover, all experiments were started at 7 a.m.

Norepinephrine Determination. Heart, submaxillary gland, spleen, hypothalamus and medulla oblongata were quickly removed, frozen at −70°C, weighed and homogenized in 0.4 N HCl0₄. Catecholamines were adsorbed on alumina [2]. NE was determined fluorimetrically [9]. The activity of ³H-NE was measured by liquid scintillation spectrometry with the scintillator system, described by de CHAMPLAIN et al. [6].

Statistical Analysis. Half-lives of NE were calculated from the slope of the decline in endogenous NE after inhibition of the synthesis or the decline in specific activity after administration of ³H-NE [17]. For estimating the significance of the difference between regression lines, the data were expressed as logarithms, plotted according to the method of least squares and weighed for the number of animals, the actual difference between the two slopes, the standard deviation of both the line and the values of each group and the range of time-values. The half-lives are expressed as the means with 95% confidence limits instead of ± standard error, since the distribution is asymmetrical.

RESULTS

Time Course of the Development of Hypertension. In SHR the systolic blood pressure rose continuously until the 12th to 14th week of age, when the blood pressure approached its

Table 1 Relationship between the development of hypertension and endogenous NE content.

SHR (n=8)	NE content	6 weeks (age)		12 weeks (age)	
		Control	SHR	Control	SHR
Systolic B.P.	(mm Hg)	131± 2	135± 6	126± 2	201± 7**
Heart	ng/heart	427±50	373±20	565± 35	472±28
	ng/g	989±85	812±41	834± 64	613±36**
Hypothalamus	ng/g	1527±79	1508±68	1781±315	1919±71
Medulla-pons	ng/g	466±25	439±18	792± 53	845±71
Residual brain	ng/g	188±13	194± 5	271± 24	261±27

DOCA-Salt (n=6)		2 weeks		4 weeks	
		Control	Hypertensive	Control	Hypertensive
Systolic B.P.	(mm Hg)	126± 3	164± 2**	126± 4	234± 11**
Heart	ng/heart	560±37	440± 31*	646± 69	505± 42
	ng/g	921±59	711± 52*	1065±105	689± 57*
Hypothalamus	ng/g	1761±12	1791±147	1883± 61	2016±160
Medulla-pons	ng/g	652±17	667± 35	496± 27	622± 13**
Residual brain	ng/g	—	—	334± 23	353± 27

The data represent the mean±S.E.M.

* P<0.05; ** P<0.001 when compared with corresponding control values.

highest levels between 200 and 210 mm Hg. In contrast, in control animals the blood pressure changed only slightly during the whole period of observation from the 6th to the 12th week of age (Table 1).

In the DOCA-salt experiments with rats the implantation of DOCA-pellets alone produced no significant rise in blood pressure during the observation time of 4 weeks. When the animals were supplied with 1% saline in place of tap water in addition to DOCA-implantation there was an elevation of the blood pressure to 148 $\pm$ 12 mm Hg after 2 weeks and to 159 $\pm$ 14 mm Hg after 4 weeks. The development of hypertension was further enhanced with chronic DOCA-saline treatment was supplemented by encapsulation of the left kidney. Thereby, the blood pressure reached 164 $\pm$ 2 mm Hg after 2 weeks and 234 $\pm$ 11 mm Hg after 4 weeks (Table 1). Encapsulation of the kidney alone had no effect on blood pressure.

Relationship between the Development of Hypertension, Organ Weights and Their NE Content. Although the systolic blood pressure of 6 weeks old SHR was not yet significantly (P> 0.05) higher than that of the corresponding controls, the difference in heart weight reached already a statistically significant level (P<0.05). There was also a statistically significant correlation (r=0.791, P<0.001) between the level of blood pressure and the heart weight [17]. This is in disagreement with previous reports [15] indicating no difference between the heart weights of controls and SHR. The heart NE content of SHR at the

Table 2 Relationship between the development of hypertention and NE turnover in heart and submaxillary gland.

SHR age in weeks			Heart		Submaxillary Grand	
			Control	Hypertensive	Control	Hypertensive
			decline of NE after blockade of synthesis			
6	T 1/2	(hr)	8.9 (8.1–9.9)	8.0 (7.1–9.3)	6.9 (6.1–8.1)	8.4 (6.9–11.1)
12	T 1/2	(hr)	7.7 (6.7–8.6)	11.3 (9.0–16.2)**	5.2 (4.6–5.8)	6.6 (5.6–8.1)*
			decline of specific activity following ³H-NE			
6	T 1/2	(hr)	8.8 (6.3–11.3)	11.2 (8.7–14.1)	7.3 (5.7–8.8)	11.3 (8.4–14.7)**
12	T 1/2	(hr)	8.4 (7.2–9.7)	11.1 (9.4–13.3)**	4.8 (4.2–5.4)	9.0 (7.4–10.9)**
DOCA-salt wks after operation			Control	Hypertensive	Control	Hypertensive
			decline of NE after blockade of synthesis			
2	T 1/2	(hr)	12.8 (10.5–17.1)	8.0 (6.5–10.8)*	7.8 (6.6–9.5)	8.8 (6.8–11.4)
4	T 1/2	(hr)	14.1 (10.5–24.4)	7.2 (6.3–8.3)***	9.0 (7.6–11.4)	10.7 (9.1–13.3)
			decline of specific activity following ³H-NE			
4	T 1/2	(hr)	9.4 (8.0–11.2) .... 7.8 (6.8–8.8)*		7.6 (6.1–9.2)	7.6 (6.4–9.4)

The values represent half-life of NE and 95% confidence limits.
0.05<*P<0.10; **P<0.015; ***P<0.01 when compared with controls.

age of 6 weeks was slightly smaller than that of age-matched controls. However, at the age of 12 weeks, when both systolic blood pressure and heart weight of the SHR had risen markedly, the heart NE content (ng/g) decreased significantly (P<0.001) and there was also a corresponding inverse correlation (r=0.345, P<0.01) between the level of systolic blood pressure and the endogenous NE content. The NE content of hypothalamus, medulla-pons and the residual parts of the brain did not differ significantly (P> 0.05) between SHR and controls both at the age of 6 and 12 weeks (Table 1).

In the DOCA-salt hypertensive rats, there was a significant correlation (r=0.296; P<0.01) between the rise in systolic blood pressure and the increase in heart weight (Table 1). The heart NE content of hypertensive rats was significantly (P<0.05) diminished both expressed in terms of ng/organ and ng/g. There was a statistically significant

Table 3 Turnover of NE in hypothalamus, medulla-pons and the residual parts of the brain.

SHR			Hypothalamus		Medulla-pons		Residual parts of the brain	
age in weeks			Control	Hypertensive	Control	Hypertensive	Control	Hypertensive
			decline of NE after blockade of synthesis					
6	T 1/2	(hr)	3.8(3.3–4.2)	4.6(3.8–5.6)	3.6(3.1–4.2)	3.8(3.2–4.5)	3.5(3.0–4.1)	3.5(3.0–4.0)
12	T 1/2	(hr)	3.5(2.6–4.2)	3.4(2.9–3.8)	4.4(3.1–6.4)	5.0(4.0–6.3)	3.4(2.9–4.3)	3.6(3.1–4.8)
			decline of specific activity following ^{3}H-NE					
6	T 1/2	(hr)	3.8(3.4–4.5)	4.1(3.6–4.7)	3.3(3.0–3.7)	3.2(2.5–4.0)	3.0(2.7–3.4)	3.3(2.7–4.0)
12	T 1/2	(hr)	4.0(3.7–4.4)	4.5(4.0–5.3)	3.1(2.7–3.7)	3.0(2.8–3.2)	2.8(2.3–3.3)	3.0(2.2–3.9)
DOCA-salt weeks after operation			Control	Hypertensive	Control	Hypertensive	Control	Hypertensive
			decline of NE after blockade of synthesis					
2	T 1/2	(hr)	5.2(4.8–5.7)	6.4(5.5–7.7)	4.0(3.6–4.6)	4.6(4.1–5.3)	—	—
4	T 1/2	(hr)	3.8(3.4–4.3)	5.1(4.5–5.7)**	2.4(1.9–2.8)	3.2(2.8–3.6)***	—	—
			decline of specific activity following ^{3}H-NE					
4	T 1/2	(hr)	2.5(1.9–2.9)	4.6(3.9–5.6)***	2.1(1.7–2.4)	2.5(2.1–2.8)*		

The values represent half-life of NE and 95% confidence limits

*$0.05 < P < 0.10$;   **$P < 0.05$;   ***$P < 0.01$ when compared with controls.

inverse correlation between the level of blood pressure and the endogenous NE content (r=0.367; P<0.001)

Relationship between Changes in Systolic Blood Pressure and NE Turnover in Peripheral and Central Adrenergic Neurons. In contrast to DOCA-salt hypertensive rats, there was an inverse relationship between the height of the systolic blood pressure and the rate of NE turnover, *i.e.*, the higher the blood pressure, the slower was the NE turnover. In prehypertensive animals of 3 and 6 weeks of age, the heart NE turnover was not yet significantly (P>0.05) delayed. However, at the age of 12 weeks, a statistically significant (P<0.05) reduction in NE turnover was present, both when determined by inhibition of tyrosine hydroxylase and by labelling the NE stores with ^{3}H-NE. In the submaxillary gland the relationship between the level of blood pressure and changes in NE turnover was similar to that in the heart (Table 2). In contrast to the periphery, in any part of the brain the changes in blood pressure were neither reflected by changes in NE content nor changes in NE turnover (Table 1 and 3).

In DOCA-salt hypertension, an increased NE turnover in all peripheral organs except the salivary gland has been reported previously [7]. In spite of some differences between the procedures of inducing hypertension in the experiments of DE CHAMPLAIN et al. [7] and ours (different strains of rats, encapsulation of the left kidney versus nephrectomy, implantation of DOCA-pellets versus repeated injection of DOCA), we confirmed the increased turnover in the heart and unchanged turnover in the submaxillary gland (Table 2). There was an increased turnover already 2 weeks after DOCA implantation and renal encapsulation. A further increase in the NE turnover occurred after 4 weeks, when the systolic blood pressure had reached a level of 234 ± 11 mm Hg. Concomitantly with the increased turnover in the heart, there was a pressure-dependent delay in hypothalamus and medulla-pons (Table 3). In addition to the delayed turnover, there was a statistically significant (P<0.001) increase in the NE content of the medulla-pons (Table 1). There was no change in the residual parts of the brain as compared to the reduced turnover in medulla-pons and hypothalamus (Table 3).

In order to decide whether the reduction in NE turnover in the brain stem is the consequence of an increased turnover in the periphery, we studied the effect of chlorisondamine, a quaternary ganglionic-blocking agent which does not cross the blood-brain barrier. From previous experiments [6] it is known that chlorisondamine, given to DOCA-salt hypertensive rats, brings down both blood pressure and peripheral NE turnover to the level of normotensive animals. Using the same experimental schedule, we confirmed the effect of chlorisondamine on the NE turnover in the periphery. In contrast to the normalization of the NE turnover in the heart, the delay in hypothalamus and medulla-pons persisted, showing that these changes were not a consequence of the turnover changes in the periphery but occured independently.

The results presented so far have shown that there is an inverse relationship between the changes in NE turnover in the heart and those in the brain-stem. However, it could be assumed that DOCA produces changes in the NE turnover in the brain-stem independent of the rise in blood pressure, since it is known that corticosteroids affect the electrical activity of hypothalamic neurons (for references, see 17). Therefore, we studied the effect of DOCA alone, which produces no elevation of systolic blood pressure. DOCA alone did not produce a statistically significant (P<0.05) change in NE turnover neither in the periphery nor in the central nervous system.

DISCUSSION

The results of the present experiments have shown that the systolic blood pressure of 3–6 week old rats of a spontaneously hypertensive strain is only slightly higher than that of age-matched normotensive Wistar controls. However, the systolic blood pressure rises steeply in the following weeks and reaches a plateau of 200–210 mm Hg when the animals become 12–14 weeks old. In these SHR, concomitantly with the rise in blood pressure, a gradually increasing reduction in NE turnover occurs in peripheral sympathetically innervated organs. However, both NE content and turnover in medulla-pons, hypothalamus and the residual parts of the brain do not differ significantly from that of age-matched Wistar controls at any time of observation, *i. e.*, 3, 6 and 12 weeks of age. Thus, there is good evidence that the functional state of peripheral and central adrenergic neurons of controls and SHR is very similar at an early time of development when the factors which determine the rise in blood pressure have not yet found their functional expression in the hypertensive strain. The inverse correlation between the level of blood pressure and the rate of NE turnover in peripheral sympathetically innervated organs of SHR raises the question whether there is a causal relationship between these two parameters. The reduction of NE turnover in peripheral sympathetic neurons seems to represent the biochemical correlate to a decreased sympathetic nervous activity. This decreased sympathetic activity may represent an attempt to compensate an increased peripheral vascular resistance to maintain the homeostasis of blood pressure. It is noteworthy that changes in peripheral blood pressure involving also change in presso-receptor activity seem not to be reflected by changes in the activity of adrenergic neurons in the brain-stem or residual parts of the brain. This is in accordance with observations in DOCA-salt hypertensive rats, in which after administration of a quaternary ganglionic blocking agent (which does not cross the blood-brain barrier) both blood pressure and heart NE turnover approached normal levels, whereas the changes in brain-stem NE turnover persisted. In the spinal cord, however, the activity of the peripheral presso-receptors seem to influence the activity of the adrenergic neurons, since after transsection of the carotid sinus and aortic nerves of rabbits there was an increase both in the NE turnover and tyrosine hydroxylase activity in the thoracolumber segments of the spinal cord [4].

SHR and DOCA-salt hypertension represent two experimental models of hypertension in which the function of both the peripheral and central adrenergic neurons is completely different and of varying importance for the development of hypertension. The reciprocal changes between the NE turnover in the heart and the brain-stem in DOCA-salt hypertension were taken to indicate that under normal conditions the activity of adrenergic neurons in the brain-stem depresses the activity of the peripheral sympathetic nervous system and that in DOCA-salt hypertension the decreased activity of the adrenergic neurons in the brain-stem was casually related to the increased activity of the peripheral sympathetic nervous system. This increased activity of the peripheral sympathetic neurons seems to be responsible—at least partially—for the development of hypertension. The assumption of a depressing effect of central adrenergic neurons on the peripheral sympathetic activity is further supported by the observation [1] that clonidinc produces its hypotensive effect by stimulating central adrenergic receptors resulting in a decreased peripheral sympathetic activity. Also the recent observations of HAEUSLER et al. (1970) [12] that the hypotensive effect of intraventricularly administered 6-hydroxy-dopamine (which releases NE) can be blocked by phentolamine but not be propranolol speak in favour of a depressing effect of NE and that α-adrenergic receptors are involved. Furthermore, the administration of l-DOPA in combination with a peripheral inhibition of DOPA decarboxylase, which leads to a marked increase in the cerebral catecholamine content, has also a hypotensive effect [14]. This speaks also in favour of the assumption that an accumulation of NE at particular central receptor sites leads to a depression of the peripheral sympathetic nerve activity and thus to hypotension. In SHR, neither the peripheral nor the central adrenergic nervous system seems to play a primary role in the development of hypertension. It seems to be more probable that the genetically determined alterations are located in the peripheral vascular system resulting in an increased vascular resistance, and thus to hypertension. It will be the task of future studies to establish the detailed mechanism of this increased vascular resistance and to delineate the possible implications for the pathogenesis of human essential hypertension.

SUMMARY

In DOCA-salt hypertensive rats (DOCA-implantation, 1% saline as drinking water, encapsulation of the left kidney) and spontaneously hypertensive rats (SHR) the NE turnover of peripheral and central adrenergic neurons was determined either by measuring the rate of decline of endogenous NE after inhibition of tyrosine hydroxylase or by measuring the decay of the specific activity after labelling the stores by intravenous or intraventricular injection of ^{3}H-NE. In SHR the NE turnover in the periphery was delayed in proportion to the rise in systolic blood pressure, whereas in brain-stem and residual parts of the brain the NE turnover did not differ from that of normotensive controls. In contrast, in DOCA-salt hypertensive rats the cardiac NE turnover was enhanced in proportion to the rise in blood pressure and reciprocally delayed in brain-stem (medulla-pons, hypothalamus) but not residual parts of the brain. Administration of chlorisondamine, a quaternary ganglionic blocking agent which does not cross the blood-brain barrier, resulted in a normalization of both blood pressure and cardiac NE turnovers, whereas the changes in brain persisted. Encapsulation of the kindey and implantation of DOCA alone produced neither a rise in blood pressure nor changes in NE turnover. It is concluded that in this form of experimental hypertension the changes in NE turnover in the brain-stem is causally related to the increased activity of the peripheral sympathetic nervous system which normally is depressed by the activity of the adrenergic neurons in the brain-stem. In SHR, neither the peripheral nor the central adrenergic nervous system seems to play a primary role in the development of hypertension. The delay in the peripheral NE turnover, which is the biochemical correlate of a decreased sympathetic activity, may represent an attempt to compensate an increased peripheral resistance resulting from changes in the reactivity of vascular smooth muscles or changes in vascular geometry.

REFERENCES

1. ANDEN, N. -E., CORRODI, H., FUXE, K., HOKFELT, B., HOKFELT, T., RYDEN, C. and SVENSSON, T. (1970): Life Sci, **9**, 513.
2. ANTON, A. H. and SAYRE, D. F. (1962): J Pharmacol Exp Ther, **138**, 360.
3. BRODIE, B. B., COSTA, E., DLABAC, A., NEFF, N. H. and SMOOKLER, H. H. (1966): J Pharmacol Exp Ther, **154**, 493.
4. CHALMERS, M. B. and WURTMANN, R. J., (1971): Circ Res, **28**, 480.
5. CHAMPLAIN, J. de, KRAKOFF, L. R. and AXELROD, J. (1967): Circ Res, **20**, 136.
6. CHAMPLAIN, J. de, KRAKOFF, L. R. and AXELROD, J. (1968): Circ Res, **23**, 479.

7. CHAMPLAIN, J. de, MUELLER, R. A. and AXELROD, J. (1969):   Circ Res, **25**, 85.

8. COSTA, E., BOUILLIN, D. J., HAMMER, W. VOGEL, W. and BRODIE, B. B. (1966): Pharmacol Rev, **18**, 577.

9. EULOR, U. S. von and LISHAJKO, F. (1961):   Acta Physiol Scand, **51**, 348.

10. GEROLD, M. and TSCHIRKY, H. (1968):   Arzneimittel-Forsch, **18**, 1285.

11. GLOWINSKI, J. and IVERSEN, L. L. (1966):   J Neurochem, **13**, 655.

12. HAEUSLER, G., GEROLD, M. and THOENEN, H. (1970):   Arch Pharmakol, **266**, 345.

13. HAYDEN, J. F., JOHNSON, L. R. and MAICKEL, R. P. (1966):   Life Sci, **5**, 1509.

14. HENNING, M. and RUBENSON, A. (1970):   J Pharm Pharmacol, **22**, 241.

15. LOUIS, W. J., SPECTOR, S., TABEI, R. and SJOERDSMA, A. (1969):   Circ Res, **24**, 85.

16. MONTANARI, R., COSTA, E., BEAVEN, M. A. and BRODIE, B. B. (1963):   Life Sci, **4**, 232.

17. NAKAMURA, K., GEROLD, M. and THOENEN, H. (1971):   Arch Pharmakol, **268**, 125.

18. NAKAMURA, K., GEROLD, M. and THOENEN, H. (1971):   Arch Pharmakol, **271**, 157.

19. OKAMOTO, K. and AOKI, K. (1963):   Jap Circ J, **27**, 282.

20. SPECTOR, S., SJOERDSMA, A. and UDENFRIEND, S., (1965):   J Pharmacol Exp Ther, **147**, 86.

ORGAN DIFFERENCE OF CATECHOLAMINE METABOLISM IN SPONTANEOUSLY HYPERTENSIVE RATS*

Y. YAMORI**

A great number studies on catecholamine metabolism in SHR were reported up to the present and some discrepancies were noted among the data about an increase or a decrease in the catecholamine turnover of the peripheral organs. Such discrepancies are mainly attributable to (1) the difference in the control animals used, as reported by Sjoerdsma and his coworkers [7], (2) the difference in the age of SHR used, for the state of autonomic nervous system or its innervated organs may be variable before and after the development of hypertension [12], and also to (3) the difference in the organ examined as revealed by the present study.

Detailed studies on catecholamine metabolism of the heart in SHR [5–7] were already reported, but the heart does not seem to be the best organ to study as to the hypertension, for cardiac output was observed to be decreased in accordance with the increase in the total peripheral vascular resistance after the development of hypertension in SHR [2]. Therefore, in order to study a possible pathogenetic role of peripheral catecholamine metabolism in relation to hypertension, peripheral resistance vessels should be given special attention. Although the enzymes involved in catecholamine metabolism of the mesenteric arteries were examined [10], these available arteries from the root of superior mesenteric artery to the branches into the intestinal loop are not mainly the resistance vessels, therefore, still not the suitable samples for study.

On the other hand, the examination of SHR's kidneys by the fluorescence histochemical technique [3] confirmed that the norepinephrine (NE) fluorescence was mainly distributed along the vessels as reported previously in other animals [8]. Consequently, NE metabolism in the kidney is supposed to reflect the metabolism of the peripheral vessels if the extraneural NE can be excluded, and the kidney may be an appropriate organ for studying the catecholamine metabolism of the peripheral vessels. In this study, extraneural accumulation of NE was estimated by the turnover study in the rats with unilaterally denervated kidney, and the net neural binding or turnover of NE was deducted from the difference between the innervated and denervated kidneys. So far as renal excretory function is not greatly affected by the denervation [9], this method is supposed to be valid for estimating the neural NE turnover of the vasculature in the kidney.

MATERIALS AND METHODS

The left renal nerves of 20 SHR's and 25 normotensive rats of Wistar/NIH strain (NR) at the age of 14 weeks were exposed carefully by using cotton cubes and cut from the splanchnic nerve. The renal plexus was removed as neatly as possible and the left renal artery and vein were completely painted with 10 per cent phenolic alcohol solution [4]. The preliminary study confirmed that the NE content of the left denervated kidney was undetectable or nearly zero 2 weeks after the denervation. Consequently, these rats were used for turnover study 2 weeks after left renal denervation. Tritiated NE (DL-7-³H-NE,

* This work was done by the author when he was a visiting scientist at Experimental Therapeutics Branch (Lab. Chief, Dr. ALBERT SJOERDSMA), National Heart and Lung Institute, NIH, Bethesda, MD, U.S.A.

** Department of Pathology, Faculty of Medicine, Kyoto University, Kyoto, Japan

7.45 c/mmole, New England Nuclear, Boston, Massachusetts) was purified on almina columns and 25 μC of it was injected intravenously via a tail vein. The rats were sacrificed 5 min., 30 min., 1, 2, 8 and 24 hours after the injection. Heart and kidney were immediately extirpated, weighed, kept frozen and homogenized in 10 ml of 0.4 N perchloric acid for NE extraction. The supernatant was used for NE assay as previously reported [6, 7]. The amount of ^{3}H-NE was determined by counting the radioactivity in a scintillation mixture to estimate the turnover (synthesis) rate [1, 6, 7].

RESULTS

The disappearance rate of ^{3}H-NE was observed in innervated and denervated kidneys in SHR and in NR. As shown in Fig. 1., the initial accumulation in denervated kidneys 5 min. after injection was not much different from that in innervated kidneys. However,

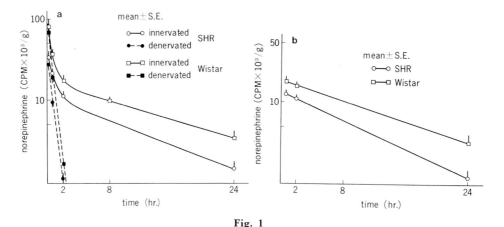

Fig. 1

a.   Disappearance curve of radioactive NE in the innervated and denervated kidneys in SHR and control Wistar.

b.   Net neural accumulation of radioactive NE in the kidney of SHR and control Wistar.

the denervated kidneys could not hold ^{3}H-NE and rapidly lost almost all of it in 2 hours or so. On the other hand, innervated kidneys showed a steep decrease in ^{3}H-NE within the initial 2 hours and then gradually released the residual ^{3}H-NE in 24 hours. Consequently, ^{3}H-NE disappearance curve consists of two components, an initial rapid decrease mainly in extraneurally bound ^{3}H-NE, and a slow decrease mainly in neurally bound ^{3}H-NE from 2 to 24 hours. The net neural binding was estimated from the difference in the ^{3}H-NE accumulation between innervated and denervated kidneys. The neurally bound ^{3}H-NE disappearance curve thus obtained in SHR was slightly steeper than that in NR, and the rate constant was significantly (p<0.01) larger, NE turnover time was shorter, and synthesis rate was greater in SHR than in NR as shown in Table I. These findings on the NE metabolism of the kidney in SHR exhibited a striking contrast to that of the heart in SHR. The turnover rate of ^{3}H-NE in the heart of SHR was significantly delayed in this study (Table I), and the data were quite similar to those reported previously [6, 7].

A preliminary study showed that the turnover rate derived from the disappearance curve from 2 to 24 hours after ^{3}H-NE injection was accelerated in the kidneys of neurogenic hypertensive rats produced by sino-aortic denervation [4, 11]: Rate constant 0.069±0.015 hr⁻, NE turnover time 14.4 hr, turnover rate 12.6 ng/hr/g. Thus, the dis-

Table 1 NE level and turnover in the heart and kidney of SHR and control Wistar (NR).

	Heart		Kidney	
	SHR	NR	SHR	NR
Endogenous NE level (ng/g)	504±42 (13)	556±20 (13)	164±5 (24)	206±8 (19)
³H-NE Accumulation (CPM × 10³/g)	671±17 (10)	614±24 (7)	18.6±1.0* (9)	25.5±2.7 (8)
Rate constant (hr⁻¹)	0.047±0.006**	0.074±0.008	[0.048±0.008]**	[0.032±0.005]
NE turnover time (hr)	21.3	13.5	[20.8]	[31.3]
Synthesis rate (ng/hr/g)	23.7	41.4	[7.9]	[6.6]

Mean±S.E.   ( ) Number of rats
[   ] Values calculated from the difference between innervated and denervated kidneys.
Significant difference from the values in Wistar
* $p < 0.05$ ** $p < 0.001$,

appearance of neurally bound NE from the kidney is supposed to be well paralleled to sympathetic vasomotor tone.

SUMMARY

The study on NE turnover of the innervated and denervated kidneys in SHR as well as in NR, showing an organ difference in NE metabolism in SHR, raised a question as to whether the heart should be regarded as a standard organ of cardiovascular system in the case of hypertension, and indicated a possibility of increased NE turnover in the peripheral vasculature in the kidney of SHR.

REFERENCES

1. BRODIE, B. B., COSTA, E., DIABAC, A., NEFF, N. H. and SMOOKLER, H. H. (1966): J Pharmacol and Exp Ther, **154**, 493.
2. DENCKLA, D.: Personal communication.
3. FALK, B. and OWMAN, C. (1965): Acta Univ. Lund, Sect II, **7**, 1.
4. KRIEGER, E. M. (1964): Circ Res, **15**, 511.
5. LOUIS, W. J., KRAUS, K. R., KOPIN, I. J. and SJOERDSMA, A. (1970): Circ Res, **27**, 589.
6. LOUIS, W. J., SPECTOR, S., TABEI, R. and SJOERDSMA, A. (1969): Circ Res, **24**, 85.
7. LOUIS, W. J., TABEI, R. SPECTOR, S. and SJOERDSMA, A. (1969): Circ Res, **24** and **25**, Suppl. I, 93.
8. NILSSON, O. (1965): Lab Invest, **14**, 1392.
9. QUINBY, W. C. (1916): J Exp Med, **23**, 535.
10. TARVER, J. H. and SPECTOR, S. (1970): Fed Proc, **29**, 278.
11. THANT, M., YAMORI, Y. and OKAMOTO, K. (1969): Jap Circ J, **33**, 501.
12. YAMORI, Y., OOSHIMA, A., NOSAKA, S. and OKAMOTO, K. (1972): In "Spontaneous Hypertenson" (K. OKAMOTO, ed.) p. 73, Igaku Shoin, Ltd. Tokyo.

LOW ACTIVITY OF DOPA DECARBOXYLASE IN CEREBRAL VESSELS OF SPONTANEOUSLY HYPERTENSIVE RATS*

C. TANAKA**

It has been demonstrated by Bertler et al. [1] that dopadecarboxylase and mono-amine oxidase are present in the walls of the brain capillaries, and these enzymes form a specific barrier mechanism for L-dopa at the capillary level. Yamori et al. [3] demonstrated that there were low levels of norepinephrine and low activity of dopa decarboxylase in SHR brainstem. It is difficult to relate the decreased norepinephrine concentration in the brainstem to the low activity of dopa decarboxylase, as tyrosine hydroxylase activity, considered to be the rate-limiting enzyme, is not significantly different in the brainstem of SHR and normotensive rats. The low activity of dopa decarboxylase in the brainstem may not be present only in neural structures.

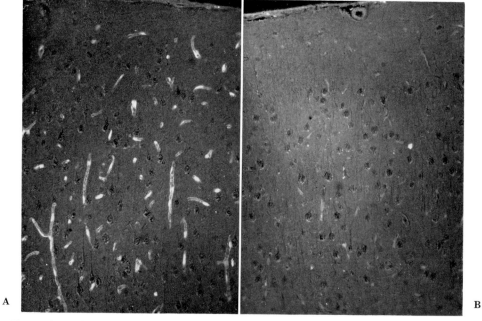

A   B

Fig. 1 Frontal section of cerebral cortex in rats treated with nialamide and L-dopa. Magnification × 160 A. Wistar-Kyoto strain rat. B. SHR.

To examine extraneuronal dopa decarboxylase activity histochemically, the cellular localization of catecholamines was studied using the fluorescence method of Falck and Hillarp [2]. Four to 26-week old SHR and normotensive Kyoto Wistar strain rats were intraperitoneally injected with L-dopa 100 mg/kg 2 hr after the administration of nial-

* This work was partly supported by research grants (No. 87514, 58417) from the Ministry of Education, Japan.
** Department of Pharmacology, Faculty of Medicine, Kyoto University, Kyoto, Japan.

amide 300 mg/kg. One hour following the injection the animals were sacrificed by decapitation. The brain was removed, freeze-dried and treated with formaldehyde gas. The tissues were embedded in paraffin in vacuo, sectioned, and studied in a fluorescence microscope.

As shown in Fig. 1, A, after treatment with nialamide and L-dopa, the parenchyma of the brain exhibited a weak green fluorescence with an intense green fluorescence in the brain capillary walls. This fluorescent material accumulated in the endothelial cells and the pericytes of the capillary walls. This demonstrates that L-dopa had been taken up by these cells and decarboxylated to dopamine by decarboxylase located in the capillary walls.

A striking feature, however, was that dopamine fluorescence did not develop in the capillary walls of SHR, (Fig. 1 B). and that an increase in green fluorescence was seen in the brain parenchyma, such as the caudate nucleus, hypothalamus and brainstem. These results show that low activity of dopa decarboxylase in the brain of SHR can be attributed to the low activity of extraneuronal decarboxylase, and that the specific barrier mechanism for L-dopa is weak or lacking in SHR.

REFERENCES

1. BERTLER, A., FALCK, B. and ROSENGREN, E. (1964): Acta Pharmacol Toxicol, **20**, 317.
2. FALCK, B., HILLARP, N. -A., THIEME, G. and TROP, A. (1962): J Histochem Cytochem, **10**, 348.
3. YAMORI, Y., LOVENBERG, W. and SJOERDSMA, A. (1970): Science, **170**, 546.

MODIFICATION OF CATECHOLAMINE METABOLISM IN SPONTANEOUSLY HYPERTENSIVE RATS

Y. UEBA*, K. MORI* and T. TOMOMATSU*

The role of the sympathetic nervous system in the control mechanism of cardiovascular dynamics is very important. This mechanism is often modified in cardiovascular diseases. For example, in some cardiovascular diseases, such as congestive heart failure, the catecholamine level in the myocardium [1, 3, 7] is decreased with an increasing of plasma [5] and urinary [4] level of catecholamine. In the present study, the changes of catecholamine distribution in various organs of spontaneously hypertensive rats is treated.

Spontaneously hypertensive male rats (SHR), and Kobe Wistar normotensive male rats (NR) of three age groups; namely, 3 weeks, 3 months and 6 to 8 months after birth, were used in this experiment. The blood pressure started rising 1 month after birth and continued to rise progressively during the following 2 months. Changes of catecholamine levels according to aging process were studied in various organs which were removed immediately after decapitation at the resting state. In another experiment the blood pressure was measured in unanesthetized rats by means of carotid cannulation connected with an electromanometer. Five mililitters per kilogram of physiological saline containing 0.2% of tyramine were infused into the jugular vein for 7 minutes. Pressor responses to the tyramine infusion were observed in SHR and NR. Also, tissue catecholamine levels were measured after the tyramine infusion. The tissue catecholamine content was determined by Crout's method [2] and the catecholamine distribution in the tissue was also observed by a histochemical fluorescence method.

The tissue catecholamine content in SHR and NR 6 to 8 months after birth was measured. The catecholamine content of the heart was significantly reduced in SHR (0.71 μg/g) in comparison with that in the control group (1.66 μg/g). On the other hand, the catecholamine content of other organs, such as lungs, liver, kidneys and adrenal glands, was not significantly different from that observed in NR.

It has also been demonstrated that the catecholamine content in rabbit organs vary with the aging process [6]. An inverse relationship was observed between the catecholamine content in the adrenal glands and in the myocardium, namely, soon after birth a high level of catecholamine in the adrenal glands was evident as opposed to a low level in the myocardium. But in the adult stage, the catecholamine level in the adrenal glands decreased with the increase of the catecholamine level in the myocardium. For this reason, we examined the change of the catecholamine level in the various organs of SHR and NR in relation to the aging process.

The myocardial catecholamine content in SHR was almost equal to that in NR 3 weeks after birth. However, this level varied conversely in both groups with aging. In SHR, the catecholamine content in the myocardium decreased with the progress of hypertension that was spontaneously acquired mostly within 3 to 5 months after birth, whereas in NR, the catecholamine content increased unrelated to the blood pressure. These unique phenomena were not observed in other organs (Fig. 1).

---

* Department of Internal Medicine, Division I, School of Medicine, Kobe University, Kobe, Japan

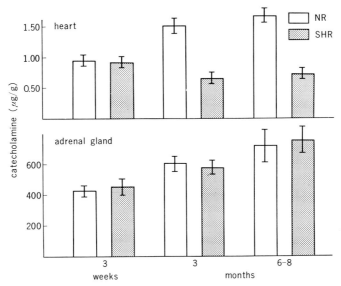

Fig. 1 Changes of catecholamine levels in the myocardium and adrenal gland
in relation to the aging process in SHR and NR.

Incidentally, catecholamine fluorescence in the heart of NR proved the distribution
of sympathetic nerves in the adventitia of vessels and myocardial space. However, the
catecholamine fluorescence in that of SHR was markedly reduced. Thus, the change of
the catecholamine level in the myocardium was also supported by a histochemical fluorescence method. These results concerning the catecholamine metabolism in SHR were
similar to those observed in congestive heart failure or hyperthyroidism, and it was
presumed that there is an acceleration of catecholamine turnover rate in sympathetic
nerve endings in SHR.

If this assumption is true, that is; if the turnover rate is actually accelerated, the
catecholamine stored in the nerve endings which is responsive to tyramine should be
reduced to some extent, and less catecholamine should be released to induce significantly
less pressor effect. To confirm this assumption, tyramine was administered to SHR and NR.

The catecholamine level in myocardium was not significantly influenced by our procedure for blood pressure recording under an unanesthetized condition (1.66 ± 0.23 μg/g
after this procedure; 1.52 ± 0.32 μg/g at resting state).

As in figure 2, the myocardial catecholamine content in NR was strikingly reduced
from 1.66 to 0.68 μg/g by the administration of tyramine. In SHR, it was also reduced
from 0.71 to 0.57 μg/g by tyramine; however, the reduction was not so significant, as
compared with that in NR. Accordingly, the reduction of the catecholamine content in
the myocardium of SHR appears to be partly due to a decrease in the catecholamine
content which is released by tyramine. Furthermore, we would like to present one typical
case of these effects in the pressor responses to tyramine in SHR and NR. In SHR, tyramine produced a marked elevation of blood pressure from 200–130 to 360–220 mm Hg,
while in NR from 120–80 to 190–140 mm Hg. Since the catecholamine release induced by
tyramine from the heart and vessels was diminished in SHR, it appeared that the difference in the pressor responses between SHR and NR was due to a varied sensitivity in
the adrenergic receptors of the cardiovascular system. In both cases, the maximum
increase in blood pressure occured within one minute after the injection of tyramine.

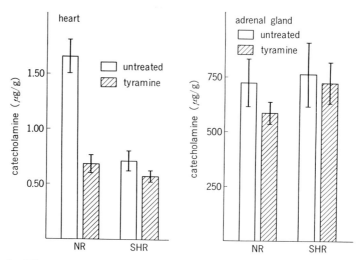

Fig. 2   Effect of tyramine on catecholamine levels of the myocardium and adrenal
gland in SHR and NR.

SUMMARY

1. As compared with that of NR a lower catecholamine content was observed in the myocardium of SHR.
2. This diminution of the myocardial catecholamine level in SHR was observed with the development of hypertension.
3. Although the catecholamine release induced by tyramine was diminished in SHR, the pressor response to tyramine was greater in SHR than NR. It is suggested that both the increased turnover rate of and hypersensitivity to catecholamine contribute to the development of hypertension.

REFERENCES

1. CHIDSEY, C. A., KAISER, G. A., SONNENBLICK, E. H., SPANN, J. F. Jr. and BRAUNWALD, E. (1964): J Clin Invest, **43**, 2386.
2. CROUT, J. R., CREVELING, C. R. and UDENFRIEND, S. (1961): J Pharmacol Exp Ther, **132**, 269.
3. ITO, Y. (1968): Jap Circ J, **32**, 761.
4. TOMOMATSU, T., UEBA, Y., MATSUMOTO, T. IKOMA, T. and KONDO, Y. (1963): Jap Heart J, **4**, 13.
5. TOMOMATSU, T., UEBA, Y., KONDO, Y., ODA, M., IJIRI, Y., KOGAME, H., ITO, Y. and YAO, T. (1967): Jap Heart J, **8**, 242.
6. TOMOMATSU, T. and UEBA, Y. (1970): Jap J Geriatr, **7**, 36.
7. TOMOMATSU, T. (1971): Jap Circ J, **35**, 979.

Chapter III

NEURAL FACTOR AND BEHAVIOR

NEURAL FRACTION OF PERIPHERAL VASCULAR RESISTANCE AND VASCULAR REACTIVITY IN THE SPONTANEOUSLY HYPERTENSIVE RAT

S. NOSAKA*, Y. YAMORI*, T. OHTA** and K. OKAMOTO*

It has generally been accepted that the sympathetic nervous system plays an essential role at least in the maintenance of hypertension. This has been supported by results of immunological sympathectomy [3, 12], administration of sympatholytic drugs [8, 10, 11] or ganglion blocking agents [8, 10, 12], and mechanical sympathetic decentralization [7, 9, 10, 14].

Two factors, however, should be taken into account in analyzing the sympathetic participation in hypertension. One is the tonic sympathetic discharges onto receptor sites of the cardiovascular system, and the other the reactivity of the effector system to norepinephrine (NE) released at the receptor sites by the sympathetic discharges. Conventional approaches, as mentioned, have not been able to evaluate the degree of contribution of each factor but have yielded simply a sum, more properly a product, of these two factors.

Therefore, many researchers are reluctant to accept the view that sympathetic activities are increased in hypertension though they admit the importance of neural tone. If blood vessels in hypertensive subjects react more to endogenous NE, the hypertension necessarily has an increased dependence on neural tone even though the latter be normal. Indeed, a large number of studies suggested that vascular reactivity is increased in hypertension [13].

The present study was designed and carried out to estimate the neurogenic fraction of hypertension of SHR. Another purpose was to evaluate the role of vascular reactivity in the formation of the neural component.

We used a vascularly isolated but neurologically intact hind limb prepared according to a modification of the method of LAVERTY and SMIRK [6] and that of BRODY [2]. The advantage of this method lay in the fact that with the aid of a motor pump we could observe changes in peripheral resistance uninfluenced by simultaneously occuring cardiac changes which sometimes obscure or exaggerate results.

MATERIALS AND METHODS

Male animals 3 to 4 months of age were anesthetised with intravenous chloralose, 40 mg/kg. Incision was made on the lower abdominal wall, and the left femoral artery and

* Department of Pathology, Faculty of Medicine, Kyoto University, Kyoto, Japan
** Department of Neurosurgery, Osaka City University School of Medicine, Osaka, Japan

the right iliacal artery were prepared for the following cannulations (Fig. 1). The left lumbosacral plexus was exposed by section of the overlying muscles. The right femoral vein was cannulated with polyethylene tubing for later intravenous injection of drugs. After complete hemostasis was assured, 1,000 units of heparin was given intravenously and two short pieces of polyethylene tubing were introduced into the prepared arteries.

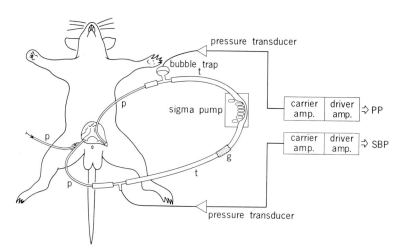

Fig. 1 Diagrammatic representation of hind limb perfusion.
SBP: systemic blood pressure, PP: hind limb perfusion pressure,
g: rubber tubing, p: polyethylene tubing, t: Tygon tubing

They were immediately connected to a third piece of polyethylene tubing so that temporary circulation was effected before the artificial perfusion began. After an interval of 20 min., necessary for minimizing reflex due to the above operation, the third tube was removed and the other two were connected to the perfusion system which contained about 1.0 ml of Ringer's solution. A metal finger type motor pump delivered blood at a constant rate of flow, 0.4 ml/min./100 gm. Perfusion pressure and systemic blood pressure were monitored through pressure transducers. The perfusion pressure, thus recorded, gave the proportional index of vascular resistance of the hind limb because the flow rate was kept constant throughout the experiment. A short piece of rubber tubing was placed in the perfusion system so that drugs (NE and angiotensin) could be injected directly into the perfused artery. The volume of drugs injected was restricted to 1 μl/100 gm of body weight.

All the results were statistically analysed by Student's small sample 't' test.

RESULTS

Neurological Intactness. Our preperations were neurologically intact. This was proved by an increase in perfusion pressure in response to bilateral carotid occlusion; and by a decrese in perfusion pressure in response to the blood pressure rise which was elicited by means of systemic administration of norepinephrine (Fig. 2A).

Absence of Significant Collateral Circulation. Collateral circulation was almost negligible in our preparation. This was proved by the fact that after sympathetic denervation a drug-induced rise or fall in blood pressure did not significantly alter the perfusion pressure until the drug reached the perfused artery through the perfusion system (Fig. 2B).

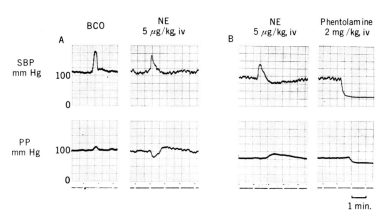

Fig. 2 Effects of bilateral carotid occlusion and systemic administration of norepinephrine on hind limb perfusion pressure before sympathetic denervation (A) and effects of systemic blood pressure rise and fall on the perfusion pressure after the denervation (B). BCO: bilateral carotid occlusion, NE: norepinephrine, PP: hind limb perfusion pressure, SBP: systemic blood pressure.

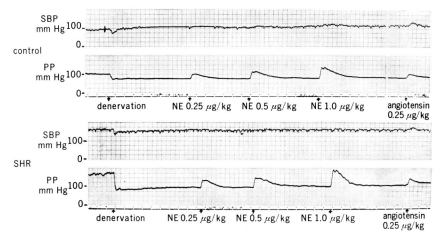

Fig. 3 Effect of sympathetic denervation on hind limb perfusion pressure and responses to norepinephrine and angiotensin after the denervation. Abbreviations: same as in figure 2.

Initial Perfusion Pressure. About thirty minutes after the beginning of perfusion, the perfusion pressure became stable (initial perfusion pressure). The initial perfusion pressure was found to be higher in SHR (152±5 mm Hg, Mean±S. E.) than in controls (102±2 mm Hg) (Table I, Fig. 3).

Effect of Sympathetic Denervation. Working on the principle that sympathetic postganglionic fibers run to the extremities via spinal nerves, we achieved complete sympathetic denervation by total section of the already exposed lumbosacral plexus. After the denervation the perfusion pressure dropped rapidly. The fall was greater in SHR (51±4 mm Hg) than

Table 1 Effects of sympathetic denervation and subsequent administration of norepinephrine and angiotensin on hind limb perfusion pressure.

No. of Animals	Systemic BP (mm Hg)			Perfusion pressure (mm Hg)						
	Systolic	Diastolic	Mean	Initial	Denervation		Norepinephrine			Angiotensin
					Floor	Fall	0.25 µg/kg	0.5 µg/kg	1.0 µg/kg	0.25 µg/kg
Control 11	126±4+	90±4	105±3	102±2	72±3	22±1	22±1	32±2	54±4	23±1
SHR 11	186±2*	141±4*	158±5*	152±5*	100±4*	51±4*	34±1*	53±1*	80±3*	35±2*

* Significant difference with p<0.01, + Mean ± S. E.

in controls (22± 1 mm Hg) (Table I, Fig. 3). Also, the basal perfusion pressure was higher in SHR (100 ± 4 mm Hg) than in controls (72±3 mm Hg).

Response to Norepinephrine and Angiotensin. Eight to ten minutes after the denervation, various amounts of NE (0.25 µg, 0.5 µg, 1.0 µg/kg of body weight) were injected into the perfused artery through the rubber tubing. Each injection of NE elicited a greater response in SHR than in controls (Table I, Fig. 3). Determination of the threshold dose was not attempted in this study. At the same time, the peak of each response was compared with the initial perfusion pressure level, i.e., the level before denervation. In controls 0.25 µg/kg of NE usually compensated for the effects of the denervation by restoring the lowered perfusion pressure to the original level, whereas 0.5 µg/kg was needed in SHR. Finally, the response to angiotensin (0.25 µg/kg) was greater in SHR.

DISCUSSION

According to ALBRECHT [1], cardiac output is slightly increased in young SHR, but it is rather decreased in the stage of their established hypertension (DENCKLA, D.: personal communication). Therefore, one expects total peripheral vascular resistance to be much greater in SHR; otherwise, it would be impossible for the blood pressure, a product of cardiac output and total vascular resistance, to be high in SHR. Indeed, our experiment showed that the peripheral resistance of the hind limb was definitely greater in SHR.

Sympathetic denervation was found to reduce the peripheral resistance of the hind limb much more in SHR than in controls. In other words, the increased peripheral resistance in SHR is more dependent on neural tone. The increased neurogenic component of blood pressure was also reported by SMIRK [12] in his genetically hypertensive rats of New Zealand strain. Similarly, the maintenance of chronic renal hypertension has been known to depend on the sympathetic nervous system. In SHR the dependence of hypertension on the nervous system has also been suggested from the results of pithing [7, 9, 10], decerebration [9] and administration of sympatholytic or ganglion blocking agents [8, 10].

As mentioned before, the increased neurogenic fraction of the peripheral vascular resistance was effected either through increased sympathetic activities, through increased vascular reactivity, or through both of these mechanisms. The second half of our experiment was aimed at an evaluation of the part vascular reactivity plays in neural fraction, and at the same time, at an inference regarding the sympathetic tonic discharges to the blood vessels of the hind limb from the amount of NE, a biochemical equivalent of sympathetic discharges, which was required to compensate for the effects of denervation.

The blood vessels of the hind limb of SHR showed a definitely increased reactivity to every suprathreshold amount of NE though this hyperreactivity was not specific for NE alone. However, the amount of NE which compensated for the effects of denervation was twice as much in SHR as in controls. This means that the increased vascular reactivity alone does not explain the much more increased neural component. The fact that substitution of the latter was achieved by a greater amount of NE in SHR necessarily leads to the assumption that there must be an increase in NE release to the vascular receptor sites in SHR. The same assumption was reached by SHIBAYAMA et al. [7] from their study of cardiovascular reactivity in pithed animals. An underlying mechanism of the increased NE liberation may be either increased sympathetic activities or increased NE release in response to a unit quantity of sympathetic discharges. The results of our previous studies, electrophysiological [9, 10] and morphological [10], support the former possibility.

The basal perfusion pressure was slightly but definitely higher in SHR. Most likely, the higher basal peripheral resistance reflects a structural vascular change, such as the adaptive medial hypertrophy of FOLKOW [4] which was affirmed electron-microscopically by HAZAMA et al [5]. It is obvious that such a structurally based narrowing of arteries leads to an increased vascular reactivity even if hyperreactivity of individual effector cells is absent. It is likely that the vascular hyperreactivity of SHR is actuated on the basis of such a mechanism.

A controversial problem in our present study was whether exogenous NE could adequately substitute for sympathetic discharges. However, endogenous NE induced by tyramine or sympathetic nerve stimulation will not give reliable results if peripheral catecholamine turnover is not equal between two groups of animals.

SUMMARY

Artificial perfusion of a neurologically intact hind limb with the animal's own blood revealed that peripheral vascular resistance was higher in the Spontaneously Hypertensive Rat (SHR). Sympathetic denervation of the perfused limb resulted in a greater fall of the peripheral resistance in SHR. Various amounts of norepinephrine (NE), given directly into the perfused artery after the denervation, elicited a greater increase of peripheral resistance in SHR. However, the amount of NE which was required to compensate for denervation effects and restore peripheral resistance to its initial state was greater in SHR.

From these results it is concluded that peripheral vascular resistance is high in SHR, being more dependent on sympathetic tone. This greater neural component is partly due to an increased vascular reactivity to NE which is tonically released from sympathetic nerve terminals. However, this increased vascular reactivity alone does not explain the greatly increased neural component. Another factor involved is likely the increased sympathetic activities.

REFERENCES

1. ALBRECHT, I., VÍZEK, M. and CŘEČEK, J. (1972):   *In* "Spontaneous Hypertension" (K. OKAMOTO, ed.), p. 121, Igaku Shoin Ltd., Tokyo.
2. BRODY, M. J., SHAFFER, R. A. and DIXON R. L. (1963):   J Appl Physiol, **18**, 645.
3. DORR, L. D. and BRODY, M. J. (1966):   Proc Soc Exp Biol Med, **123**, 155.
4. FOLKOW, B. (1971):   Clin Sci, **41**, 1.
5. HAZAMA, F., TANAKA, T. OOSHIMA, A., HAEBARA, H., AMANO, S., YAMAZAKI, Y. and OKAMOTO, K. (1972):   *In* "Spontaneous Hypertension" (K. OKAMOTO, ed.), p. 134, Igaku Shoin, Ltd., Tokyo.

6. LAVERTY, R. and SMIRK, F. H. (1961): Circ Res, **9**, 455.
7. SHIBAYAMA, F., MIZOGAMI, S. and SOKABE, H. (1971): Jap Heart J, **12**, 68.
8. OKAMOTO, K., HAZAMA, F., TAKEDA, T., TABEI, R., NOSAKA, S., FUKUSHIMA, M., YAMORI, Y., MATSUMOTO, M., HAEBARA, H., ICHIJIMA, K. and SUZUKI, Y. (1966): Jap Circ J, **30**, 987.
9. OKAMOTO, K., NOSAKA, S., YAMORI, Y. and MATSUMOTO, M. (1967): Jap Heart J, **8**, 168.
10. OKAMOTO, K. (1969): *In* "International Review of Experimental Pathology" (G. W. RICHTER and M. A. EPSTEIN, eds.), Vol 7, p 227, Academic Press, New York.
11. REED, R. K., SAPIRSTEIN, L. A., SOUTHARD, F. D., Jr. and OGDEN, E. (1941): Am J Physiol, **141**, 707.
12. SMIRK, F. H. (1970): *In* "Hypertensive Mechanisms" (R. READER, ed.), p. II-55, American Heart Association, New York.
13. SOMLYO, A. P. and SOMLYO, A. V. (1970): Pharmacol Rev, **22**, 249.
14. TAQUINI, A. C., (1963): Circ Res, **12**, 562.

METABOLIC BASIS FOR CENTRAL BLOOD PRESSURE REGULATION IN SPONTANEOUSLY HYPERTENSIVE RATS

Y. YAMORI*, A. OOSHIMA*, A. NOSAKA*, and K. OKAMOTO*

Central catecholamine metabolism in hypertension has attracted more attention since YAMORI, LOVENBERG and SJOERDSMA [11] reported the low norepinephrine (NE) level and concomitant decrease of aromatic L-amino acid decarboxylase activity in the brainstem of spontaneously hypertensive rats (SHR). The NE level in SHR was slightly low in the whole brainstem and 80 per cent of the control level in the anatomically discrete areas of hypothalamus and pons plus medulla (Fig. 1). As NE synthesis from labelled

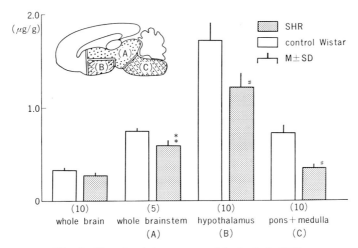

Fig. 1 Norepinephrine content of the brain in SHR.
The extent of whole brainstem, hypothalamus and pons plus medulla is indicated as the dotted area (A), straped areas (B) and (C), respectively, in the upper left scheme. Data cited from YAMORI, LOVENBERG and SJOERDSMA's article [11].
( ); Number of Rats
Statistically significant difference from the control   ♯ p<0.001   ✳ p<0.01
Method: Modification of von EULER and LISHAJKO's method

tyrosine was also decreased [4], two NE synthesizing enzymes were examined. Although nonpurified tyrosine hydroxylase in the brainstem of SHR showed no difference in activity from that in control Wistar rats, aromatic L-amino aciddecarbox ylase activity in SHR was markedly decreased, nearly half of the control level in Wistar-NIH. This decrease was still apparent after dialysis of the enzyme in the buffer containing the coenzyme and the decarboxylase activity was not affected by various experimental conditions, such as the induction of acute DOCA-salt or renal hypertension, cortisone treatment and adrenalectomy. These facts tempted us to attribute the decreased NE synthesis in the

* Department of Pathology, Faculty of Medicine, Kyoto University, Kyoto, Japan

brainstem of SHR to the genetic abnormality of this enzyme. Consequently, various trials were done to compensate for the supposed genetic metabolic lesion at DOPA decarboxylation as summarized in Fig. 2 [10]. For example, intraperitoneal or oral administration of DOPA or α-methyl DOPA with peripheral decarboxylase inhibitor decreased blood pressure and this blood pressure lowering effect seemed to be related to an increase in the level of NE or its analogue, α-methyl NE. MAO inhibitor, pargyline, also decreased blood pressure and concomitantly increased the brain NE level. Generally speaking, various procedures for increasing brain NE or NE analogues decreased the blood pressure. This inverse relationship between brain NE level and blood pressure indicated that the central noradrenergic mechanism might play a sympatho-inhibitory role. The most interesting topic on this line was that it seemed to be possible to depress

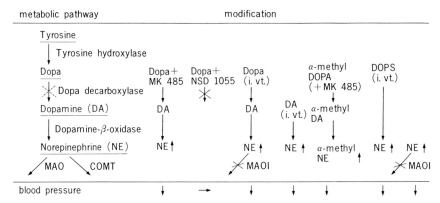

Fig. 2 Catecholamine metabolism in the brainstem and effects of its modification on blood pressure.
    ✳: supposed metabolic lesion in SHR,
    MAO: monoamine oxidase, MAOI: monoamine oxidase inhibitor (pargyline),
    COMT: catechol-O-methyl transferase
    MK 485: peripheral   decarboxylase   inhibitor   (DL-(3,4-dihydroxyphenyl)-2-hydrazino-2-
            methylpropionic acid),
    NSD 1055: decarboxylase inhibitor (4-bromo, 3-hydroxybenzyloxylamine),
    i. vt.: intraventricular injection,
    other treatments: intraperitoneal injection unless especially described

the development of hypertension by increasing NE level in the brainstem. Among the various treatments, such as DOPA alone or peripheral decarboxylase inhibitor alone, only the combination of DOPA plus peripheral decarboxylase inhibitor in the drinking water for one week significantly increased the NE level in the brainstem and also efficiently delayed the development of hypertension [10].

Therefore, firstly, NE metabolism was investigated in 6-week-old SHR at the very initial stage of hypertension to clarify the role of catecholamine (CA) metabolism in the development of hypertension. These SHR showed blood pressure around 140 mm Hg, already a little higher than that in controls. The content of tritiated NE was assayed 2 and 24 hours after the intravenous injection of 10 μc/kg of ^{3}H-NE. Our preliminary study showed that exogenous tritiated NE disappeared more rapidly from the heart in SHR than in two groups of age-matched normotensive rats, Wistar-Mishima and Wistar-Kyoto [13]. This was rather in contrast to what had been observed in the heart of adult SHR which showed a clear delay in NE turnover [5]. The same tendency as observed in the heart was also noted in the kidney and spleen of SHR. The disappearance from the salivary gland, however, was not significantly accelerated in SHR in comparison with two control groups. Although the endogenous NE level in these peripheral organs did not correlate to hypertension when SHR was compared to two normotensive groups, the rate constant of the regression equation of NE disappearance curve was significantly increased in the heart, kidney and spleen of SHR. On the other hand, tritiated NE content was assayed 2 and 24 hours after the injection (2 μc/20 μl per rat) into the lateral ventricle. By contrast to the acceleration of ^{3}H-NE disappearance from the peripheral organs in SHR, the disappearance was obviously delayed in the brainstem, but not in telencephalon when SHR was compared to two normotensive groups. This delay was significant, and especially marked when compared to Wistar-Mishima. The endogenous NE level in the brainstem as a whole showed no difference from the levels in two controls in this stage, but the rate constant of the regression equation of NE disappearance curve was significantly decreased in the brainstem of SHR. Fig. 3 shows the summary of these findings. NE

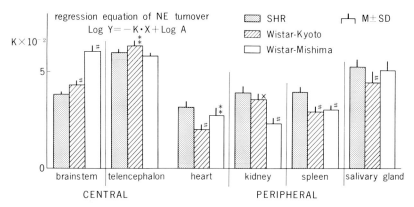

Fig. 3 ^{3}H-NE turnover in young SHR and control rats.
Statistically significant difference from SHR   ♯ p<0.001,   * p<0.01,   × p<0.05
See the text for the details.

disappearance rate was significantly decreased in the brainstem of young SHR, as compared to two normotensive strains, but in most of the peripheral organs examined, these rates were increased at least at the very initial stage of hypertension. This fact suggested that such an inverse relationship between central and peripheral NE metabolism might be involved in the pathogenesis, the development of hypertension in SHR.

Therefore, secondly, the role of central NE in blood pressure regulation was studied mainly by observing the effect of intraventricularly injected NE precursor or related substances. L-DOPA (0.07–0.7 mg/20 μl), dopamine (0.1 mg/20 μl) and NE (1–30 μg/20 μl) injected into the lateral ventricle decreased the blood pressure and also decreased the heart rate. The pretreatment of MAO inhibitor (pargyline, 0.5–0.7 mg/20 μl, i. vt.) intensified these depressor effects. 6-hydroxy dopamine (0.2–0.8 mg), which depletes NE from nerve endings, caused acute pressor response when injected intravenously. Conversely, it gradually decreased the blood pressure when injected intraventricularly. The central depressor effect may be due to the fact that central noradrenergic receptor is exposed to much exogenous NE or endogenous NE which is accumulated after MAO inhibition or released by 6-hydroxy dopamine.

    In order to clarify which one is important, NE or dopamine, for the central depressor effect, fusaric acid, a potent dopamine β-hydroxylase inhibitor was injected intraventricularly. This substance decreases the blood pressure in SHR as reported by Drs. NAGATSU, UMÉZAWA et al. [7]. A rather large dose (0.5 mg/20 μl) of this substance increased the blood pressure when injected intraventricularly and the depressor effect of L-DOPA (0.07 mg/20 μl, i. vt.) was no longer observed after the inhibition of dopamine β-hydroxylase by fusaric acid. This fact showed the importance of NE, not dopamine, in the central depressor response.

The depressor effect of L-DOPA (0.07 mg/20 μl, i. vt.) was also arrested after the intraventricular administration of α blocker, phentolamine (0.1 mg/20 μl). According to ANDÉN et al. [1], depressor effect of clonidine (2-(2,6-dichlorphenylamino)-2-imidazoline hydrochloride, St 155, Catapresan®) is ascribed to the stimulation of central α-receptor and this agent (2–20 ug/20μl) induced a greater prolonged depressor effect when injected intraventricularly in SHR than in control Wistar. These experiments indicate that the central depressor effect of NE is mediated through α-receptor.

Moreover, the sympathetic and vagal discharges were recorded after injection of 50 μg of L-DOPA into the IVth ventricle under the condition of cramping blood pressure at a constant level to avoid the influence of baroceptor reflux. L-DOPA itself seemed to decrease the firing rate of sympathetic discharge. MAO inhibitor, pargyline (100 μg, i. vt.), also decreased the firing rate. Especially L-DOPA after pargyline markedly decreased the rate, but no change was observed in the vagal discharge. Consequently, centrally administered DOPA was confirmed to inhibit the sympathetic discharge to the periphery.

Thirdly, we analyzed the genetic abnormality of the brainstem decarboxylase activity in the various cross and backcross generations obtained by the mating between SHR and Wistar-Mishima. The hybrid F_1 showed the intermediate enzyme activity and blood pressure between both parental strains. The analysis of the activity in F_2 and 2 backcross generations showed that the abnormality seemed to be transmitted to the offspring in an additive mode of inheritance and that the enzyme activity was reverse to the blood pressure level of each generation. The correlation between the brainstem decarboxylase activity and blood pressure level was further examined in the individual rats of F_2 generation which showed a wide variation of blood pressure from normotensive to hypertensive level [9]. A weak inverse correlation was observed ($r = -0.24 \pm 0.14$) and the regression equation was as follows: $Y = 162.7 - 1.4X$ ($Y =$ blood pressure in mm Hg, $X =$ specific activity, mμM/h.mg.protein) [12]. The F_2 with the low brainstem decarboxylase activity corresponding to SHR level (6.7 ± 0.6, $M \pm 2SD$) showed a significantly ($p < 0.05$) higher blood pressure (157 ± 12 mm Hg) than the F_2 (146 ± 12 mm Hg) with high decarboxylase activity in the range of normotensive controls (13.3 ± 1.3, $M \pm 2SD$).

However, in the course of this genetic analysis it was found that the brainstem decarboxylase activity of Wistar-Kyoto was also low and not so greatly different from that in SHR except for the midbrain plus the thalamus. On the other hand, Wistar-Mishima, the authentic Wistar strain from the U.S. showed as high a level as in Wistar-NIH or Sprague-Dowley in Japan. Consequently, Wistar-Kyoto, the antecedent colony of SHR, is a kind of mutant as to the brainstem decarboxylase. As some descendants of this colony still show a mild high blood pressure sporadically, they might be readily susceptible to the development of hypertension. The genetic abnormality of the brainstem decarboxylase activity seen in this colony might be related to the supposed insufficiency of the central sympatho-inhibitory mechanism and also to their susceptibility to hypertension.

In summary of the CA metabolism of the brainstem in SHR, tritiated NE turnover was decreased in comparison with those in both Wistar-Mishima and -Kyoto. The decarboxylase activity of SHR was also lower than that of Wistar-Mishima, but close to that of Wistar-Kyoto. Therefore, it is necessary to clarify at least one more abnormality in order to explain the difference in the tritiated NE turnover between SHR and Wistar-Kyoto.

Moreover, our trials to induce a sustained experimental hypertension in control rats by depleting central NE after the intraventricular injection of 6-hydroxy dopamine (100–800 μg/20 μl) was not so successful [15]. The treated SHR developed hypertension and the treated Wistar rats kept normal blood pressure level except for some sporadic cases with relatively high blood pressure after the treatment. Although the denervation supersensitivity of central α-receptor after NE depletion should be taken into consideration, this experiment partially indicated the limitation of the insufficiency of central noradrenergic mechanism as the sole cause of genetic hypertension.

Therefore, fourthly, the possible roles of other neurotransmitters in the central blood pressure regulation in SHR was investigated [14]. Aromatic L-amino acid decarboxylase is also involved in the metabolism of serotonin, and serotonin as well as its precursor 5HTP induced depressor response mainly when injected intraventricularly. For these reasons, the level of 5HIAA, the metabolite of serotonin was assayed in the brain of SHR, but in so far as examined no significant difference was detected.

Cholinergic agents, such as carbachol (5 μg/20 μl) caused sympathetic excitation in SHR as well as in normotensive rats when injected intraventricularly. And the intraventricular injection of eserine (5 μg/20 μl), cholinesterase inhibitor, caused a rather prolonged rise in blood pressure. Therefore, two main enzymes of cholinergic mechanism, acetylcholinesterase [2] and choline acetylase [6] activities were examined in the whole brainstem, hypothalamus, midbrain plus pons and telencephalon in 40-day-old young and 3 to 6 month-old adult SHR. In comparison with normotensive Wistar-Kyoto, a slight but significant increase in acetylcholinesterase activity was noted in the whole brainstem of SHR, and such increase was also detected in choline acetylase activity in young SHR. Moreover, it is noteworthy that the total acetylcholinesterase activity of sympathetic cervical ganglion was increased in both young and adult SHR. As the sympathetic impulses are conducted by cholinergic mechanism in sympathetic ganglion and acetylcholinesterase activity is decreased after the decentralization of the ganglion, this increase in acetylcholinesterase might be an indicator of increased cholinergic activity and may be coincident with the increased activity of sympathetic nervous system.

Centrally administered glutamic acid (100 μg/20 μl, i. vt.) induced a short pressor response and gamma aminobutylic acid (GABA) (100 μg/20 μl, i. vt.) decreased the blood pressure in SHR. Glutamic acid, a pressor agent, is converted into GABA, a depressor agent by glutamic acid decarboxylase, which is also a pyridoxal phosphate requiring enzyme as well as aromatic L-amino acid decarboxylase. Consequently, glutamic acid decarboxylase activity [8] was examined, but was not substantially changed in SHR.

Among several other enzymes assayed, glucose-6-phosphate dehydrogenase activity [3], which was mainly localized in neurons histochemically, showed an increase in the total and specific activity in the sympathetic ganglia of SHR and this finding seemed to support the aforementioned view speculated from the findings of cholinergic mechanism.

In summary, noradrenergic mechanism of the brainstem which may play a sympatho-inhibitory role, is inadequate in SHR and this inadequacy might be partially explained by the genetic abnormality of aromatic L-amino acid decarboxylase in this rat. Among the other neurotransmitters, cholinergic mechanism which may be sympatho-excitatory in the central nervous system and evidently in the sympathetic ganglion, might be activated in SHR as was indicated by the increase in acetylcholinesterase and choline acetylase activity. This kind of metabolic imbalance between the central pressor and depressor mechanisms might be involved in the pathogenesis, at least in the initiation of hypertension.

REFERENCES

1. ANDÉN, N. E., CORRODI, H., FUXE, K., HÖKFELT, B., HÖKFELT, T., RYDIN, C. and SVESSON, T. (1970): Life sci, **9**, Part I, 513.

2. KLINGMAN, G. I., KLINGMAN, J. D. and POLISZCZUK, A. (1968): J Neurochem, **15**, 1121.

3. KORNBERG, A. and HORECKER, B. L. (1955): In "Methods in Enzymology" (S. P. COLOWICK and N. O. KAPLAN eds.), Vol 1, p. 323, Academic Press, New York.

4. LOUIS, W. J., KRAUSS, K. R., KOPIN, I. J. and SJOERDSMA, A. (1970): Circ Res, **27**, 589.

5. LOUIS, W. J., TABEI, R., SPECTOR, S. and SJOERDSMA, A. (1969): Circ Res, **24** and **25**, Suppl. I, 93.

6. McCAMAN, R. E. and HUNT, J. M. (1965): J Neurochem, **12**, 253.

7. NAGATSU, T., MIZUTANI, K., NAGATSU, I., UMEZAWA, H., MATSUZAKI, M. and TAKEUCHI, T. (1972): In "Spontaneously Hypertenson" (K. OKAMOTO ed.), p. 31, Igaku Shoin Ltd., Tokyo.

8. ROBERTS, E. and SIMONSEN, D. G. (1963): Biochem Pharmacol, **12**, 113.

9. TANASE, H., SUZUKI, Y., OOSHIMA, A., YAMORI, Y. and OKAMOTO, K. (1970): Jap Circ J, **34**, 1197.

10. YAMORI, Y., DEJONG, W., YAMABE, H., LOVENBERG, W. and SJOEDSMA, A. (1972): J Pharmacol and Pharm, in press.

11. YAMORI, Y., LOVENBERG, W. and SJOEDSMA A. (1970): Science, **170**, 544.

12. YAMORI, Y. OOSHIMA, A. and OKAMOTO, K. (1972): Jap Circ J, in press.

13. YAMORI, Y. OOSHIMA, A. and OKAMOTO, K. (1972): Jap Circ J, in press.

14. YAMORI, Y. OOSHIMA, A. and OKAMOTO, K. (1972): Jap Circ J, in press.

15. YAMORI, Y., YAMABE, H., DEJONG, W., LOVENBERG, W. and SJOEDSMA, A. (1972): Eur J Pharmacol, **17**, 135.

BAROCEPTOR REFLEX FUNCTIONS IN THE
SPONTANEOUSLY HYPERTENSIVE RAT

S. NOSAKA*[a] and S. C. WANG*

Many investigations have been accumulated in regards to baroceptor participation in hypertension. They may be divided into two categories: studies on neurogenic hypertension induced by disrupting buffer nerves and studies on baroceptor functions in otherwise induced hypertension.

Sustained hypertension was successfully produced by bilateral denervation of carotid sinus and aortic baroceptors in the dog by Novak [12] in 1940. Similarly, compression of carotid sinus areas [16] or constriction of common carotid arteries [16] or brachiocephalic and left subclavian arteries [3] is known to elicit hypertension, possibly by reducing the impulses in carotid sinus nerve traffic either through restricting sinus distension against normal intrasinus pressure or decreasing intrasinus pressure itself. However, the hypertension produced by these means is not regarded as a model of human essential hypertension, mainly because its hemodymanics are characterised by tachycardia and increased cardiac output [1]. In addition, neurogenic hypertension is known to fluctuate and is not usually very severe.

The second group of investigations has been aimed at baroceptor functions in hypertension initiated by other mechanisms. From the effects of procaine block of carotid sinus areas, Kezdi [5] presented evidence that baroceptor functions in human hypertensive patients were not either supressed to cause increased sympathetic outflow as in neurogenic hypertension or activated to reduce the sympathetic outflow as in acute blood pressure elevation, but rather the baroceptors adapted to the high blood pressure level. This so-called resetting mechanism was later confirmed by a series of electrophysiological studies in chronic renal hypertensive dogs by McCubbin et al. [8, 9] and Kezdi [6]. Another implication of this mechanism is that baroceptors in hypertension are not working at their full capability, which has led to a practical application of a 'baropacer' for the treatment of human hypertension [14].

Heyman and Neil [4] suggested that changes in arterial distensibility in baroceptor areas might be the cause of essential hypertension. A hereditary-determined deficit of distensibility of Windkessel system was postulated by Volhard [15] as a mechanism for initiation of the hypertension, making it prone to function at a higher set level. Recently, however, most, if not all, researchers agreed that the shift of baroceptor functions is secondary to hypertension. This is based on Kezdi's clear demonstration [6] that 'protected' sinus was never reset in chronic renal hypertension, and on McCubbin's observation [8, 9] that resetting always lagged behind hypertension. Indeed, convincing evidence is lacking for the baroceptor shift as a primary mechanism to cause hypertension.

In the Spontaneously Hypertensive Rat (SHR), an experimental model of human essential hypertensive patients, a few attempts have been made to elucidate the baroceptor functions. Thant et al. [13] evaluated the total amount of tonic inhibition by baroceptors in SHR by means of acute mechanical and chemical denervation and found that the resultant blood pressure response was greater in young SHR than in young controls

---

* Department of Pharmacology, College of Physicians and Surgeons, Columbia University, New York, N.Y., U.S.A.

a) Present adress: Department of Pathology Faculty of Medicine, Kyoto University, Kyoto, Japan.

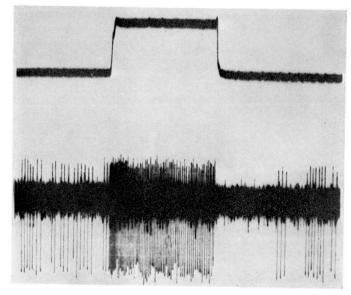

Fig. 1 Transient response of a sinus baroceptor.
Top tracing is the carotid sinus perfusion pressure which shows a stepwise increase in pressure (40 mm Hg) from 100 mm Hg, and the bottom a single fiber activity of rat carotid sinus nerve.

but not different in adult animals. Though they interpreted the greater response in young SHR to be due to increased sympathetic activities, the finding may suggest that the tonic baroceptor discharges are increased in total number in SHR than in controls at their young age. A shift of baroceptor function range was also suggested in SHR by an electrophysiological study on the aortic baroceptors [10].

We investigated further functions of baroceptors in SHR and, this time, of the carotid sinus using techniques that we developed for rat carotid sinus perfusion and carotid sinus nerve recordings. A detailed description of the techniques was made elsewhere [11].

Baroceptors have a static function, which is 'proportional' to the magnitude of pressure, and a transient state function, which is concerned with a rate of change in pressure. Figure 1, a unit recording obtained by teasing sinus nerve into a single fiber, clearly shows that a baroceptor fires instantly in response to a change in pressure but adapts rapidly, reaching a new steady state. We studied such a steady state function and a transient function separately. Most of the previous studies did not specify which component they dealt with.

Carotid sinuses were isolated and perfused artificially. The carotid sinus perfusion pressure (CSPP) was either kept constant for a long time at various levels (steady state) or was changed stepwisely (transient state). The resultant baroceptor responses, as evaluated by reflex blood pressure responses or by electrophysiologically recorded sinus nerve activities, were compared between SHR and controls (6 to 8 months of age). The results from blood pressure responses were substantially similar to those from nerve recordings. On the base of these results baroceptor behaviors in steady state and transient state were summarised in a schematic fashion in Fig. 2 and 3, respectively.

A curve of steady state relationship between CSPP and baroceptor response showed a shift to higher CSPP in SHR: both the threshold pressure (a minimum pressure to elicit a response) and the pressure to bring about a maximum response were significantly elevated in SHR as compared with controls (Fig. 2).

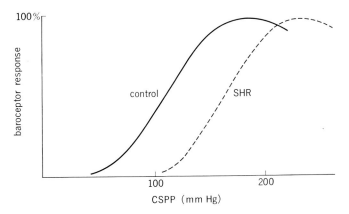

Fig. 2 Steady state relationship between carotid sinus perfusion pressure and baroceptor response. CSPP: carotid sinus perfusion pressure

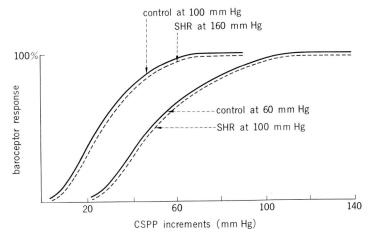

Fig. 3 Baroceptor response to step change of carotid sinus perfusion pressure. CSPP: carotid sinus perfusion pressure

Baroceptors, after they adapt to a steady state, are said to fire constantly without diminution in the firing rate for a long time [2].   Therefore, the shift in this steady state sensitivity in SHR is likely concerned with maintenance of the hypertension: if a disturbance is added to SHR circulatory system, antihypertensive drugs for example, which lowers the elevated blood pressure, baroceptors will counteract this hypotensive action and try to keep the high blood pressure by increasing sympathetic outflow.

Transient state sensitivity was found to be dependent on basal CSPP level (Fig. 3). For example, in controls a stepwise increase of 20 mm Hg elicited a remarkable baroceptor response when the basal CSPP was 100 mm Hg, but the response to the same increment was negligible when the basal CSPP was 60 mm Hg.   Also, a greater increment was required to bring about a maximum response at the basal CSPP of 60 mm Hg than at 100 mm Hg.   In other words, baroceptor sensitivity was high at 100 mm Hg but low at 60 mm Hg in controls.   In SHR, however, baroceptors were not sensitive at 100 mm Hg but the sensitivity was definitely high at 160 mm Hg.   Therefore, it is clear that the transient state function of baroceptors of SHR was also shifted to high sinus pressure.

The shift in the transient state sensitivity in SHR obviously operates to stabilize the hypertension. Neurogenic hypertension is known to fluctuate markedly, whereas the hypertension of SHR is quite stable. This is likely bacause in SHR the rate sensitive component of baroceptor functions is operating effectively around the elevated blood pressure.

We have no clear understanding as to whether these baroceptor changes are primary or secondary to hypertension. We cannot rule out the possibility that these changes may exist on the base of a genetical structural change of the arterial wall of baroceptor area, elevating the blood pressure level through an increase in sympathetic activities to the level which matches the higher 'preset' barostatic level. However, the resultant hypertension should share specific hemodynamic features with neurogenic hypertension, which SHR does not have. Also, the fact that the set level of baroceptors change in a short time when they are exposed to abnormal pressure [7], may reduce the possibility that baroceptors are so potent a guide for developing high blood pressure.

The mechanism underlying these baroceptor changes remains unknown. However, our results showed that SHR baroceptors behave just normally at high CSPP. Therefore, it is possible to postulate that a reduction of sinus wall distensibility, which could be compensated by increasing CSPP, may be a factor responsible for the functional changes of SHR baroceptors.

REFERENCES

1. BING, J. R., THOMAS, C. B. and WAPLES, E. C. (1945): J Clin Invest, **24**, 513.
2. BRONK, D. W. and STELLA, G. (1934): Am J Physiol, **110**, 708.
3. HAWTHORNE, E. W. and MANDAL, A. K. (1962): Circ Res, **11**, 153.
4. HEYMANS, C. and NEIL, E. (1958): "Reflexogenic Areas of the Cardiovascular System", Little, Brown and Co., Boston.
5. KEZDI, P. (1953): Arch Int Med, **91**, 26.
6. KEZDI, P. (1962): Circ Res, **11**, 145.
7. KRIEGER, E. M. (1970): Am J Physiol, **218**, 486.
8. McCUBBIN, J. W. (1958): Circulation, **17**, 791.
9. McCUBBIN, J. W., GREEN, J. H. and PAGE, I. H. (1956): Circ Res, **4**, 205.
10. NOSAKA, S. and OKAMOTO, K. (1970): Jap Circ J, **34**, 685.
11. NOSAKA, S. and WANG, S. C. (1972): Am J Physiol, in press.
12. NOVAK, S. J. G. (1940): Ann Surg, **111**, 102.
13. THANT, M., YAMORI, Y. and OKAMOTO, K. (1969): Jap Circ J, **33**, 501.
14. TUCKMAN, J., REICH, T., LYON, A. F., GOODMAN, B., MENDLOWITZ, M. and JACOBSON, J. H. (1968): In "Hypertension, XVI" (J. E. WOOD, ed.), p. 23, American Heart Association, New York.
15. VOLHARD, F. (1948): Schweiz Med Wochschr, **78**, 1189.
16. WAKERLIN, G. E., CRANDALL, E., FRANK, M. H., JOHNSON, D., POMPER, L. and SCHMID, H. E. (1954): Circ Res, **2**, 416.

CENTRAL HYPOTHERMIC EFFECT OF L-DOPA IN SPONTANEOUSLY HYPERTENSIVE RATS*

C. TANAKA**, S. TAKAORI** and K. OKAMOTO***

A possible explanation to pathogenesis of hypertension by central catecholamine deficiency has been shown on the basis of findings that norepinephrine content and L-aromatic amino acid decarboxylase activities in the lower brainstem and hypothalamus of spontaneously hypertensive rats (SHR) are lower than those in normotensive Wistar rats [9]. Central hypotensive effects of L-dopa have been reported in Parkinsonian patients [3], in SHR [10] and also in normotensive rats treated with peripheral decarboxylase inhibitor [7]. A concept has been proposed by FELDBERG and MYERS [6] that balance in the release of monoamines from the cells of anterior hypothalamus could be the mechanism in central thermoregulation. Moreover, the fluorescence of norepinephrine surrounding nerve cells in the nucleus preopticus medialis was reported to be stronger in SHR than in normotensive controls [8]. If there is any change in catecholamine metabolism of the anterior hypothalamus, a disorder in thermoregulation may be present in SHR as a result of the unblance in brain monoamine levels.

The present experiments were, therefore, set up to examine the effect of L-dopa on body temperature in unrestricted normotensive Wistar-Kyoto rats and SHR, 4–26 week-old of both sexes. Rectal temperature was recorded using an electrical thermometer (Kyoto Keisokuki Co. Kyoto, Japan). All body temperature measurements were carried out in a room with a controlled temperature of $23 \pm 1 °C$. L-dopa (Daiichi Seiyaku) and N-(DL-seryl)-N'-(2,3,4-trihydroxybenzyl)-hydrazine (Ro 4-4602, Hoffmann-La Roche) which had been dissolved in pyrogen-free 0.9% NaCl solution were used. Norepinephrine content in the brain was assayed according to the method of ANTON and SYARE [1].

Body temperature of 4–26 week-old SHR which were measured at 2: 30 to 3: 30 p.m. was approximately higher $1.0 °C$ than that of the age-matched normotensive rats. There are two possible explanations that thermoregulation in SHR is very labile to exogenous influences such as handling or that the set-point of body temperature is higher than that in the normotensive controls. Norepinephrine content in the brainstem was slightly lowered in male SHR as compared to the age-matched Wistar-Kyoto rats. This decrease, however, was not statistically significant. A direct correlation could not be found between brain norepinephrine levels and hyperthermia in SHR.

Intraperitoneal administration of L-dopa (100 mg/kg) produced a transient hyperthermia in the normotensive rats. This rise on body temperature reached maximum 45 min. after injection of L-dopa and recovered to the pre-injection level 2–3 hours after treatment. Many investigators have used Ro 4-4602, a peripheral dopa decarboxylase inhibitor, as a valuable tool in dissociating central and peripheral effects of L-dopa [2, 7]. Three doses of Ro 4-4602 (30, 50 and 500 mg/kg i.p.) were administered to five rats in each group. Higher doses produced pronounced hypothermic responses, however, lower doses did not significantly influence body temperature. When L-dopa in a dose of 100 mg/kg was injected intraperitoneally to rats with Ro 4-4602 (30 mg/kg), a significant fall

* This work was partly supported by a research grant (No. 7020) from the Ministry of Education, Japan.
** Department of Pharmacology** and Department of Pathology***, Faculty of Medicine, Kyoto University, Kyoto, Japan

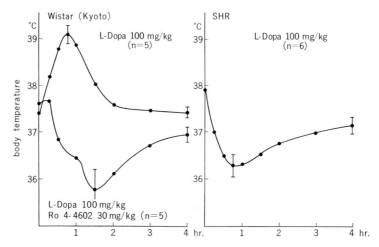

Fig. 1 Effects of L-dopa on rectal temperature in male SHR and normotensive rats. *Left panel*: normotensive Wistar-Kyoto rats were administered L-dopa (100 mg/kg i.p.) alone and Ro 4-4602 (30 mg/kg i.p.) with L-dopa (100 mg/kg). *Right panel*: SHR were given L-dopa in a dose of 100 mg/kg. Vertical bars show standard errors of means. n: Number of animals.

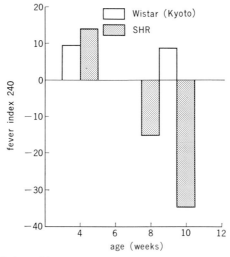

Fig. 2 Effects of L-dopa (100 mg/kg i.p.) on rectal temperature in female SHR and normotensive Wistar-Kyoto rats. Histograms show fever indices with area beneath rectal temperature curve in cm², measures by planimetry up to 240-min. point.

in body temperature was observed within 30 min. and a maximum fall appeared 90 min. after injection (Fig. 1).

The effects of norepinephrine applied into the cerebral ventricle on body temperature have been reported to vary among animal species [4, 5, 6]. For intraventricular injection of drugs a cannula was implanted into the lateral ventricle under pentobarbital anesthesia. After injection of norepinephrine (2.5 μg, volume of 0.02 ml), a transient fall in rectal temperature was observed in the normotensive rats. Intraventricular injection of L-dopa in doses of 25 and 50 μg also produced a long-lasting fall in rectal temperature.

When L-dopa (100 mg/kg) was administered intraperitoneally to SHR, a significant fall in rectal temperature was observed, as shown in right panel of Fig. 1. This hypothermic response of L-dopa in SHR was potentiated by treating with Ro 4-4602. In comparing the response to L-dopa, fever indices, areas beneath body temperature curves in cm², were measured by planimetry up to 240-min. point. Hyperthermia induced by intraperitoneal injection of L-dopa (100 mg/kg) appeared in 4 week-old SHR as well as in the normotensive controls. Conversely, in 8 week-old SHR, L-dopa produced a slight hypothermia and in those of 10 weeks, marked hypothermia was found with a rise in blood pressure (Fig. 2).

Hyperthermia induced by L-dopa is probably due to a peripheral mechanism, as intraperitoneal injection of norepinephrine also produced hyperthermia in the normotensive rats. On the other hand, hypothermic response of L-dopa which appeared in SHR and the normotensive rats treated with Ro 4-4602, is considered to be centrally mediated. These results also suggest a possibility that a disturbance of the blood brain barrier mechanism for L-dopa may be present in SHR.

REFERENCES

1. ANTON, A. H. and SYARE, D. F. (1962): J Pharmacol Exp Ther, **138**, 360.
2. BUTCHER, L. L. and ENGEL, J. (1969): Brain Res, **15**, 233.
3. CALNE, D. B. and SANDLER, M. (1970): Nature, **226**, 21.
4. COOPER, K. E. CRANSTON, W. I. and HONOUR, A. J. (1965): J Physiol London, **181**, 852.
5. FELDBERG, W. and LOTTI, V. J. (1967): Br J Pharmacol Chemother, **31**, 152.
6. FELDBERG, W. and MYERS, R. D. (1964): J Physiol London, **173**, 226.
7. HENNING, M. and RUBENSON, A. (1970): J Pharm Pharmacol, **22**, 553.
8. OKAMOTO, K. (1969): In "International Review of Experimental Pathology" (G. W. RICHTER and M. A. EPSTEIN, eds.), Vol 7, p 227, Academic Press, New York.
9. YAMORI, Y., LOVENBERG, W. and SJOERDSMA, A. (1970): Science, **170**, 546.
10. YAMORI, Y., LOVENBERG, W. and SJOERDSMA, A. (1971): Jap J Const Med, **34, 36**.

BEHAVIORAL AND PHARMACOLOGICAL CHARACTERISTICS OF THE SPONTANEOUSLY HYPERTENSIVE RAT

K. SHIMAMOTO* and A. NAGAOKA*

It is postulated that the level of blood pressure and rate of cardiac automaticity are regulated by the activities of autonomic centers located in the hypothalamus and medulla, where noradrenaline is regarded as one of the possible transmitters controlling their activities. Recently, from the studies in relation to the brain catecholamine of the spontaneously hypertensive rat (SHR), YAMORI et al. [7, 8] concluded that the decreased level of noradrenaline in these brain structures conditioned the development and maintenance of the hypertension. Since a correlation between the brain level of catecholamine and the behavior patterns in the experimental animals has been established by a number of investigations, the SHR and control Wistar rats in the present experiments were compared in regard to their emotionality in an open field test, the aggressive behavior produced by keeping the animals in the isolated living condition, and the behavioral excitement in response to methamphetamine, apomorphine and L-DOPA.

The animals used in all experiments were the SHR at 20 to 23 generations and the control Wistar rats both of which were reared under specific pathogen free conditions.

Open field tests were carried out as follows. Male and female animals at 4 stages were divided into 16 groups each consisting of 10 SHR and Wistar rats. The apparatus was similar to that described by HALL [4]. The animals were exposed to the open field for 5 consecutive days, and on the 5 th day the animals were administered subcutaneously 2 mg/kg of methamphetamine.

The mean body weight in the male and female SHR was significantly less than those of the control rats. In contrast with the Wistar rats, the blood pressure in SHR rose progressively with the advance of age. Though the activity scores in both strains of animals were decreased by the repetition of trials, the scores in the female SHR and those in the male SHR at the oldest age (289 days) were significantly less than those in the control rats. The defecating behavior of rats in an open field is regarded as an autonomic response to novel or noxious stimuli [1, 2]. Percent defecation on the first trial is lower in the SHR except the females at the age of 38 days. The defecating rate in the female SHR as well as the male SHR at advanced ages was also lower during further trials. On the other hand, the defecation scores in the home cage were not significantly different between the two strains of rats. HOLLAND and GUPTA [5] reported that rearing behavior in an open field correlated with the excitement of the brain cortex. The SHR at almost all trials showed higher rearing scores than the control animals. This difference in rearing score between SHR and control rats, as described afterwards, was markedly augmented by the administration of methamphetamine. In contrast with rearing scores, the preening scores were less in the SHR than in the control ones, and the SHR at the oldest age exhibited no preening behavior. The summarized results of the open field behavior in the SHR and in the DOCA hypertensive rats showed that the mean scores of preening, defecation and urination of SHR on the first trials at all test ages were lower than those of control rats and the rearing score was higher in the SHR. However, the rearing score

* Biological Research Laboratories, Research and Development Division, Takeda Chemical Industries, Ltd. Osaka, Japan

in the DOCA hypertensive rats was rather lower than that in the control unilaterally nephrectomized rats.

The effects of methamphetamine injected subcutaneously on the open field performance were tested 30 minutes after the injection. The treated animals exhibited a marked increase in motor activity and rearing, and a decrease in defecation and preening. The rearing scores were increased more markedly in the SHR, while contrarily they were decreased in the control females at the age of 306 days. The defecation was abolished by the treatment in the SHR but it was not affected but rather increased in the control males at the advanced ages.

The aggressive behaviors produced by isolation were tested using SHR and control rats at the ages of 4.5, 19 and 42 weeks. The mouse-killing and rod-gnawing responses were assessed at 2 and 4 weeks after the isolation. Mouse-killing response in isolated animals was markedly higher in males than in females, and the aggressive behavior in the isolated SHR was much more frequent than that in the control rats. This response in grouped animals however was observed only in the old SHR. On the other hand, the results of rod-gnawing response in these animals were similar to those of mouse-killing response.

The effects of three central stimulant drugs on the behavior in the SHR and control Wistar rats were studied in the following ways. The animals were used as a group of 6 at the age of 11 to 14 weeks, and the behavioral changes were scored according to the method of QUINTON and HALLIWELL [6] and ERNST [3].

The scores of the behavioral excitement caused by 0.5, 2 and 8 mg/kg of methamphetamine were larger in the SHR than in the control Wistar rats. The excitatory action in the SHR treated with the lower two doses was marked both in the peak effect and in the duration of action. However, these behavioral excitements caused by the drug did not differ between the DOCA hypertensive and control uninephrectomized rats. Moreover, the behavioral response to 0.5 mg/kg of methamphetamine was enhanced by the previous intraperitoneal injection of imipramine (10 mg/kg) and iproniazid (150 mg/kg). The potentiation was also more marked in the SHR. The previous reserpinization (2.5 mg/kg) of the rats of either strain enhanced the onset of action and peak effect of the drug. However, the duration of action was slightly reduced and it was about 120 minutes in both strains. On the other hand, the behavioral excitement in both strains of rats was completely inhibited by the pretreatment of alpha-methyl tyrosine (250 mg/kg as DL-compound).

The stereotyped gnawing behavior caused by the subcutaneous injection of 2 and 5 mg/kg of apomorphine was almost the same in both strains of rats. It has been reported by ERNST [3] that the action of apomorphine, just as that of dopamine, is directly on the receptor in corpus striatum.

L-DOPA in the doses of 12.5, 25 and 50 mg/kg on the animals previously treated with iproniazid produced marked piloerection and exophthalmos dose-dependently, and after the latency about 90 minutes it also produced impulsive running, intermittent and ataxic movement. Such behavioral abnormalities were slightly less frequent in the SHR. The increased motor activity caused by the largest dose of L-DOPA was followed by a coma. The time required for the coma to develop was almost the same in both strains of rats.

These findings suggest low emotionality in an open field, high aggressiveness, and a susceptible release of dopamine from corpus striatum in the SHR.

ACKNOWLEDGMENT

We would like to thank Professor K. OKAMOTO for suggesting this project and for stimulating our interest in it.

REFERENCES

1. BROADHURST, P. L. (1969): Ann N Y Acad Sci, **159**, 806.
2. DENENBERG, V. H. (1969): Ann N Y Acad Sci, **159**, 852.
3. ERNST, A. M. (1967): Psychopharmacologia, **10**, 316.
4. HALL, C. S. (1934): J Comp Psychol, **18**, 385.
5. HOLLAND, H. C. and GUPTA, B. D. (1966): Anim Behav, **14**, 574.
6. QUINTON, R. M. and HALLIWELL, G. (1963): Nature, **200**, 178.
7. YAMORI, Y., LOVENBERG, W. and SJOERDSMA, A. (1970): Science, **170**, 544.
8. YAMORI, Y., LOVENBERG, W. and SJOERDSMA, A. (1971): Jap J Const Med, **34**, 36.

RELATIONSHIP BETWEEN BEHAVIOR AND BRAIN MONOAMINES IN SPONTANEOUSLY HYPERTENSIVE RATS

S. TAKAORI*, C. TANAKA* and K. OKAMOTO**

The role of brain monoamines in the pathogenesis of hypertension has been discussed by several investigators [3, 6, 11]. The present experiment was designed to analyse the relationship between brain monoamine levels and animal behavior in both normotensive Wistar-Kyoto strain rats and spontaneously hypertensive rats. Studies were done on blood pressure and Sidman-type avoidance response in rats whose brain serotonin or catecholamines were reduced by treatment with p-chlorophenylalanine or α-methyl-p-tyrosine. In addition, the effects of L-5-hydroxytryptophan and L-dopa on the avoidance responses in both control and spontaneously hypertensive rats were studied.

Table 1 Brain contents of serotonin in normotensive Wistar rats and spontaneously hypertensive rats (SHR).

		Age (days)	No. of rats	Blood pressure (mm Hg)[a]	Telencephalon (μg/g)[a]	Brainstem (μg/g)[a]
Male	Wistar	90–120	10	133.0 ± 3.4	0.48 ± 0.01	0.69 ± 0.02
	SHR	90–120	5	184.3 ± 5.4**	0.51 ± 0.01	0.66 ± 0.02
	Wistar	180–210	7	135.4 ± 3.6	0.53 ± 0.02	0.75 ± 0.03
	SHR	180–210	7	200.7 ± 3.6**	0.68 ± 0.02**	0.85 ± 0.03*
Female	Wistar	90–120	5	118.6 ± 2.9	0.44 ± 0.01	0.64 ± 0.01
	SHR	90–120	5	177.0 ± 4.0**	0.55 ± 0.01**	0.76 ± 0.02**
	SHR	180–210	5	170.2 ± 3.0	0.60 ± 0.02	0.69 ± 0.04

a: Results are mean ± standard error.
* $P < 0.05$, ** $P < 0.01$ (Significantly different from the control values of the age-matched normotensive rats).

The content of brain serotonin in normotensive Wistar and spontaneously hypertensive rats are shown in Table 1. The rats were killed by decapitation. The brain was quickly removed and divided into two portions: the telencephalon and the brainstem. The cerebellum, the pineal body and most of the meninges were excluded. Serotonin was assayed according to the method of BOGDANSKI et al [2]. The brain tissues were homogenized in 0.1 N HCl and the fluorescence in acidified aliquots of the butanol-heptane extraction was measured in a spectrofluorophotometer. The serotonin levels in the telencephalon and brainstem of spontaneously hypertensive male rats aged 90 to 120 days were not clearly different from those normotensive rats of the same age. At 180 to 210 days of age, however, the serotonin levels in the telencephalon and brainstem were significantly increased in the spontaneously hypertensive rats as compared with those in the other group. In the females, the contents of brain serotonin in the spontaneously hypertensive rats was clearly higher than those of the normotensive controls.

The content of brain norepinephrine in male normotensive control and spontaneously hypertensive rats aged 90 to 120 days was determined according to the method of ANTON and SYARE [1]. The norepinephrine content in the brainstem was 0.56 ± 0.03 μg/kg

* Department of Pharmacology and ** Department of Pathology, Faculty of Medicine, Kyoto University, Kyoto, Japan

(mean±standard error) in the normotensive rats (number of rats=6; blood pressure, mean ± standard error, 135.2±2.6 mm Hg), while the level of the spontaneously hypertensive rats (number of rats=5; 215.2±6.3 mm Hg) was slightly reduced, 0.51±0.01 μg/g.

p-Chlorophenylalanine is known to produce a selective reduction of serotonin content in the brain by inhibition of tryptophan hydroxylase [4, 5]. In the present experiments, a single oral administration of 300 mg/kg of p-chlorophenylalanine markedly lowered the brain serotonin in both normotensive and spontaneously hypertensive rats. Twenty-four hours after the administration of p-chlorophenylalanine, the serotonin levels in the telencephalon and brainstem of the spontaneously hypertensive rats dropped to 25 and 23% of the respective control levels. Four days after administration, the brain serotonin level in the normotensive rats was still markedly reduced, and after 10 days the level in the telencephalon and brainstem was 57 to 70 % of the respective controls.

In our laboratory, we have measured systolic blood pressure in the tail artery of rats by using a phototransducer, DC amplifier and ink-writing oscillograph, this method has the advantages of high sensitivity and simplicity. The systolic blood pressure corresponds to the onset of the pulse wave. A single oral administration of 300 mg/kg of p-chloro-phenylalanine produced an obvious increase in the blood pressure of both normotensive and spontaneously hypertensive rats for several days. The time-course of the blood pressure after administration of p-chlorophenylalanine was as follows: In the normotensive rats, the initial level was 134.8±3.3 mm Hg (mean±standard error, number of rats=8), and the levels at 1, 3, 5 and 7 days after administration were 143.1±4.2, 155.1±3.5 (significantly higher than the initial level; p<0.01), 144.1±1.3 (p<0.05) and 135.1±2.7 mm Hg, respectively. In the spontaneously hypertensive rats, the initial level was 203.3±5.7 mm Hg (number of rats=6), and the levels at 1, 3, 5 and 7 days after administration were 215.2±7.1, 219.5±6.2, 216.3±5.5 and 206.5±8.8 mm Hg, respectively. On the other hand, an intraperitoneal injection of 12.5 and 25 mg/kg of L-5-hydroxy-tryptophan markedly lowered the blood pressure, especially in the spontaneously hypertensive rats. The time-course of blood pressure after the injection of 25 mg/kg was as follows: In the normotensive rats, the initial level was 137.3±2.0 mm Hg (number of rats=7), and the levels 30 min and 24 hours after administration were 127.7±2.3 (significantly lower than the initial level; p<0.01) and 136.6±3.7 mm Hg, respectively. In the spontaneously hypertensive rats, the initial level was 205.5±3.8 mm Hg (number of rats=6), and the levels 30 min and 24 hours after administration were 173.7±10.7 (significantly lower than the initial level; p<0.05) and 207.0±3.2 mm Hg, respectively.

For behavioral tests, a non-discriminated avoidance apparatus devised by SIDMAN [7] was utilized. Each rat was housed in a Skinner box for 30 min a day, and frequencies of lever-presses and electroshocks were recorded. The avoidance response-shock interval was the 40 sec and the shock-shock interval was 10 sec. Shock duration was fixed at 1 sec. In other words, whenever the animal pressed the lever, the onset of the shock was postponed for 40 sec. When the animal did not press the lever during the 40 sec following the last lever-press, a shock was given through the floor rods. A more detailed description of the experimental procedures is found in the previous papers [9, 10].

The normotensive control Wistar rats which underwent more than 15 test training sessions were classified into three groups: good-, poor- and non-performance. According to our experiments of the last 5 years, the good-performance rats included 40% of the total trained animals, with the poor- and non-performance rats covering the remaining 60%. Conversely, most of the spontaneously hypertensive rats belonged to the good-performance group after undergoing the training tests. Fig. 1 shows the time-course of the average avoidance response rate/min in the normotensive and the spontaneously hyper-

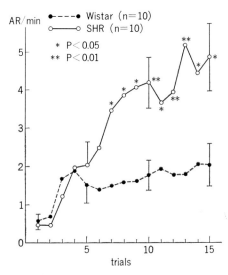

Fig. 1 Time-course of mean avoidance response rate/min (AR/min) in normotensive Wistar rats and spontaneously hypertensive rats (SHR). Each point represents the mean rate of 10 animals. Vertical lines represent the standard error.

tensive rats during the first 15 test sessions. The average avoidance response rate/min of the spontaneously hypertensive rats rapidly rose after the 5th test and maintained more than 4 even after the 10th test, although it was only approximately 2 in the normotensive controls. The average avoidance response rate of the spontaneously hypertensive rats was significantly higher than that of the control after the 7th trial. The average number of shocks/min of the spontaneously hypertensive rats was significantly lower than that of the control Wistar rats after the 7th trial.

In the normotensive rats undergoing more than 20 sessions of training trials, p-chlorophenylalanine in oral doses of 100 and 300 mg/kg resulted in a marked and long-lasting elevation of the avoidance response rate with a decrease in number of shocks for several days. In spontaneously hypertensive rats, the increase in the avoidance response rate caused by p-chlorophenylalanine was slight as the initial level of the avoidance response rate was higher than the control.

In the normotensive control rats, an intraperitoneal injection of 25 mg/kg of L-5-hydroxytryptophan did not affect the avoidance response rate, while 50 mg/kg produced a considerable reduction of the avoidance response rate 30 min after administration. In the spontaneously hypertensive rats, both 25 and 50 mg/kg of L-5-hydroxytryptophan markedly lowered the frequency of the avoidance responses.

α-Methyl-p-tyrosine is known to be an inhibitor of tyrosine hydroxylase and a cause of selective lowering of the brain catecholamine level without a concomitant decrease in brain serotonin [8]. When 100 mg/kg of α-methyl-p-tyrosine was administered twice at a time interval of 12 hours (total dose: 200 mg/kg i.p.), the avoidance response rate decreased in both the normotensive and the spontaneously hypertensive rats six hours after the last injection.

An intraperitoneal injection of 100 mg/kg of L-dopa did not change the avoidance response rate in either the normotensive or the spontaneously hypertensive rats. 200 mg/kg produced a slight increase in the avoidance response rate of the normotensive animals. The same dose of L-dopa, however, brought about a marked decrease in the avoidance response rate of the spontaneously hypertensive rats.

It can be concluded that the brain serotonin content of the spontaneously hypertensive rats was higher than that of the normotensive control group, although the norepinephrine content in the brainstem slightly decreased in the spontaneously hypertensive rats. p-Chlorophenylalanine, a specific serotonin depletor, produced an obvious increase in blood pressure in both the normotensive and the spontaneously hypertensive rats for several days. On the other hand, L-5-hydroxytryptophan considerably lowered the blood pressure, especially in the spontaneously hypertensive rats. In Sidman-type avoidance behavior, most of the spontaneously hypertensive rats undergoing training tests belonged to the good-performance group, as opposed to only 40% of the total trained normotensive rats. The effects of p-chlorophenylalanine, L-5-hydroxytryptophan and L-dopa on the avoidance behavior varied somewhat between the normotensive and the spontaneously hypertensive rats. An increase in the avoidance response rate caused by p-chlorophenyl-alanine was more marked in the normotensive rats than in the spontaneously hypertensive rats. L-5-hydroxytryptophan markedly decreased the avoidance response rate in the spontaneously hypertensive rats. L-dopa produced a slight increase in the avoidance re-sponse rate of the normotensive rats. In the spontaneously hypertensive rats, however, the same dose of L-dopa lowered the avoidance response rate.

REFERENCES

1. ANTON, A. H. and SYARE, D. F. (1962): J Pharmacol Exp Ther, **138**, 360.
2. BOGDANSKI, D. F., PLETCHER, A., BRODIE, B. B. and UDENFRIEND, S. (1956): J Pharmacol Exp Ther, **117**, 82.
3. HENNING, M. and RUBENSON, A. (1970): J Pharm Pharmacol, **22**, 553.
4. JÉQUIER, E., LOVENBERG, W. and SJOERDSMA, A. (1967): Mol Pharmacol, **3**, 274.
5. KOE, B. K. and WEISSMAN, A. (1966): J Pharmacol Exp Ther, **154**, 499.
6. OKAMOTO, K. (1969): *In* "International Review of Experimental Pathology" (G. W. RICHTER and M. A. EPSTEIN, eds.), Vol. 7, p. 227. Academic Press, New York.
7. SIDMAN, M. (1953): J comp physiol Psychol, **46**, 253.
8. SPECTOR, S., SJOERDSMA A. and UDENFRIEND, S. (1965): J Pharmacol Exp Ther, **147**, 86.
9. TAKAORI, S., YADA, N. and MORI, G. (1969): Jap J Pharmacol, **19**, 587.
10. TAKAORI, S. and TANAKA, C. (1970): Jap J Pharmacol, **20**, 607.
11. YAMORI, Y., LOVENBERG, W. and SJOERDSMA, A. (1970): Science, **170**, 544.

Chapter IV

CARDIOVASCULAR DYNAMICS

CARDIOVASCULAR REACTIVITY TO NOREPINEPHRINE OF THE SPONTANEOUSLY HYPERTENSIVE RAT

H. SOKABE* and S. MIZOGAMI*

The term "cardiovascular (CV) reactivity" was defined as "the degree with which the heart and peripheral vascular system respond to quantitated stimuli" [10, 11]. The stimulus used in this paper was norepinephrine (NE), since determination of CV reactivity to NE, chemical transmitter of the sympathetic nervous system, in the hypertensive states after eliminating the sympathetic neural innervation furnishes a basic information concerning the mechanism of blood pressure elevation.

(1) If CV reactivity were increased, the increased sensitivity of CV system to NE would explain hypertension.

(2) If CV reactivity were not increased, high blood pressure must be explained by increased activity in the sympathetic nervous system.

A schematic explanation is given in Fig. 1. In the first situation CV reactivity is in-

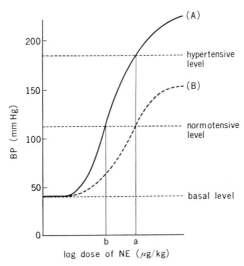

Fig. 1 Schematic explanation of the relationship between CV reactivity and amount of NE available at the receptor sites of the CV system in the hypertensive and normotensive states. See text for details.
(i) H=(A), N=(B), H(NE)=N(NE)=a; (ii) H=N=(A), H(NE)=a, N(NE)=b

---

* Department of Pharmacology, Toho University School of Medicine, Tokyo, Japan

creased in the hypertensive (H) state. Dose-response (DR) curve of NE in H state follows course (A), and that in normotensive (N) state follows (B). Dose of NE which elicits a response equal to H and N levels (mm Hg) is the same, and corresponds to dose a (μg/kg). In the second situation CV reactivity is not increased in H states. DR curse in H and N states follows the same course (A). Dose of NE which elicits a response equal to H level is a, and that to N is b. Dose a is larger than b.

In the above consideration, no humoral factor responsible for blood pressure regulation was assumed. This is particularly based on the fact that elimination of the central nervous system (CNS) lowers blood pressure to an equal basal level in normotensive and hypertensive animals [13]. This would not be absolutely true in our data, and the differences became greater after cocainization [7]. However, the differences may not be of sufficient magnitude to explain the blood pressure elevation in hypertension. And we would like to proceed on this assumption that a humoral factor primarily responsible for blood pressure elevation would not exist.

In order to obtain reliable results on CV reactivity based on the above consideration and assumption, it is necessary: (i) to eliminate the CNS completely to remove the sympathetic neural innervation from the CV system, (ii) to start at the same basal blood pressure level in H and N states, (iii) to obtain the full DR curve of NE, and (iv) without anesthesia, which might modify the condition of the CV system.

We have devised a preparation of the rat which meets these requirements by pithing, decerebration, and vagotomy [13]. Under ether anesthesia the trachea and the femoral artery and vein were cannulated. The rat was pithed by inserting a steel rod through the orbital fossa to the end of the spinal canal. The tracheal cannula was connected to a positive-pressure respirator. Cerebral tissue was further destroyed by cotton balls pressed into the cranial cavity through an opening in the cranium. The vagosympathetic trunks were cut bilaterally. The DR curve to NE was determined 20 min. after removal of ether.

Two series of experiments were carried out [7, 13]. In series 1 male rats were used throughout. SHR were F12-17 and 17 to 23 weeks of age. The DR curves of NE (9 doses, ca. 0.01–100 μg as l-NE base/kg, i.v.) in SHR were compared with those of normotensive Wistar rats, from which the SHR had been derived. Mean blood pressure determined by the direct femoral artery cannulation ranged 140–185 and 125–140 mm Hg in SHR and Wistar rats, respectively. DR curves to NE of SHR showed the same course as those of Wistar rats, although they reached higher levels at the largest 2 doses in hypertensive rats than in the controls. High blood pressure levels of SHR correspond to 2–4 μg NE on the DR curves. Normal blood pressure levels of Wistar rats correspond to 0.4–2 μg NE.

Essentially the same results were obtained in hypertensive rats induced by clipping the left renal artery and removing the right kidney. Rats of Donryu strain, 8 to 9 weeks of age, were used and studied 4 to 8 weeks after clipping. Normal rats of Donryu strain were used as controls. Essentially the same results were also obtained in deoxycorticosterone (DOC) hypertension. The Donryu rats, 8 to 9 weeks of age, were unilaterally nephrectomized and given 1% saline instead of drinking water. They were studied after DOC treatment for 4 to 6 weeks. Mean blood pressure ranged 160–230, 170–200 and 110–130 mm Hg in hypertensive rats made by clipping, DOC hypertensive and normal Donryu rats, respectively.

Thus CV reactivity to NE was essentially unchanged in SHR, and also other two types of renal and adrenal hypertension. The results indicate that the observed high blood pressure is not due to increased sensitivity to NE in the hypertensive rats.

A possibility remains that uptake of NE by the sympathetic nerve endings might participate in the observed CV reactivity, since exogenous NE acts on both the receptor sites and the so-called transfer sites in the nerve terminals. Hence overall reactivity to NE is determined by both sensitivity of the receptors and degree of the uptake. Therefore, CV reactivity was reexamined in series 2 after pretreatment with cocaine (5 mg/kg, i.v.) which blocks the uptake process, or using methoxamine, a directly acting sympathomimetic amine, predominantly α-type, and not taken up by adrenergic nerve endings.

Female rats were used in series 2. SHR were F21 and 17 to 20 weeks of age. Systolic blood pressure ranged 160–200 and 110–140 mm Hg in SHR and normal Wistar rats, respectively. The DR curve of NE (9 doses, 0.0123–123 μg as l-NE base/ kg, i.v.) in SHR followed the same course of the Wistar rats, except in higher doses confirming the results in series 1, and served as a control for further study. The DR curve of NE after cocainization shifted to left in both SHR and normal Wister rats. Sensitivity to NE was equally increased with cocaine in both cases. Relationship between the two DR curves was unchanged after cocainization. It may be said that the uptake mechanism of NE is the same between SHR and controls, and that the receptor sites are not modified in SHR, although the uptake block has not been considered the sole mechanism for potentiation of the action of NE with cocaine. The DR curves to methoxamine (8 doses, 5–640 μg as salt/ kg, i.v.) were obtained in SHR and normal Wistar rats. They followed essentially the same course except at higher doses. It is concluded that neither uptake nor receptor is responsible for the high blood pressure of the SHR.

Essentially the same results were obtained in rats rendered hypertensive by clipping or DOC. Rats of Donryu strain, 10 to 12 weeks of age, were subjected to the treatments, and used for the study 6 to 10 weeks after the treatments. Systolic blood pressure ranged 150–230, 170–210 and 100–130 mm Hg in hypertensive rats made by clipping, DOC hypertensive and normal Donryu rats, respectively. DR curves to NE confirmed the results of series 1. The DR curves of NE after cocainization in hypertension by clipping and with DOC followed approximately the same course as those of normal Donryu rats. Neither uptake nor receptor mechanism of the sympathetic nerve endings is responsible for these types of experimental hypertension. CV reactivities to methoxamine in clipping and DOC hypertension were essentially the same, and not large enough to explain the blood pressure differences between hypertensive and normotensive rats. The results indicate again that neither uptake mechanism nor sensitivity of the receptor sites is responsible for the elevated blood pressure in these types of hypertension.

Table 1 shows the doses of NE and methoxamine which correspond to the original blood pressure levels before the CNS destruction on the DR curves in series 2. It is clearly shown that larger doses of NE or methoxamine are necessary to reach the high blood pressure levels in the hypertensive rats.

Previous works on CV reactivity to NE in SHR have shown some inconsistency. The work has been initiated by OKAMOTO's group in 1966 in a whole animal preparation anesthetized with α-chloralose [9]. In the isolated aortic strip, reactivity to NE seemed not to be increased [1, 6, 14]. In the peripheral vascular beds, hindquarter and mesentery, the reactivity was increased [4, 5], but it was not large enough to explain the high blood pressure in SHR [8]. In the entire CV system the results were not consistent [7, 9, 12, 13]. The CV reactivity in other types of hypertension determined in preparations similar to ours, utilizing the pithing procedure, has also been reported [3, 12]. The details were different, and the results did not accord with each other.

Our results indicated that CV reactivity to NE in SHR was unchanged. It was also unchanged in hypertension induced by clipping or with DOC in the rat. Sensitivity of the receptor sites and uptake of the nerve endings remained unchanged. The results do not always accord with the previous works on CV reactivity, probably because of the

Table 1 Analyses of dose-response curves in series 2.

	Dose of NE which Corresponds to Original BP Level (μg/kg)
Wistar	1.6– 2.7*
SHR	7.4–11.0
Donryu	1.6– 2.4
Clipping	9.2–21.0
DOC	17.0–34.0
(Cocaine Pretreatment)	
Wistar	0.72–0.96
SHR	1.9 –2.9
Donryu	0.27–0.36
Clipping	0.9 –2.9
DOC	2.9 –4.8

	Dose of Methox which Corresponds to Original BP Level (μg/kg)
Wistar	124–144
SHR	180–210
Donryu	72– 92
Clipping	140–250
DOC	180–280

* confidence limit L ($\alpha = 0.05$)

differences in methodology: type of the assay preparation, age of the animals, severity of the hypertensive states, selection of the control, etc. The concept that elevated blood pressure may be due to supersensitivity to a pressor factor is not compatible with the fact that an increased activity in the sympathetic nervous system is observed in hypertensive state [2, 15]. Although our results are consistent with the view that hypertension may be due to increased activity of the sympathetic nervous system, further studies are necessary to clarify the problems on CV reactivity in hypertension.

REFERENCES

1. CLINESCHMIDT, B. V., GELLER, R. G., GOVIER, W. C. and SJOERDSMA, A. (1970): Eur J Pharmacol, **10**, 45.
2. DeCHAMPLAIN, J., KRAKOFF, L. and AXELROD, J. (1969): Circ Res, **24–25**, I–75.
3. FINCH, L. (1971): Br J Pharmacol, **42**, 56.
4. FOLKOW, B., HALLBÄCK, M., LUNDGREN, Y. and WEISS, L. (1970): Acta Physiol Scand, **80**, 93.
5. HAEUSLER, G. and HAEFELY, W. (1970): Naunyn-Schmiedebergs Arch Pharmackol Exp Pathol, **266**, 18.
6. HALLBÄCK, M., LUNDGREN, Y. and WEISS, L. (1971): Acta Physiol Scand, **81**, 176.
7. MIZOGAMI, S., SUZUKI, M. and SOKABE, H. (1972): Jap J Const Med, in Press.
8. NOSAKA, S., YAMORI, Y., OHTA, T. and OKAMOTO, K. (1972): In "Spontaneous Hypertension" (K. OKAMOTO, ed.), p. 67, Igaku Shoin Ltd., Tokyo.
9. OKAMOTO, K., HAZAMA, F., TAKEDA, T., TABEI, R., NOSAKA, S., FUKUSHIMA, M., YAMORI, Y., MATSUMOTO, M., HAEBARA, H., ICHIJIMA, K. and SUZUKI, Y. (1966): Jap Circ J, **30**, 987.
10. PAGE, I. H. and BUMPUS, F. M. (1961): Physiol Rev, **41**, 331.
11. PAGE, I. H., KANEKO, Y. and McCUBBIN, J. W. (1966): Circ Res, **18**, 171.
12. SCHOLTYSIK, G. and UNDA, R. (1971): Arzneimittel-Forsch, **21**, 891.
13. SHIBAYAMA, F. MIZOGAMI, S. and SOKABE, H. (1971): Jap Heart J, **12**, 68.
14. SPECTOR, S., FLEISCH, J. H., MALING, H. M. and BRODIE, B. B. (1969): Science, **166**, 1300.
15. YAMORI, Y., LOVENBERG, W. and SJOERDSMA, A. (1971): Jap J Const Med, **34**, 36.

VASCULAR RESISTANCE AND REACTIVITY TO VARIOUS VASOCONSTRICTOR AGENTS IN HYPERTENSIVE RATS

G. HAEUSLER* and L. FINCH*

INTRODUCTION

From a great number of experimental observations (for references see DOYLE's [4], LAVERTY et al.'s [13], and SOMLYO and SOMLYO's [15] papers) the conclusion may be drawn that increased reactivity to various vasoconstrictor stimuli is a common feature of arterial blood vessels in hypertensive patients and animals. However, there are some reports, though much less numerous, which indicate a normal or even a decreased vascular reactivity in hypertension.

As far as the positive reports on an increased vascular reactivity in hypertension are concerned, two major possibilities exist, which may explain the increase in responsiveness. Some observations are compatible with the view that the individual vascular smooth muscle cells become supersensitive to vasoconstrictor stimuli [1, 2, 3, 9, 12, 13].

A different explanation was put forward by FOLKOW and his collaborators [6, 7]. They claim that hypertension leads to an adaptive structural change of the vessel wall resulting in an increase of the wall/lumen ratio. According to FOLKOW et al. [8], an increase of the wall/lumen ratio strikingly alters the shape of the dose-response curve for a vasoconstrictor agent. Compared with normal arteries, the slope of the dose-response curve becomes steeper and a higher maximum is attained. However, the vasoconstrictor threshold dose does not change. This concept implies that increased vascular reactivity cannot initiate hypertension but is rather the result of it.

In the course of our studies on several types of hypertensive rats we often found an increased vascular reactivity. In the current paper an attempt is made to analyse these observations in respect to the two aforementioned theories on vascular hyper-reactivity.

METHODS

The majority of the experiments was carried out in rats of either sex from a closed randomized colony (Wistar descent) which in the following are referred to as "normotensive rats". At the age of 6 weeks these rats were used for the induction of DOCA/NaCl and renal hypertension performed according to conventional methods [5]. Six to eight weeks later hypertension was usually fully developed. If not otherwise stated, these 12 to 14-week-old DOCA/NaCl and renal hypertensive rats were used for the experiments and compared with age-matched normotensive controls and with spontaneously hypertensive rats. The latter originated as a hypertensive mutant of a Wistar strain in Japan [14] brother-sister mating being continued in our breeding unit.

Vascular resistance was measured in a whole animal preparation [7], in isolated perfused hindquarters, in isolated perfused mesenteric [11] and renal arteries. In the latter three preparations full dose-response curves for the vasoconstrictor effect of NE and 5-HT were obtained; the contractile response to Ca^{++} was measured in depolarized mesenteric arteries. Oxygenated Tyrode solution (37 °C, containing as a plasma substitute 3–4% w/v FICOLL®) was used for the perfusion of the whole rat preparation and

---

* Department of Experimental Medicine of F. Hoffmann-La Roche & Co., Ltd., Basle, Switzerland.

of the isolated hindquarters and oxygenated Krebs-Henseleit solution (37°C) for that of the isolated mesenteric and renal artery preparations. For Ca^{++} dose-response curves the isolated mesenteric arteries were perfused with a depolarizing solution of the following composition (mM): KCl 10, K_2SO_4 76, $KHCO_3$ 16, $MgCl_2$ 1.2, KH_2PO_4 1.2, glucose 5.6. Each dose of the agonists (NE, 5-HT, $CaCl_2$) was contained in a volume of 0.1 ml and was injected within 7 sec in order to avoid an injection artifact in the pressure recordings. The injections were given 1–2 cm apart from the blood vessels.

RESULTS AND DISCUSSION

Vascular resistance

The existence of structural changes of the arterial wall in hypertensive animals can be derived from the finding that during complete vascular relaxation the vascular resistance is elevated. Therefore, pressure-flow diagrams were obtained in normotensive and three types of hypertensive rats using a whole-animal preparation. From a cannula introduced into the ascending aorta the animal was perfused with increasing volumes of Tyrode solution containing a plasma substitute and the resistance to flow was measured. In this way the total vascular resistance was determined with the exception of those of the pulmonary and coronary vascular beds. Several technical variations were tried in order to obtain maximal vasodilatation. Perfusion was carried out in pithed rats and in rats anesthetized with pentobartitone. In the latter group an additional pretreatment with either 10 mg/kg reserpine or guanethidine was given or calcium-free Tyrode solution was used for perfusion instead of the normal one. The most satisfactory results were obtained in rats anesthetized with pentobarbitone (50 mg/kg i.p.) and given 10 mg/kg guanethidine i.v. In these animal preparations the addition to the perfusion solution of papaverine, sodium nitrite, sodium nitroprusside, isoproterenol or acetylcholine did not yield a further decrease in perfusion pressure. Therefore, the vessels were considered to be in a state of maximal dilatation and this method was used for all further experiments.

While DOCA/NaCl and renal hypertensive rats showed a significantly increased vascular resistance when compared with normotensive rats, no difference could be detected between normotensive controls and spontaneously hypertensive rats (Fig. 1). Very similar results were obtained when vascular resistance was measured in isolated perfused hindquarters under the conditions of maximal vasodilatation. The pressure-flow diagram indicated a marked increase of vascular resistance in DOCA/NaCl hypertensive and a less pronounced but statistically significant increase in renal hypertensive rats. As in the whole-animal preparation, the pressure flow curves of normotensive and spontaneously hypertensive rats were virtually identical. The latter finding does not agree with results obtained by FOLKOW et al. [7, 8]. They reported an elevated vascular resistance in spontaneously hypertensive rats measured both in the whole animal preparation and in isolated perfused hindquarters. Since FOLKOW et al. [7] used spontaneously hypertensive rats at an age of 7 months or more, we repeated the perfusion experiments in the isolated hindquarters with 7-month-old spontaneously hypertensive rats. In these older animals a statistically significant increase in vascular resistance was found.

Complete pressure-flow diagrams were not constructed in isolated perfused mesenteric and renal arteries. Both preparations were perfused *in vitro* at a constant rate of 6 ml/min resulting in a mean basal pressure of 32–34 mm Hg and 40–42 mm Hg, respectively. This basal perfusion pressure could not be lowered by vasodilatating agents indicating that under these conditions the preparations were maximally dilated. The mean basal

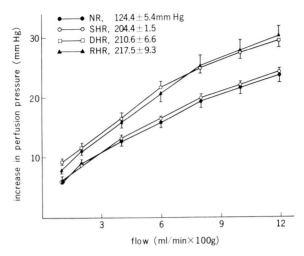

Fig. 1 Vascular resistance (with the exception of those of the pulmonary and coronary vascular beds) of a whole-rat preparation under the condition of maximal vasodilatation. From a cannula introduced into the ascending aorta the rats were perfused with increasing volumes of Tyrode solution containing a plasma substitute and the resistance to flow was recorded. Normotensive rats (NR), spontaneously hypertensive rats (SHR), DOCA/NaCl hypertensive rats (DHR) and renal hypertensive rats (RHR). The mean values (±S.E. as vertical bars) of 8 experiments in each group are shown. The blood pressure values ±S.E. given for each group at the top of the figure were obtained with a tail-cuff method in conscious animals one day before the experiemnt.

perfusion pressure of the mesenteric arteries did not differ significantly in normotensive and the three types of hypertensive rats; nor was there any difference when isolated perfused renal arteries of normotensive and spontaneously hypertensive rats were compared.   Resistance of the renal arteries of DOCA/NaCl hypertensive rats was significantly lower, which probably reflects the compensatory dilatation after unilateral nephrectomy. These results show that an increased vascular resistance could be demonstreated (1) only in DOCA/NaCl and renal hypertensive rats and (2) only when preparations were used which contained all segments of an arterial vascular bed.   This is true for 12 to 14-week-old rats.   In spontaneously hypertensive rats an increased resistance was found at an age of 7 months.   In the isolated perfused renal and mesenteric arteries, which represent preparations consisting exclusively or mainly of conductance vessels, a resistance increase could not be detected.

Vascular reactivity

Using the same type of hypertensive animals and the same organ preparations as for the measurement of vascular resistance, the reactivity of the arterial blood vessels to NE, 5-HT and Ca^{++} was determined.

Dose-response curves for the vasoconstrictor effect of NE in isolated perfused hindquarter preparations were steeper and attained a higher maximum in the hypertensive animals.   In DOCA/NaCl and renal hypertensive rats threshold responses could be elicited with lower doses of NE.   Adopting a definition of FOLKOW et al. [8], a threshold response was considered to be a 25% rise in resistance from the state of maximal vasodilatation.   Normotensive controls and spontaneously hypertensive rats showed an equal vasoconstriction to NE in the threshold range.   With increasing doses of NE, however, the dose-response curve of the spontaneously hypertensive rats diverged from that of the normotensive controls. Using 5-HT as an agonist, the same differences of the shape of the dose-response curves between normotensive controls and DOCA/NaCl and renal hypertensive rats were observed as described for NE. In contrast to the results obtained with NE the dose-response curves for 5-HT were equal for normotensive and spontaneously hypertensive rats.

The pressure-flow diagrams indicated that the vascular resistance in isolated perfused hindquarters of renal and DOCA/NaCl hypertensive rats is increased. In these animals the dose-response curves for both NE and 5-HT were similarly steeper and attained similarly increased maxima Therefore, the dose-response curves have the characteristics which could be predicted from an increase of the wall/lumen ratio of the vessels. However, there was, in addition, a lowering of the vasoconstrictor threshold dose for both agonists suggesting an increased sensitivity of the individual smooth muscle cells. Furthermore, it is worthy of note that the correlation between increase in vascular resistance and reactivity is rather poor for these two types of hypertensive rats. While both renal and DOCA/NaCl hypertensive rats showed a similarly increased reactivity to the vasoconstrictor agents, vascular resistance was markedly higher in DOCA/NaCl than in renal hypertensive rats.

The vascular resistances of hindquarter preparations from normotensive and spontaneously hypertensive rats did not differ from each other. In spite of this, the reactivity to NE in the spontaneously hypertensive rats was increased. This could be explained with the theoretically possible case that in the spontaneously hypertensive rats the wall/lumen ratio was increased without any narrowing of the lumen. What remains to be explained is why the reactivity to one agonist (NE) was increased, while to the other (5-HT) is was not.

Furthermore, some of the results obtained in the isolated mesenteric artery preparation cannot be adequately explained merely on the basis of an increased wall/lumen ratio. Though it is unlikely that in this preparation the vascular resistance is altered in hypertensive animals, the reactivity to NE was increased and the maxima of the dose-response curves were similarly elevated in both spontaneously and DOCA/CaCl hypertensive rats. The corresponding experiments in renal hypertensive rats are lacking. Thus, the shape of the NE dose-response curves could be explained by the assumption that an increased muscle mass acts on an unchanged vascular lumen.

However, different results were obtained when 5-HT was used as an agonist (Fig. 2). The most prominent finding was a clear-cut lowering of the vasoconstrictor threshold dose of 5-HT for all three types of hypertensive rats. Furthermore, depending on the type of hypertension the 5-HT dose-response curves were much steeper and their maxima were considerably elevated as compared with normotensive rats [10]. Apart from the lowering of the 5-HT vasoconstrictor threshold dose, another observation seems to question the validity of the concept that merely a change of the wall/lumen ratio is responsible for the increased vascular reactivity. From a change of the wall/lumen ratio it could be predicted that for any given vasoconstrictor agent the increase in the maximum response should be the same. This is not borne out in the current results. For instance, in DOCA/NaCl hypertensive rats the increase in the maximum response to NE and 5-HT differed markedly, it was 30 and 420%, respectively.

The vasoconstrictor response to NE and 5-HT of renal arteries isolated from spontaneously and DOCA/NaCl hypertensive rats was virtually the same as in normotensive controls.

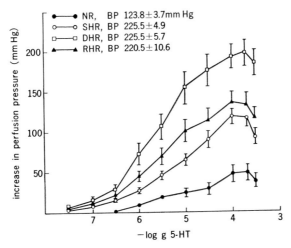

Fig. 2 Dose-response curves for the vasoconstrictor effect of 5-HT in isolated perfused mesenteric artery preparations of NR (n=15), SHR (n=10), DHR (n—10) and RHR (n=10). The mean values (±S.E. as vertical bars) are shown.

For further clarification of vascular hyper-reactivity, Ca^{++}-induced vasoconstriction was studied in completely depolarized mesenteric arteries.   In paired experiments equal Ca^{++} does-response curves were obtained for normotensive and all three types of hypertensive rats.   These results are surprising since it was expected that alterations of the dose-response curves for vasoconstrictor agents, which are related to an increase of the wall/lumen ratio, should remain apparent also in this type of experiment.   On the other hand, changes in vascular reactivity due to an alteration of excitation-contraction coupling should have disappeard.   Although these findings tend to invalidate the concept of an increased wall/lumen ratio being responsible for the vascular hyper-reactivity, it seems too early at the moment to overemphasize these results.   Differences between normotensive and hypertensive arteries with regard to the extend of unspecific Ca^{++} binding and to the velocity of Ca^{++} penetration could well have masked the expected differences of the shape of the Ca^{++} dose-response curves.   Furthermore, damage to the arteries due to the complete dopolarization could have influenced the results.

CONCLUSION

Six to eight weeks after the induction of DOCA/NaCl and renal hypertension, vascular resistance measured under the condition of maximal vasodilatation was higher in whole-animal preparations and in isolated perfused hindquarters of 12 to 14-week-old hypertensive rats than in the age-matched normotensive controls.   At the same age spontaneously hypertensive rats showed a normal vascular resistance, but it was elevated in 7-month-old animals.   An increased vascular reactivity to norepinephrine and 5-hydroxytryptamine was observed in isolated perfused hindquarter and mesenteric artery preparations of all three types of hypertensive rats.   For DOCA/NaCl and renal hypertensive rats this hyper-reactivity cannot be adequately explained merely on the basis of an increased wall/lumen ratio of the hypertensive vessel wall since under some, though not all experimental conditions, the vasoconstrictor threshold doses of norepinephrine and 5-hydroxytryptamine were lower in the hypertensive arteries.   Further objections are given by the different maximum response to norepinephrine and 5-hydroxytryptamine in the mesenteric arteries of the hypertensive rats and by the equality of Ca^{++} dose-response curves obtained in depolarized mesenteric arteries of normotensive and hypertensive rats. Therefore, in addition to a change of the wall/lumen ratio, an increase in the sensitivity of the individual vascular smooth muscle cells seems to occur in DOCA/NaCl and renal hypertensive rats. Indications for such a supersensitivity were less numerous in spontaneously hypertensive rats, suggesting that differences between several types of hypertension may exist at the level of the vascular smooth muscle cells.

REFERENCES

1. BANDICK, N. R. and SPARKS, H. V. (1970): Am J Physiol, 219, 340.
2. BOHR, D. F. and SITRIN, M. (1970): Circ Res, 26 and 27, Suppl II, 83.
3. DAHL, L. K., HEINE, M. and TASSINARI, L. (1964): Criculation, 29 and 30, Suppl II, 11.
4. DOYLE, A. E. (1968): N Z Med J, 67, 295.
5. FINCH, L. and LEACH, G. D. H. (1970): Br J Pharmacol, 39, 317.
6. FOLKOW, B. (1971): Clin Sci, 41, 1.
7. FOLKOW, B., HALLBÄCK, M., LUNNGREN, Y. and WEISS, L. (1970): Acta physiol scand, 79, 373.
8. FOLKOW, B., HALLBÄCK, M., LUNDGREN, Y. and WEISS, L. (1970): Acta physiol scand, 80, 93.
9. GORDON, D. B. and NOGUEIRA, A. (1962): Circ Res, 10, 269.
10. HAEUSLER, G. and FINCH, L. (1971): Experientia, 27, 15.
11. HAEUSLER, G. and HAEFELY, W. (1970): Naunyn-Schmiedeberg's Arch Pharmakol, 266, 18.
12. HINKE, J. A. M. (1965): Circ Res, 17, 359.
13. LAVERTY, R., McGREGOR, D. D. and McQUEEN, E. G. (1968): N Z Med J, 67, 303.
14. OKAMOTO, K. and AOKI, K. (1963): Jap Circ J, 27, 282.
15. SOMLYO, A. P. and SOMLYO, A. V. (1970): Pharmacol Rev, 22, 249.

THE IMPORTANCE OF ADAPTIVE CHANGES IN VASCULAR DESIGN FOR THE ESTABLISHMENT AND MAINTENANCE OF PRIMARY HYPERTENSION, AS STUDIED IN MAN AND IN SPONTANEOUSLY HYPERTENSIVE RAT

B. FOLKOW*, M. HALLBÄCK*, Y. LUNDGREN*,
R. SIVERTSSON* and L. WEISS*

Few research fields exhibit as much controversy as that of primary hypertension, but there is *one* key point where most authorities seem to agree: In the well-established phase of this important "disorder of regulation" systemic flow resistance is raised largely in proportion to the pressure rise [27, 28]. Furthermore, this resistance increase is widely assumed to reflect a raised level of vascular smooth muscle activity. The vivid controversy mainly concerns the *background* of this assumed increase of smooth muscle activity; *i.e.* whether it is a consequence of nervous, hormonal or myogenic factors, or/and due to an increased sensitivity of the vascular effectors, enhancing their responses to extrinsic excitatory influences.

However, this widely accepted assumption—that the key solution to the raised resistance in well-established primary hypertension should be an increased smooth muscle activity—can, indeed, be seriously challenged. Not only does this concept lack reliable experimental support; if anything, the available experimental evidence rather seems to speak *against* this concept (see *e.g.* Table VII of Sivertsson's article [28]). This no doubt important problem, touching the very background of chronic hypertension, will below be illuminated, first from a theoretical point of view and then by experimental studies. These studies (see also [8]) have been performed both on man with primary ("essential") hypertension and on the spontaneously hypertensive rat (SHR [25, 26]) which, together with the New Zealand strain of hypertensive rat [24], seems to offer the best animal model so far of primary hypertension in man. We all owe much to Professor OKAMOTO and to Professor SMIRK and their coworkers for providing hypertension research with these important biological tools.

Let us start with a simple statement that is selfevident to anyone who, for example, intends to compare the activity of two muscle strips, allowed to contract isotonically in an organ bath. The prevailing activity levels of these strips can be appreciated by means of their length, only if one estimates the respective *ratios* between their resting and active lengths. The active length alone is obviously meaningless, because it is a function of the resting length which, again, is structurally determined and may well differ in the two strips.

The same simple relationship must obviously be true also when muscles encircle cylindrical tubes, such as blood vessels. Concerning the resistance vessels, the key point in established primary hypertension, resistance to flow (R) is here commonly used as an index of the average internal radius (r_i) of the resistance vessels, assuming the other factors in the Poiseuille relationship—tube length and blood viscosity—to be relatively constant. It then follows that r_i, in the given case and situation, is also a useful expression for the average length of the vascular smooth muscles (l) that encircle the lumen.

Also from a practical point of view this relationship between R and l is a most useful

---

* Department of Physiology, University of Göteborg, Göteborg, Sweden.

one in haemodynamic studies, both because R is easily calculated as the ratio between the pressure drop (P_A–P_V) and flow (Q), and because any change in l, and consequently in ri, becomes greatly amplified when expressed as R, R being inversely proportional roughly to the *fourth* power of ri. In such a system the resistance at *complete* vascular smooth muscle relaxation *($Rmin$)* would be an expression of the resting length of the encircling muscle elements. $Rmin$ must, however, then be measured at a well defined trans-mural pressure, simply because relaxed vascular walls are fairly distensible, at least at lower transmural pressures [18]. Under standardized conditions $Rmin$ would thus con-stitute the structurally defined "resting" baseline, from which current levels of vascular smooth muscle activity can be judged as the *ratio* between the prevailing R level and $Rmin$.

However, such a correlation is only valid for a given vascular bed in acute experiments where the structural design, and hence $Rmin$, can be safely assumed to remain constant. In *all* other cases—even in one and the same circuit of a given individual when restudied after some time—it is necessary to carefully measure $Rmin$ each time. The reason is that $Rmin$ may well differ considerably as a result of *e.g.* a structural adaptation of the resistance vessels. It is, of course, still more important to measure, for each individual, both $Rmin$ and the current level of R if one intends to compare normotensive and hypertensive sub-jects concerning the respective levels of smooth muscle activity in the resistance vessels. Also here the current level of R cannot be alone relevant; it is obviously only the respec-tive *ratios* between this level and $Rmin$ that can reveal anything about the extent of smooth muscle shortening. Actually, as will be further outlined below, the entire dynamics of resistance vessels are bound to become remarkably changed whenever their structurally determined wall/lumen ratio becomes changed.

It is, in a way, remarkable that such fairly selfevident relationships have hardly at all been applied to vascular dynamics until our group some 20 years ago utilized them for evaluations of "vascular tone" (*i.e.* the average activity level of the vascular smooth muscles) in different systemic circuits [8] and, a few years later, for similar comparisons in identical vascular beds from normotensive and hypertensive subjects [6, 9, 28]. Up to this day, however, most investigators of the haemodynamics in hypertension seem to have taken it more or less for granted that the "resting" level of flow resistance should directly reflect the level of vascular smooth muscle activity, whether subjects are normotensive or hypertensive. One has even used the arterial pressure levels for such purposes, despite the fact that pressure is a function also of another key variable, the cardiac output.

The essence of this problem is schematically illustrated in Fig. 1 [see also 8, 9, 28]. For *normal* resistance vessels the relationship between the degree of active smooth muscle shortening—considered to be initiated from their outer muscle sheath where no doubt the vasoconstrictor fibres exert their primary impact—and the extent of resistance incre-ase is given by the "resistance curve" N. For such normal resistance vessels a change from their "resting" equilibrium of smooth muscle tone at point A to maximal vasodilata-tion means a shift along curve N to its intersection with the ordinate, at which point the vascular smooth muscles are completely relaxed. Likewise, an intensification of smooth muscle activity, beyond the "resting" equilibrium at point A, is given by a shift along curve N up to *e.g.* point B. This latter shift, from A to B along curve N, illustrates in principle the generally assumed viewpoint concerning the background of the increased resistance in hypertension: R is thought to be raised primarily as a result of an enhanced activity level of the vascular smooth muscles.

However, in a situation of chronic hypertension it cannot be assumed *a priori* that the "normal" curve N should still be relevant for the haemodynamic situation, since the resistance vessels are likely to have changed their design. It should here be remembered that pathologists for nearly a hundred years have described how hypertensive vessels, just like the left ventricle of the heart, appear to display thickened walls, which presumably starts as a simple media hypertrophy. Because of technical difficulties, this latter type of adaptive structural change could, however, not be precisely measured in the resistance vessels, until quite recently (see below). Probably in part for such reasons, its possible haemodynamic consequences have been almost entirely neglected until it became of interest to us in a series of haemodynamic studies that started in the early fifties.

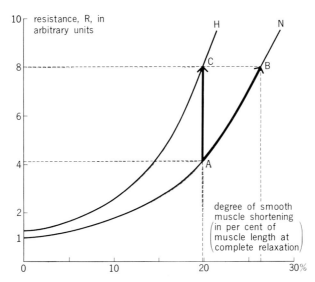

Fig. 1 Diagram illustrating the relationship between degree of vascular smooth muscle shortening and resistance in a "normal" resistance vessel (N) and in a "hypertensive" resistance vessel (H), where an increase in wall/lumen ratio has taken place, of such a nature that the thickened wall encroaches on the lumen even at maximal vasodilatation. Modified from SIVERTSSON's article[28], with kind permission.

Fig. 1 illustrates, by the resistance curve H, the haemodynamic consequences of a media hypertrophy which is so organized that it partly encroaches upon the lumen even at maximal dilatation [8, 9, 28]. Thus, compared with the "normotensive" resistance curve N the structurally enhanced wall/lumen ratio implies in this very case not only a raised resistance that is present even at maximal vasodilatation. Because of the enlarged wall mass in relation to the lumen, it also implies a throughout steeper resistance curve; *i.e.* an enhanced *vascular* reactivity which does not necessitate any enhanced *smooth muscle* reactivity or sensitivity. A raised resistance can now be maintained at an essentially *normal* level of smooth muscle activity (compare point *A* on curve *N* with point *C* on curve *H*), thanks to the changed structural design of the hypertensive resistance vessels. It is also clear from curve *H* that this changed design still allows for a perfectly normal, perhaps even increased range of vasodilatation-vasoconstriction. The important thing is, however, that the resistance vessels in this example *are structurally "reset" to operate around a raised resistance equilibrium* that does *not* necessitate any raised activity level of the contractile elements.

It should in this context be stressed that, in case a media hypertrophy should be so organized as to leave the lumen unchanged, or even decreased, at maximal dilatation—which is, of course, theoretically entirely possible [9]—R_{min} would remain normal, or even reduced. However, also in such a case of vascular wall hypertrophy (which seems to apply for the SHR *renal* vessels; see below) the resistance curve would be throughout steeper than curve N because of the larger bulk of media tissue, implying a proportionally higher resistance level for any given level of smooth muscle activity. In other words, also here a vascular hyperreactivity would be present without necessitating any smooth muscle hyperreactivity.

So much about theoretical considerations; let us now see what experimental studies may reveal. Our first studies were performed in man, utilizing the forearm [6, 9] and hand [28] vascular beds in comparisons between normotensive "control" subjects and patients with essential hypertension. In essence, the resistance vessels of the hypertensive subjects proved to differ from those of the normotensive controls just as curve H differs from curve N in Fig. 1. In other words, resistance was indeed considerably raised even at maximal vasodilatation in the hypertensive subjects, while their "resting" level of vascular smooth muscle activity was *largely normal*, as judged by the ratio between "resting" R and R_{min}. Further, their resistance vessels displayed a pronounced hyperreactivity, while their vascular smooth muscle reactivity, as judged in terms of threshold sensitivity to noradrenaline, appeared to be largely normal [28].

All these findings strongly suggest the presence of a structural change of the regional resistance vessels, so organized that a hypertrophied wall partly encroaches upon the lumen. Further, in case these regional changes in vascular design were more or less generalized throughout the systemic circulation, they were marked enough to largely *alone* explain the raised blood pressure level, without necessitating any enhanced vascular smooth muscle activity, at least not during "rest". This does, of course, by no means exclude that during daily life conditions vascular tone may be considerably enhanced in hypertensive subjects, at least intermittently, and as a result of *e.g.* neuro-hormonal excitatory influences.

The mentioned results have been strongly supported by studies performed by CONWAY and his coworkers [4, 5]. Moreover, in recent, most important studies by Japanese investigators the extent of media hypertrophy of the resistance vessels in hypertension has been measured quantitatively by an ingenious technique [20, 29]. In principle, just like the well-known hypertrophy of the left ventricle of the heart, the systemic arteries and most sections of the precapillary resistance vessels were found to display a media hypertrophy that seems to be closely proportional to the average pressure level. Only the smallest resistance sections, placed just proximally to the capillaries, appear to exhibit little or no hypertrophy, probably a result of such a large pressure drop along proximally placed resistance sections that the more distal ones are not exposed to any raised pressure. Thus, the mentioned haemodynamic and morphologic studies go closely hand in hand, but the haemodynamic studies have, in addition, revealed that even during maximal vasodilatation the regional flow resistance is increased in hypertensive man, and almost in proportion to the raised pressure level.

The question then arose: What initiates the structural changes that had been traced in hypertensive subjects and which appeared to be pronounced enough as to largely alone explain the raised blood pressure during rest? It is well known that primary hypertension exhibits a strong hereditary element and, to judge from *e.g.* population studies, there seem to be several genetically linked factors that predispose for this type of hypertension [27]. The initiation of the observed structural vascular changes in all likelihood calls for some functional "trigger" factor, in terms of *e.g.* a pressure load that may well be intermittent if it only raises the *average* pressure for a long enough period. It is, however, unlikely that such a pressure load would be of *renal* origin in primary hypertension, though a secondary renal involvement in later stages may be common. Our interest was instead directed to the central nervous system, where the hypothalamic defence area integrates a most characteristic cardiovascular response, normally elicited by a variety of psychogenic stimuli in daily life. This response, found in virtually all animals, including man [3, 7, 18, 19, 22], implies centrally induced increases of both arterial pressure and cardiac output, which preferentially favours the skeletal muscles at the expense of the gastrointestinal tract, the kidneys, the skin, etc.

Against such a general background it was proposed [7] that primary hypertension in man might be due to a complex interaction between such centrally elicited pressure and output increases and a gradual structural adaptation of heart and precapillary vessels to this functionally elicited pressure load, if this was repeated often enough. The proposed functional "trigger" mechanism, as well as the structurally based "maintenance" factor, would be per se perfectly "normal" as to their basic nature but either, or both, might perhaps be *quantitatively* somewhat exaggerated in a genetically linked way in subjects predisposed to primary hypertension. It is evident that the proposed type of functional trigger mechanism is likely to be greatly influenced also by "stressful" environmental factors, so that genetical and environmental factors would constitute a complexly intertwined relationship that may vary from individual to individual.

So far we had not experimentally explored hypertension in animals; the renal and hormonal types of hypertension, available at that time, appeared to us to be too dissimilar, concerning origin, to primary hypertension in man. We explored, however, what would happen in normotensive rats—thus lacking any genetically linked predisposal to

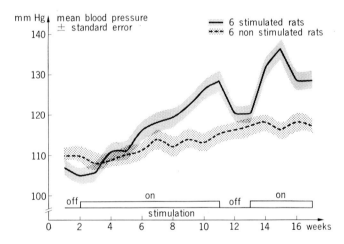

Fig. 2 Diagram illustrating the gradual change of resting mean blood pressure in otherwise normotensive rats, which for a prolonged period were exposed to intermittent weak stimulations of the hypothalamic defence area. The control rats were identically treated with exception of the hypothalamic stimulations. From Folkow and Rubinstein's article [19], with kind permission.

primary hypertension— if the central neuro-hormonal influences on the cardiovascular system were artificially reinforced. This was produced by means of weak but often repeated stimulations of the hypothalamic defence area via chronically implanted electrodes and the stimulations were continued for several months [19]. This type of chronic, intermittent stimulation gradually brought about a moderate degree of fairly sustained hypertension (Fig. 2). Likewise, in most interesting studies Henry and his group [22] have exposed mice, living in closed "mouse societies", to "social stress". These results illustrate very convincingly how such factors, conveying their cardiovascular influence mainly via the hypothalamic defence area, can largely alone precipitate sustained hypertension and also most of its lesional complications. It is likely, however, that the situation would be aggravated in animals with a "latent" predisposition for hypertension.

This was the situation when we about four years ago could start studies on SHR which, according to the excellent studies by Окамото, Аокі and their coworkers [25, 26], appeared to exhibit a multigenetical background of hypertension. It appeared, for example, that the cardiovascular system of these animals was exposed to an increased neuro-hormonal discharge pattern, which in many respects seemed to mimic that known to be induced from the hypothalamic defence area. Incidentally, such a view was strongly supported by quite recent experiments, where we compared awake SHR and NCR with respect to their defence reactions, as provoked under identical control situations by graded "stressful" stimuli in the form of sudden light, sound and vibration [16]. Blood pressure and heart rate were continuously recorded and vibration proved particularly efficient for eliciting a reproducible defence reaction, with its characteristic blood pressure rise and heart rate increase, the latter known to involve both an intensified accelerans fibre discharge and a centrally supressed vagal tone [18].

To all sudden stimuli, SHR tended to respond stronger than NCR, both in pressure and heart rate. With the help of β-adrenergic blocking drugs and atropine the adrenergic and vagal influences on the heart could be selectively explored and it became clear that SHR responded significantly stronger than NCR to these stressful stimuli, also with respect to e.g. the extent of central supression of vagal tone. In general, these findings strongly suggest a true "hyperreactivity" in SHR of those central autonomic structures that mediate emotional behaviour during alertness and mental stress. Such a central mechanism may thus well serve as a potent, though perhaps intermittent "trigger" mechanism for eliciting gradually the structural vascular changes mentioned above.

Further, this promising "model" of primary hypertension in man was likely to offer excellent possibilities to further explore the haemodynamic consequences of the vascular structural adaptation discussed above. It would, for example, be far more easy than in man to find out whether the structural changes were generalized, how rapidly they developed, whether they could be prevented or brought to regression, etc. It might also be possible to explore whether they constituted one of the genetically linked predisposing factors in SHR, in the sense that they might be more easy to establish than in ordinary rats. To this end we started to perfuse the entire systemic circuit (with exception for the coronaries which were excluded for technical reasons) of SHR and matched normotensive control rats (NCR) with plasma substitute after induction of a generalized maximal dilatation [11]. The animals were about 7 months old, which means that SHR were in the "well-established" phase of hypertension. It was found that R_{min} was higher in SHR than in NCR at all perfusion pressures studied and almost in proportion to their higher "resting" blood pressure, just as was the case when hypertensive and normotensive human subjects were compared.

To determine the dose-response curves of vasoconstrictor agents, acting on the resistance vessels of SHR and NCR, we turned for technical reasons to another preparation, using a paired, constant-flow perfusion of the isolated hindquarters from one SHR and one matched NCR, identically prepared and treated and about 7 months old [12]. Theoretically, in case an enhanced smooth muscle sensitivity to constrictor agents was the only difference between SHR and NCR, it would reveal itself as a lowered threshold dosage and as a parallel shift of the SHR dose-response "resistance curve" towards the left. On the other hand, the presence of an enlarged bulk of contractile wall mass in the

SHR resistance vessels would reveal itself as an unchanged threshold but a subsequently steeper resistance curve, as combined with a raised maximal pressor response, the latter being a consequence of the enhanced contractile strength that could be expected by the larger bulk of contractile tissue.

We started from complete vascular relaxation and then gave graded infusions of vaso-constrictor agents (usually noradrenaline but occasionally angiotensin, vasopressin and barium ions in the form of $BaCl_2$) from subthreshold amounts up to overwhelmingly high concentrations. These supramaximal concentrations forced the resistance vessels to exhibit their maximal contractile strength when facing the ultimately very high perfusion pressures created during constant flow perfusion. In this direct comparison between SHR and matched NCR it was found, as in man, that resistance was higher in SHR than in NCR, even at maximal vasodilatation and almost in proportion to the raised "resting" blood pressure in SHR. As in the human hand, however, SHR and NCR did not differ as to "threshold" sensitivity to vasoconstrictor agents. On the other hand, once sub-stantial vasoconstrictions were elicited, where any difference in wall/lumen ratio between the SHR and NCR resistance vessels would express itself as a difference in steepness of the resistance curves, the SHR resistance curves were indeed much steeper throughout. Furthermore, the maximal contractile strength was higher in SHR and largely in propor-tion to their higher "resting" arterial blood pressure (Fig. 3 left part).

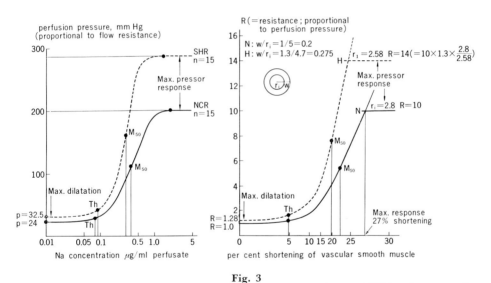

Fig. 3

Left part: Average "resistance curves" for spontaneously hypertensive rats (SHR) and normotensive control rats (NCR), based on the results of fifteen paired experiments.
Right part: Mathematically deduced "resistance curves" for two hypothetical resistance vessels, H and N, where H differs from N only in the respect that its media thickness is supposed to be increased 30%, encroaching on its lumen even at complete smooth muscle relaxation. w/r=ratios of wall thick-ness to internal radius. From FOLKOW et al.'s article[12], with kind permission.

The right part of Fig. 3 illustrates the computed responses during constant-flow per-fusion of two hypothetical resistance vessels, one normotensive, *N*, and one hypertensive, *H*. These two vessels were assumed to differ *only* in the respect that the media of *H* was 30 per cent thicker due to hypertrophy, and in such a way that it encroached upon the lumen of *H* also at maximal dilatation. Thus, if the ratio of wall-thickness to internal radius (w/r) is set to 1:5 at maximal dilatation in N, which seems to be reasonable figures [30], it would be 1.3:4.7 in H. Then *identical* smooth muscle shortenings were assumed for N and H up to the maximal possible ones, where only the mentioned difference in vascular design, with the consequent difference in contractile strength, were allowed to affect the characteristics of the computed resistance curves.

When the relationship between these computed resistance curves is compared with that of the experimental NCR-SHR resistance curves, a surprising similarity is revealed in all important points. Some types of vascular changes, proposed to be involved in hypertension, such as smooth muscle supersensitivity, are directly incompatible with the observed characteristics of the resistance curves, and comparisons of isolated arterial strips from NCR-SHR also refute such a type of mechanism. As to other mechanisms proposed, several of these would have to be combined to fit the experimentally obtained resistance curves and, in addition, any influence of the by now well-documented media hypertrophy *would then have to be disregarded*. For such reasons it seems difficult to avoid the conclusion that the haemodynamic change in SHR is mainly constituted by an adaptive increase of the wall/lumen ratio of the resistance vessels, essentially caused by a media hypertrophy that encroaches upon the lumen even at maximal vasodilatation. In fact, this structural adaptation appears to be so pronounced in SHR that it may keep up the raised resistance and pressure during "resting" steady state at a largely *normal* level of vascular smooth muscle tone. This statement by no means denies the possibility that functional factors, *e.g.* in the form of centrally elicited neurohormonal exacerbations, may more or less intermittently superimpose exaggerated resistance and pressure increases in SHR as compared with NCR. Such a type of influence is in full harmony with the earlier stated hypothesis concerning a close interrelationship between functional and structural factors in the course of primary hypertension (and probably also in other types of hypertension).

The renal vascular bed of SHR, at least when young, forms an interesting exception from the other major systemic circuits, in the sense that its resistance at maximal dilatation is, if anything, *lower* than in NCR. This surprising difference, which might after all have a fairly simple explanation [14], makes it very unlikely that any "Goldblatt mechanism" should be involved in early phases. As to other characteristics, *e.g.* the shape of the resistance curve, the SHR renal vascular bed is closely similar to *e.g.* the hindquarter vascular bed.

As to the time course of the structural vascular adaptations discussed here, the hindquarter vessels of SHR and NCR [10], or the hindlimb vessels of cats [28], were exposed to regional hypotension for only a few weeks or months. Since the mentioned type of structural vascular adaptation is in all likelihood a general phenomenon, that is related to hypertrophy versus atrophy in *e.g.* trained as compared with untrained skeletal muscles, it was expected to reveal itself also in situations of regional hypotension, where the animal could serve as its own control. Briefly, the resistance curves of these hypotensive vascular beds exhibited already after a few weeks a clearly reduced R_{min}, a decreased steepness of the resistance curve and a proportionally decreased maximal contractile strength, while smooth muscle sensitivity to constrictor agents appeared to be unchanged (Fig. 4).

Still more recent studies suggest that a substantial structural adaptation is evident already within a week, at least with respect to the *regression* of wall thickness when the pressure load is reduced. It seems probable, then, that the reverse process, the hypertrophic build-up of tissue, is a somewhat slower process, but still it is likely to be evident already within some weeks or months, if parallels are drawn to other types of muscle. Further, in quite recent experiments [21], where renal hypertension was inflicted upon otherwise normotensive rats, a comparison of their "resistance curves" with those of normotensive con-

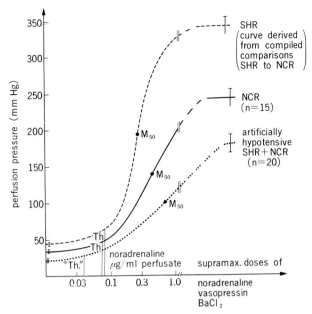

Fig. 4 Average "resistance curves" of the hindquarter vascular beds from ordinary SHR and NCR and from aorta-ligated SHR-NCR. Note how the three curves differ in terms of resistance at maximal dilatation, slope of the resistance curve and maximal contractile strength, and in due proportion to the differences in "resting" blood pressure. This is in SHR 203±8 mm Hg, in NCR 145±4 mm Hg and in the hypotensive SHR-NCR 97±12 and 80±6 mm Hg, respectively. The apparent difference in threshold to noradrenaline in the hypotensive hindquarters is merely a result of a "technical artifact"[10]. From FOLKOW et al.'s article, with kind permission.

trols, suggests that the vascular wall hypertrophy occurs quite rapidly and is thus seen also in animals that are *not* genetically predisposed to hypertension. It is still, however, possible that normotensive rats and SHR differ *quantitatively* in this respect, and other recent experiments, comparing immunosympathectomized SHR-NCR with ordinary SHR-NCR might indicate such a quantitative difference [13], though more studies along these lines are needed.

In any case it should be stressed that the results on the regionally hypotensive SHR vessels, referred to above, suggests that the rapid structural adaptation of the resistance vessels is a strictly *local* affair, dependent primarily on the regional pressure load and, perhaps, also on the pressure-dependent autoregulatory adjustment of regional vascular tone. The hypotonic hindquarter vessels must have been exposed to largely the same neuro-hormonal influences and the same chemical environment as the vessels in the hypertensive upper part of the animal.

This by no means denies that hormones of general importance for cell growth, such as growth hormone and thyroxine, are likely to be necessary "permissive" factors for the full establishment of *e.g.* the hypertrophic vascular changes that occur as a result of an increased pressure load. The question then arises whether the *lack* of such hormonal influences, normally supporting the structural adaptation of heart and resistance vessels, etc., might explain why a truly hypertensive state can hardly be achieved in hypophysectomized or thyreodectomized animals [25].

The rapid regression of the structural changes, occurring when regional hypotension was inflicted upon the hindquarters of SHR, stimulated to some therapeutic studies with different types of antihypertensive agents in SHR. Thus, when old and severely hypertensive SHR were "normalized" as to pressure for 8–12 weeks by means of large doses of apresoline and guanethidine, given in the drinking water, signs of a considerable regression of the structural changes of the resistance vessels were obtained [15]. These animals were old and so severely hypertensive that they in all likelihood corresponded to very advanced hypertensive disease in man and, yet, regression of the structural changes was quite evident.

In another therapeutic study on young animals, starting almost at the prehypertensive age, treatment with large doses of the β-adrenergic blocking agent, propranolol, was continued for about 8 months to suppress predominantly cardiac output [17]. The reason was that other studies,earlier referred to, indicate that central neuro-hormonal influences— perhaps in the form of the defence reaction with its characteristic increase of cardiac output and hence of blood pressure—might form at least part of the functional trigger mechanisms that gradually lead to structural vascular changes and, therefore, to established hypertension. "Resting" blood pressure in these SHR stayed fairly normal throughout and subsequent explorations of the "resistance curves" of their hindquarter vessels revealed that these had remained fairly normal, while the vessels of untreated SHR of similar age exhibited the characteristic differences to NCR that have been described earlier.—Further experiments along these lines are presently carried out, as are studies where we try to explore whether the vessels of SHR might be somewhat more prone to respond with hypertrophy to a given load than those of ordinary rats.

How close are then the parallels between primary hypertension in man and that in SHR? It was earlier mentioned that SHR appear to be genetically somewhat hyperreactive as to e.g. the centrally integrated defence reaction, and perhaps also concerning other patterns. Further such neuro-hormonal pressor influences appear to constitute a functional trigger mechanism for gradually establishing structural vascular changes, whereby a stable hypertension would be achieved. The earlier mentioned experiments on normotensive rats and on mice, exposed to enforced "mental stress", also point in this general direction. Incidentally, the well known baroreceptor "resetting", by means of which the reflex homeostasis gradually so to say "accepts" the hypertensive state, also appears to be mainly, perhaps only, a consequence of such a structural vascular adaptation. Thus, an elegant analysis on rabbits, made hypertensive, strongly indicates that it is the *arterial walls*, rather than the mechano-receptors, that become gradually "reset" [1], and in a way which strongly indicates the presence of the same type of structural change as that affecting the cardiovascular system from the left ventricle down to include the main resistance vessels. To return to man, the characteristic defence reaction, often induced in most species during the "strain of daily life", causes also here considerable but transient increases of blood pressure and cardiac output [2, 3, 23]. Further, it has been repeatedly pointed out that, early, labile stages of essential hypertension often display a cardiovascular pattern closely mimicking a mild defence reaction [3] with a pressure rise that is mainly due to an increased cardiac output which particularly favours muscle blood supply; first in later "well-established" stages the increased resistance becomes the dominant feature.

In other words, in both man and SHR there might be a combination of a common cortico-hypothalamic response pattern and a secondary, though *rapidly* developed, structural adaptation of the resistance vessels, the latter being a response to the enhanced average pressure load. Both these factors, that become closely interwoven in time, must be considered as per se perfectly "normal" mechanisms but, when for environmental and/or genetical reasons exaggerated, they may together transform an initially normotensive cardiovascular system into a hypertensive one. Either or both of these factors may thus be genetically linked and it is known that both types of primary hypertension are based on several genetic elements. It is, moreover, evident that environmental factors, in the form of mental stress may greatly contribute, probably by accentuating central excitatory influences, which *e.g.* the results on mice by HENRY et al. [22] make clear.

It is still unsettled whether the structural adaptation of the resistance vessels is for genetical reasons more easily precipitated in SHR than in NCR, though some findings might, as mentioned, point in this general direction. As to man, it has been reported (for ref. see [28]) that patients with essential hypertension have a prevalence of "mesomorphic body build", which might also imply a slightly greater tendency of vessels and heart to respond by hypertrophy to a given increase of load. It should be stressed that even a small quantitative difference in this very respect may, in the long run, have important consequences, since the functional and structural factors tend to mutually reinforce each other and may even form a potential vicious circle [7, 10]. However, only future studies can definitely answer the important but, indeed, difficult questions as to which are the most important genetical factors in primary hypertension of man and SHR. The type of structural vascular adaptation here mainly discussed, no doubt seems to be a phenomenon present in *all* individuals but, like any "normal" mechanism or factor, it may for genetical reasons be somewhat more pronounced in primary hypertension in man and/or in SHR. The more pronounced such a factor would be, the less it would need in terms of a functional pressure load, due to *e.g.* environmental "stress" influences, to initiate gradually a hypertensive state.

ACKNOWLEDGEMENTS

Most of the studies discussed here have been supported by grants from the Swedish Medical Research Council (B72-14X-16-08A, K71-14R-3469) and from the Faculty of Medicine, University of Göteborg.

REFERENCES

1. AARS, H. (1969): Acta Physiol Scand, **75**, 406.
2. BEVAN, A. T., HONOUR, A. J. and STOTT, F. H. (1969): Clin Sci, **36**, 329.
3. BROD, J. (1963): Br Heart J, **25**, 227.
4. CONWAY, J. (1963): Circulation, **27**, 520.
5. CONWAY, J., JULIUS, S. and AMERY, A. (1967): Hypertension, **16**, 79.
6. FOLKOW, B. (1956): *In* "Hypotensive Drugs," p. 163, Pergamon Press, London.
7. FOLKOW, B. (1960): The joint symposium on the pathogenesis of essential hypertension; WHO and Czechoslo. Cardiol. Soc., 247. State Medical Publ. House, Prague.
8. FOLKOW, B. (1971): Clin Sci, **40**, 1.
9. FOLKOW, B., GRIMBY, G. and THULESIUS, O. (1958): Acta Physiol Scand, **44**, 255.
10. FOLKOW, B., GURÉVIC, M., HALLBÄCK, M., LUNDGREN, Y. and WEISS, L. (1971): Acta Physiol Scand, **83**, 532.
11. FOLKOW, B., HALLBÄCK, M., LUNDGREN, Y. and WEISS, L. (1970): Acta Physiol Scand, **79**, 373.
12. FOLKOW, B., HALLBÄCK, M., LUNDGREN, Y. and WEISS, L. (1970): Acta Physiol Scand, **80**, 93.
13. FOLKOW, B., HALLBÄCK, M., LUNDGREN, Y. and WEISS, L. (1971): Acta Physiol Scand, **82**, 27 A.
14. FOLKOW, B., HALLBÄCK, M., LUNDGREN, Y. and WEISS, L. (1971): Acta Physiol Scand, **83**, 96.
15. FOLKOW, B., HALLBÄCK, M., LUNDGREN, Y. and WEISS, L. (1971): Acta Physiol Scand, **83**, 280.

16. FOLKOW, B., HALLBÄCK, M. and WEISS, L. (1972):   Acta Physiol Scand, in press.
17. FOLKOW, B., LUNDGREN, Y. and WEISS, L. (1972):   Acta Physiol Scand, in press.
18. FOLKOW, B. and NEIL, E. (1971):   "Circulation", Oxford University Press, Oxford, New York.
19. FOLKOW, B. and RUBINSTEIN, E. (1966):   Acta Physiol Scand, **68**, 48.
20. FURUYAMA, M. (1962):   Tohoku J Exp Med, **76**, 388.
21. HALLBÄCK, M., LUNDGREN, Y. and WEISS, L. (1972):   Acta Physiol Scand, in press.
22. HENRY, J. P., MEEHAN, J. P. and STEPHENS, P. M. (1967):   Psychosom Med, **29**, 408.
23. HINMAN, A. T., ENGEL, B. T. and BICKFORD, A. F. (1962):   Am Heart J, **63**, 663.
24. LAVERTY, R. and SMIRK, F. H. (1961):   Circ Res, **9**, 455.
25. OKAMOTO, K. (1969):   Int Rev Exp Pathol, **7**, 227.
26. OKAMOTO, K. and AOKI, K. (1963):   Jap Circ J, **27**, 282.
27. PICKERING, G. W. (1968):   "High Blood Pressure," J. and A. Churchill, London.
28. SIVERTSSON, R. (1970):   Acta Physiol Scand, Suppl 343.
29. SUWA, N. and TAKAHASHI, T. (1971):   "Morphological and Morphometrical Analysis of Circulation in Hypertension and Ischemic Kidney," Urban and Schwarzenberg. München-Berlin-Wien.
30. Van CITTERS, R. L. (1966):   Circ Res, **18**, 199.

POSSIBLE MECHANISMS OF VASCULAR REACTIVITY DIFFERENCES IN SPONTANEOUSLY HYPERTENSIVE AND NORMOTENSIVE RAT AORTAE

S. SHIBATA* and K. KURAHASHI*

Experimental hypertension, induced by a variety of methods and in different stages of chronicity is not a single entity nor a particularly suitable model of human essential hypertension. The spontaneously hypertensive Wistar rat (SHR), alternatively developed through selective inbreeding techniques by OKAMOTO and AOKI [1] appears to be a good model for studying the mechanisms involved in the initiation and maintenance of high blood pressure.

Despite numerous studies on these animals [5], the question of vascular reactivity to norepinephrine has not been conclusively answered, and much controversy exists in the literature. OKAMOTO et al. [7] reported greater vascular responsiveness to norepinephrine in the SHR. CLINESCHMIDT et al. [2] and HALLBÄCK et al. [4] reported that the aortic strips of SHR and normotensive Wistar rats (NWR) showed equal sensitivity to norepinephrine. In contrast, SPECTOR et al. [8] and HAEUSLER and HAEFELY [3] demonstrated that the vascular smooth muscles of SHR were less responsive than those of normal rats to the contractile effects of norepinephrine, potassium and serotonin.

We recently found that the aortic strips from SHR showed less vascular reactivity to vasoconstrictive agents than those of two different strains of normotensive rats. The present report describes the results of attempts to define the possible mechanisms of the differences between the reactivities of aortic strips from SHR and normotensive rats to some vasoconstrictive agents.

Three different groups of rats of both sexes weighing 240 to 350 g (age 80–100 days) were used. The experimental group consisted of spontaneously hypertensive Wistar rats. The control groups consisted of normotensive Wistar and Sprague-Dawley rats. Furthermore, the prehypertensive SHR which had not yet developed hypertension (30–35 days after birth) were used. For this experiment, spiral aortic strips were used and tension changes were recorded by means of a strain gauge transducer and Grass polygraph.

Blood pressure: The mean systolic and disatolic blood pressures were measured by pressure transducers connected by cannulae to the femoral artery. Blood pressure of hypertensive rats was significantly higher than that of normotensive rats (Table 1).

Reactivity to norepinephrine: The contractile response of hypertensive strips to norepinephrine was significantly less than that of normotensive strips. The amplitude of the maximal contraction induced by norepinephrine (10^{-6} M) in hypertensive strips was about 40% less than that of normotensive strips (Fig. 1).

Configuration of norepinephrine response: In the normotensive strips, norepinephrine elicited two phases of contraction consisting of a fast and a subsequent slow component. On the other hand, in hypertensive strips, only the fast component was observed.

When the fast components of the total norepinephrine responses in both hypertensive and normotensive strips were compared, no significant difference was observed in dose-response curves (Fig. 1).

Although the nature of the slow component is not completely understood, BOHR (1963) proposed that the rate limiting factor for the slow component of the norepinephrine contraction is the role played by Ca^{++} in coupling the membrane excitation with the

* Department of Pharmacology, School of Medicine University of Hawaii, Honolulu, Hawaii U.S.A.

Table 1 Blood pressures of spontaneously hypertensive and normotensive rats.

	Hypertensive rat	Normotensive rat	
		Wistar	Sprague-Dawley
Systolic			
Blood Pressure (mm Hg)	250±5	175±4	165±5
Diastolic			
Blood Pressure (mm Hg)	190±4	130±4	125±6
Body Weight (g)	250–350	250–360	250–350
No. of Rats	100	159	50

The values of systolic and diastolic blood pressures of the hypertensive rats are significantly higher than those of normotensive rats (t-test, 0.001 > P).

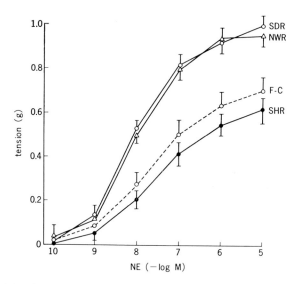

Fig. 1 The contractile action of norepinephrine on the aortic strip of the hypertensive (SHR), normotensive Wistar (NWR) and Sprague-Dawley (SDR) rats. F–C indicates the dose-response curve of the fast component for the norepinephrine response of NWR aortic strips. Each vertical bar indicates the Mean±SEM of 15 observations.

development of tension by the contractile protein. This point of view is strongly supported by our data showing the disappearance of the slow component of the noreipnephrine response either in low Ca^{++} -medium or after treatment with several cations, such as Mn^{++}, Co^{++}, or La^{+++}, which specifically inhibit Ca^{++} ion flux. It is, therefore, reasonable to assume that the absence of the slow component might be attributed to the decreased availability of Ca^{++} for the coupling process. Actually, with the absence of the slow component, the difference in the vasoconstrictor responses of hypertensive and nor motensive strips to norepinephrine disappeared.

Similar low vascular reactivity of hypertensive strips was observed on the contractile responses to nonspecific stimulants such as potassium, barium and angiotension. Previously, the decreased vascular reactivity of hypertensive rat aorta to norepinephrine and potassium was reported by SPECTOR et al. [8].

Reactivity to potassium: Dose-response curves of hypertensive strips for K^+ show less reactivity than that of normotensive strips.

Reactivity to barium and angiotensin: The dose-response curves of hypertensive strips for Ba^{++} and angiotensin showed less reactivity than that of normotensive strips.

The configuration of the total contraction produced by nonspecific stimulants was not separable into two components as was the norepinephrine response. Therefore, the presence or absence of the slow component per se may not be a suitable explanation for the difference in the vascular reactivity of hypertensive and normotensive strips. However, it is generally accepted that calcium is essential for the coupling of membrane excitation with tension development by the contractile protein. The relationship between extreme changes of Ca^{++} concentration and the contractile response follows the assumption that membrane excitation and excitation-contraction coupling constitute two consecutive processes leading to the development of tension by contractile protein. Since the contraction produced by the nonspecific stimulants is mediated by membrane depolarization, the decrease in available Ca^{++} for the coupling system of vascular smooth muscle of hypertensive rats may lead to low vascular reactivity to those stimuli.

Reactivity to Mn^{++}, Co^{++}, Sr^{++}, and La^{+++}: It is interesting to note that only the hypertensive strips were able to show the contractile response to Mn^{++}, Sr^{++}, and La^{+++}. No detectable contraction was produced by these cations in the normotensive strips.

These results were a reversal of the observation on the responsiveness to other stimuli tested. The explanation of why only the hypertensive strips were capable of developing tension following treatment with these cations is not apparent. This suggests a qualitative difference in the intrinsic musculature of both types of blood vessels.

Rhythmic contractility: When normotensive strips were subjected to certain concentrations of Ba^{++}, KCl, Sr^{++}, norepinephrine or serotonin, rhythmic activity was superimposed on the tonic contraction. However, such rhythmic contractility was not observed in any of the hypertensive strips. If rhythmicity itself indicates a single unit organization of vascular smooth muscle, the nature of hypertensive vascular smooth muscle presumably is of the multi-unit, nonpropagating type rather than the single unit type.

Reactivity to nitroglycerine and papaverine hydrochloride: The relaxant effect of nitroglycerine and papaverine on the normotensive and hypertensive strips was measured at different resting tensions (0.5, 1.5, and 3.0 g). Five strips from different animals were used for each experiment. When the normotensive and hypertensive strips were exposed to nitroglycerine (10^{-6} and 10^{-5} M) at different resting tensions, no significant difference in the relaxant response to this agent was observed.

The application of papaverine ($10^{-6} - 10^{-4}$ M) failed to cause any relaxant effect on either type of strips at different resting tensions.

Although the mechanisms of vasodilator action of nitroglycerine and papaverine are not known, these agents elicited similar responses on both the hypertensive and normotensive strips. This suggests that probably no difference exists in the relaxing systems of both types of vascular smooth muscles.

Reactivity of prehypertensive strips: One might pose the question as to whether or not the low abnormal vascular reactivity of hypertensive strips is due to the compensatory mechanisms of hypertension. In these experiments, the aortic strips were obtained from the hypertensive rat which had not yet developed hypertension (136 mm Hg, 30–35 days after birth), indicating a prehypertensive state. The dose-response curves of prehypertensive strips for norepinephrine and potassium showed less reactivity than that of matched normotensive strips.

The effect of Mn^{++}, Co^{++} or La^{+++} on the mechanical response of prehypertensive and normotensive aortic strips: As with the hypertensive strips, it can be seen that only prehypertensive strips show the contractile response to those cations, while the normotensive strips exhibited no response.

The abnormal vascular reactivity of hypertensive strips may be due to the original changes in the musculature itself rather than to the secondary changes in compensatory mechanisms, since the strips in prehypertensive state showed similar abnormal vascular response.

It is reasonable to conclude that the level of available calcium ion for the excitation-coupling process may play an important role in the possible mechanisms leading to the differences in vascular reactivity of hypertensive and normotensive rats.

REFERENCES

1. Bohr, D. F. (1963): Science, **139**, 597.
2. Clineschmidt, B. V., Geller, R. G., Govier, W. C. and Sjoerdsma, A. (1970): Eur J Pharmacol, **10**, 45.
3. Haeusler, G. and Haefely, W. (1970): Naunyn-Schmiedeberg's Arch Pharmakol, **10**, 269.
4. Hallbäck, M., Lundgren, Y. and Weiss, L. (1971): Acta Physiol Scand, **81**, 176.
5. Okamoto, K. (1969): Int Rev Exp Pathol, **7**, 227.
6. Okamoto, K. and Aoki, K. (1963): Jap Circ, J **27**, 282.
7. Okamoto, K., Hazama, F., Takeda, T., Tabei, R., Nosaka, S., Fukushima, M., Yamori, Y., Matsumoto, M., Haebara, H., Ichijima, K. and Suzuki, Y. (1966): Jap Circ J, **30**, 987.
8. Spector, S., Fleisch, J. H., Maling, H. M. and Brodie, B. B. (1969): Science, **166**, 1300.

REACTIVITY TO SYMPATHOMIMETIC AMINES OF ATRIA ISOLATED FROM NORMOTENSIVE AND SPONTANEOUSLY HYPERTENSIVE RATS

M. FUJIWARA*, N. TODA*, S. SHIBATA** and M. KUCHII**

In the spontaneously hypertensive Wistar rats (SHR) developed by OKAMOTO and AOKI [4], vascular reactivity to norepinephrine was reported from several laboratories with inconsistent results [1, 2, 3, 5, 7]. Recently, SHIBATA et al. [6] confirmed that SHR aortic strips are less reactive to specific (norepinephrine) and non-specific (potassium, barium) stimuli than are the aortic strips of inbred normotensive Wistar and Sprague-Dawley rats.

Although the change in the peripheral resistance of the vascular system is an important factor in the development of hypertension, increased cardiac output is also implicated in the etiology of the disease. To our knowledge, however, no report has appeared in literature regarding the reactivity of SHR cardiac muscle to stimulants. In the present study, the isolated atrial reactivity of SHR to isoproterenol, epinephrine, phenylephrine and potassium was compared to that of normotensive Wistar rat atria.

The animals were killed by a blow on the head, the carotids cut and the chest opened to dissect the heart. The atria were removed from the ventricles and suspended in an isolated organ bath containing Krebs-Ringer bicarbonate medium. The spontaneously beating atrial preparations were connected by a thin silk thread to a force-displacement transducer (Grass model FT 03), and the contractile movements were recorded on a six-channel Grass (model 7) polygraph.

SHR atria showed a greater amount of spontaneously developed tension than normotensive Wistar rat atria. The inotropic and chronotropic responses of SHR atria to isoproterenol were less than those of normotensive rat atria. However, SHR atria showed normal reactivity to phenylephrine. In SHR atria a high concentration of epinephrine elicited a decreased inotropic effect, in comparison to the response of normotensive rat atria, but no difference in the chronotropic effect was observed. Greater negative inotropic and chronotropic responses to potassium were observed in SHR atria, but they showed a normal negative inotropic response to acetylcholine. These results may indicate a difference in the nature of the beta-receptor of SHR and normotensive rat atria and an intrinsic, contractile abnormality of SHR atria.

Further experiments were carried out to determine whether such abnormal cardiac reactivity of SHR is attributable to a compensatory mechanism to reduce the elevated blood pressure or to original changes of the musculature. In these experiments, atria were obtained from the 30 to 35-day-old SHR which had not yet developed hypertension, indicating a pre-hypertensive state.

Essentially similar results were obtained in the pre-hypertensive rat atria. Thus, the abnormal atrial reactivity of SHR atria can not be attributed to a compensatory mechanism for attenuating hypertension. However, the greater spontaneously developed tension of SHR atria probably reflects a compensatory change to maintain a constant blood sup-

* Department of Pharmacology, Faculty of Medicine, Kyoto University, Kyoto, Japan.
** Department of Pharmacology, School of Medicine, University of Hawaii, Honolulu, Hawaii, U.S.A.

ply against the high resistance of peripheral vessels, since such an increase in the spontaneously developed tension was not observed in the pre-hypertensive rat atria.

REFERENCES

1. CLINESCHMIDT, B. V., GELLER, R. G., GOVIER, W. C. and SJOERDSMA, A. (1970): Eur J Pharmacol, **10**, 45.
2. HAEUSLER, G. and HAEFELY, W. (1970): Naunyn-Schmiedeberg's Arch Pharmakol, **266**, 18.
3. HALLBÄCK, M., LUNDGREN, Y. and WEISS, L. (1971): Acta Physiol Scandinav, **81**, 176.
4. OKAMOTO, K. and AOKI, K. (1963): Jap Circ J, **27**, 282.
5. OKAMOTO, K., HAZAMA, F., TAKEDA, T., TABEI, R., NOSAKA, S., FUKUSHIMA, M., YAMORI, Y., MATSUMOTO, M., HAEBARA, H., ICHIJIMA, K. and SUZUKI, Y. (1966): Jap Circ J, **30**, 987.
6. SHIBATA, S., KURAHASHI, K. and MORI, J. (1971): In "Vascular Smooth Muscle" of XXV International Congress of Physiological Sciences, p. 29.
7. SPECTOR, S., FLEISCH, J. H., MALING, H. M. and BRODIE, B. B. (1969): Science, **166**, 1300.

THE HEMODYNAMICS OF THE RAT DURING ONTOGENESIS, WITH SPECIAL REFERENCE TO THE AGE FACTOR IN THE DEVELOPMENT OF HYPERTENSION

I. ALBRECHT*, M. VÍZEK* and J. KŘEČEK*

Ten years after the first development of a colony of spontaneously hypertensive rats (SHR) observations on these animals by Japanese authors have shown them to be an extremely useful model for studying experimental hypertension. Comparative studies on the pathological anatomy, pharmacology and neurophysiology of these animals, recently summarised by OKAMOTO [7], have been made. These studies have again shown that hypertension is an age dependent disorder, and both severity and genesis vary as a function of time. A number of reports [3, 6, 8] on this age aspect have already been published all with a similar conclusion: young animals, before the stage of sexual maturation, are more sensitive to hypertensive stimuli. OKAMOTO and his group have divided the course of spontaneous hypertension into three stages, on the basis of a number of criteria in addition to arterial blood pressure (B.P) levels:

1. prehypertension–age levels 40–60 days
2. early hypertension–from 4 to 6 months of age
3. advanced hypertension–from 12 to 14 months of age.

In agreement with this subdivision there develop a number of changes of a morphological nature, primarily in endocrine organs, which differentiate the hypertensive animal from the normal. It would appear that the above three delimited age ranges are critical for further development of blood pressure changes. FOLKOW, B. [1], LEDINGHAM, J. and PELLING, D. [4], LEDINGHAM, J.M. [5] and GUYTON, A.C. [2] have all stressed the importance of studying hypertension in terms of haemodynamics and cardiac output, rather than only in terms of B.P. Because of the age differences in sensitivity to hypertensive stimuli and the fact that haemodynamic studies have been carried out only in adult rats [5] we decided to follow basic parameters during the course of ontogenesis. These studies will continue in as complete an analysis as possible of the haemodynamics of SHR, and only preliminary findings are presented in the present communication.

METHODS

Wistar strain rats of both sexes, in good health, were used. Measurements were made in Pentobarbital anaesthesia, 40 mg/kg. A cannula was introduced into the carotid artery and pressures were measured with an Elema strain gauge connected to an electromanometer. The same cannula was then used for cardiac output (CO) determination on the Stewart Hamilton principle with intra jugular injection of Evans Blue as the indicator. Just previous to the latter, ^{86}Rb was injected into the same vein to determine organ distribution of blood flow and CO. The dye dilution curve was obtained by allowing the animal to bleed freely into a rotating collector with rapid collection of about 30 microliter samples which were then analysed for Evans Blue content after centrifugation of the cells. Organ flows were expressed both as ml total flow per gm wet tissue and

* Institute of Physiology, Czechoslovac Academy of Sciences, Prague, Czechoslovakia.

as % of CO on the basis of gamma counts from the removed organs. Measurements on SHR were carried out in α-chloralose anaesthesia (40 mg/kg).

RESULTS AND DISCUSSION

CO was measured on 109 males between the ages of 30 and 400 days. As can be seen in Fig. 1, the period since the weaning 30–50 days, was accompanied by a small decrease in CO, whereas the following 10 days of life saw a sharp further decrease of about 30%. The age period 50–60 days was therefore the period of the greatest rate of decrease in this parameter. Fig. 2 shows that the same period is also associated with a sharp rise in total peripheral resistance and increase in B.P. At the age 55 days, in the middle of

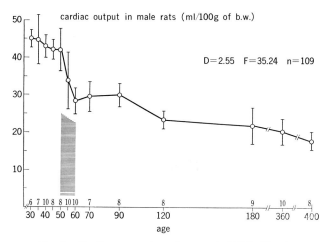

Fig. 1 Cardiac output in male rats (ml/100 of b.w.).

this period, we also found the greatest degree of scatter of values measured, which further suggests that the largest rate of change is occurring. Also, pulse rate, undoubtedly influenced by pentobarbital anesthesia, showed a falling tendency with increasing age, whereas stroke volume rapidly increased to age 50 days, with a further increase occuring only after age 60 days.

Similar results were obtained in females. Sixty four determinations of CO from 30 to 107 days of age showed decreasing values with age up to 60 days, followed by stabilisation up to age 100 days (Fig. 3). As in the males total peripheral resistance (Fig. 4) increased from age 40 days and stabilised at about age 60 days. Stroke volume in females showed maximal changes between ages 30 and 40 days, with no further significant differences up to age 55 days. The decrease in stroke volume from the 60th days and the following increase up to 107 were accompanied by changes in CO. Pulse rate showed a small but insignificant decreasing tendency over the entire period.

Thus, in males between 50 and 60 days of age, and in females between 40 and 60 days of age, there occur marked changes in CO and peripheral resistance. Since the decrease in CO relative to body weight was accompanied by a slight decrease in absolute CO, one factor to be considered is the increased rate of weight gain. As shown by JELÍNEK (1958) there is no marked increase in fat depots in this age range, rather an increase in active body mass. In other words, this is the type of body growth modulated by gonadal activity.

MANN & PARSON (1950) have shown that the weight of the seminal vesicles in males is proportional to gonadal activity. This parameter has been used here as s simple index

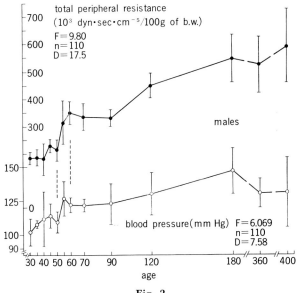

Fig. 2

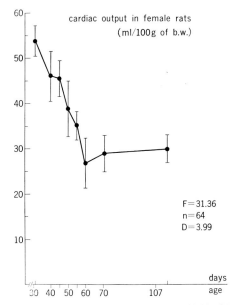

Fig. 3 Cardiac output in female rats   (ml/100 of b.w.).

of androgenic activity and has been correlated with values of CO/100 gm body wt. We studied the correlation of relative CO (ml/100 gm of b.w.) vs relative seminal vesicle wt (mg/100 g of b.w.) in the age range 40 to 60 days. There was a negative correlation ($r_{xy} = -0,7711$) which suggest an interrelation between gonads and CO during adolescence.

Males were gonadectomised at age 6 days, with sham-operated controls. The same operation was also carried out in 180 day old males. After operation at age 6 days, CO was measured at age 49 days, just before the age of maximal changes and at 60 days,

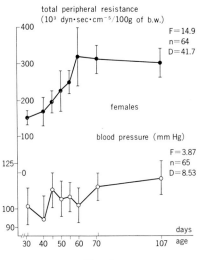

Fig. 4

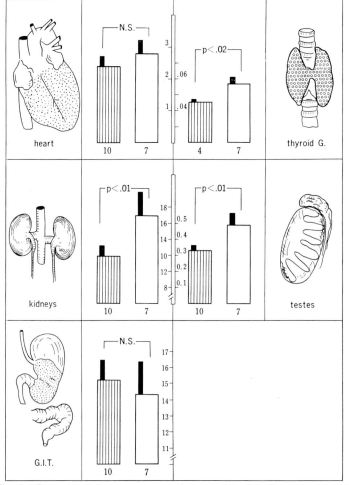

Fig. 5 Organ blood flow in male rats (flow fraction of cardiac output in %).

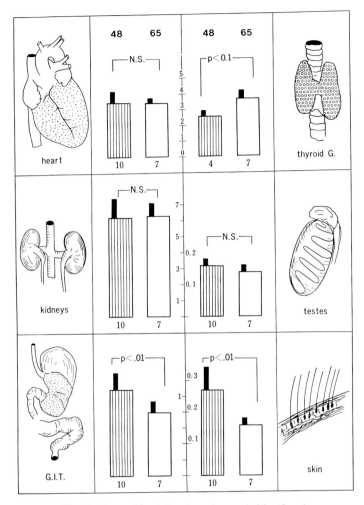

Fig. 6 Organ blood flow in male rats (ml/l g tissue).

when these changes have normally stabilised. The animals operated at 180 days were measured 60 days later. We found that the early operation produced no changes at age 49 days, but significant differences occured 11 days later, at which time the gonadectomised animals always showed higher values of CO than their sham-operated controls. Gonadectomy at age 180 days did not change haemodynamic values at all. It would appear, then, that the testes, and probably testosteroe, play a role in haemodynamic changes of adolescence.

We also tested the action of 6-OH-dopamine on the development of CO. The drug was given in two doses at ages 35 and 42 days. CO was measured at the age 63 days. The result shows that 6-OH-dopamine decreased B.P. and peripheral resistance but increased pulse rate, stroke volume and CO. It is not clear whether the treated to untreated control differences were a particular function of age range selected in these experiments, and further observations in other ranges will have to be made.

Fig. 5 shows fractions of CO flowing through the myocardium, thyroids kidneys, testes and gasrointestinal tract (GIT) in 48 (cross-hatched columns) and 65 day-old rats (empty columns). Relative myocardial and GIT flows did not change, but there was

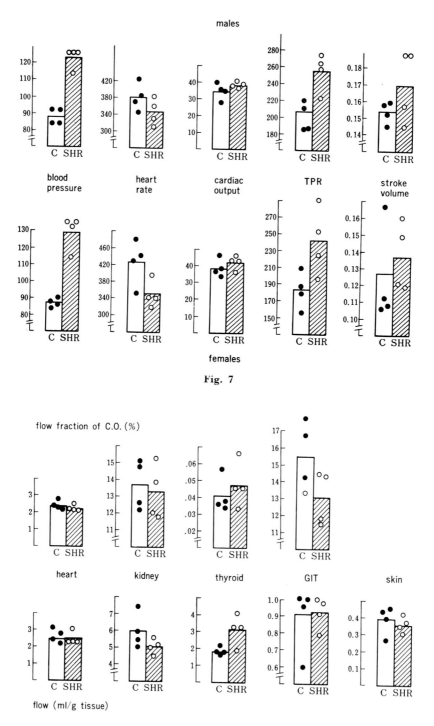

Fig. 7

Fig. 8

a significant increase in fraction to the kidneys at age 65 days, as well as to the thyroid and testes.

Absolute values of organ blood flows (Fig. 6) showed an increase only in the thyroid, with decreases in skin and GIT. These results have been useful to give us some idea of the details of haemodynamic reactions in the animal most frequently used for studies of hypertension—the rat. Adolescence is clearly a critical period for the action of hypertensive stimuli or tendencies. Results on SHR may thus be compared with our non-hypertensive baseline material.

Fig. 7 shows average values (columns) and separate ones (circles) of B.P., pulse rate, cardiac output, total peripheral resistance and stroke volume in males and females, controls and SHR, at age 50 days. The numbers were too small to permit statistical evaluation thus far. However, there are some marked differences, SHR being associated with a lower pulse rate and higher peripheral resistance. CO and stroke volume differences are not so clear. Fig. 8 shows relative organ flows, and SHR was not associated with any great difference in myocardial, renal or thyroid values. GIT flows tended to be lower. Absolute organ flow values, however, showed a marked rise in thyroid values with a tendency to a decrease in kidneys of SHR relative to controls. In this parameter GIT values were the same for both.

These results are too preliminary yet to enable us to make any definite conclusion on the haemodynamic nature of spontaneous hypertension, but we feel that our present approach and technique will give us critical information on this problem.

REFERENCES

1. FOLKOW, B. (1964): Circ Res, **24** and **25**, Suppl I, 279.
2. GUYTON, A. C., COLEMAN, T. G., BOWER, J. D. and GRANGER, H. J. (1970): Circ Res, **26** and **27**, Suppl II, 135.
3. JELÍNEK, J., ALBRECHT, I. and MUSILOVÁ, H. (1966): Physiol Bohemosolv, **15**, 424.
4. LEDINGHAM, J. M. and PELLING, D. (1967): Circ Res, **21**, Suppl II, 187.
5. LEDINGHAM, J. M. (1971): Proc Med, **1964**, 409
6. MUSILOVÁ, H., JELÍNEK, J. and ALBRECHT, I. (1966): Physiol Bohemoslov, **15**, 525.
7. OKAMOTO, K. (1969): In "International Review of Experimental Pathology" (G. W. RICHTER and M. A. EPSTEIN, eds.), Vol. 7, p. 227, Academic Press, New York.
8. SKELTON, F. R. and GUILLEBEAU, J. (1956): Endocrinology, **59**, 201.

CARDIOVASCULAR PATHOLOGY

PATHOLOGY OF DIETARY INDUCED CEREBROVASCULAR DISEASES IN SPONTANEOUSLY HYPERTENSIVE RATS*

K. OKAMOTO**, F. HAZAMA**, H. HAEBARA**, S. AMANO**,
T. TANAKA** and A. OOSHIMA**

Dietary modifications of hypertensive cerebrovascular changes were studied giving SHR 1% saline for drinking replacing tap water with and without a special high fat-cholesterol diet.

Experimental animals used were SHRs and normal Wistar rats of 2 to 4 months of age and of both sexes. They were allotted into 3 groups. Animals in the first group were fed on normal stock chow (Nihon Clea Co.) and ordinary tap water (Control group). To animals in the second group, known as the NaCl group, 1 % saline was supplied for drinking. To the third group of animals, a high fat diet which contained cholesterol and 1 % saline for drinking were supplied ad libitum. This is the Fat-Chol.-NaCl group. The composition of the special diet is as follows: 20 % tempura oil, 5 % cholesterol, 2 % bile powder (crude sodium cholate) and 73 % stock chow (Nihon Clea Co.).

After various feeding schedules, the animals were killed by decapitation. Histopathological and electron microscopical materials were taken from the brain immediately after decapitation. Animals which died spontaneously were also histologically studied. Some animals were perfused with contrast medium mixed with Berlin Blue from the femoral artery for microangiography. The perfused brain was radiographically studied using Softex. The brain was then serially sectioned and cleared to make microscopical preparations.

As stated in a separate paper [3], SHR can be classified into 3 substrains; namely A, B and C. These substrains are related to clinical and pathological findings.

Approximately 5 weeks after initiation of experimental feedings, animals in the NaCl and the Fat-Chol.-NaCl groups began to show neurological signs such as involuntary movements, disturbance in gait, paresis or paralysis of the extremities, incontinentia urinae, rage etc.

On sections, brains of the animals with and without neurological signs often revealed macroscopical changes. Some animals showed massive intracerebral hemorrhage (Fig. 1), some, infarct often with cyst formation (Fig. 2) and others, subarachnoidal hemorrhage. The brain was sometimes markedly swollen and anemic.

---

* This work was supported in part by a Grant-in-aid for Scientific Research from the Ministry of Education, Japan, and the Chiyoda Mutual Life's Subsidiary Fund for Social Welfare Works.
** Department of Pathology, Faculty of Medicine, Kyoto University, Kyoto, Japan

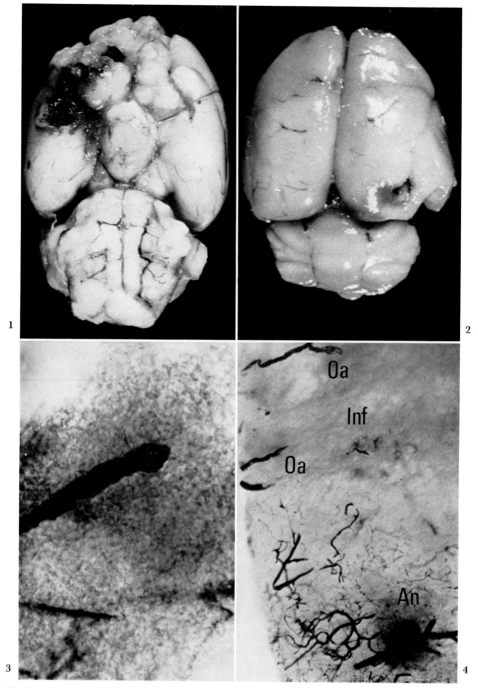

Fig. 1 An intracerebral massive hemorrhage in the temporal lobe.
Fig. 2 A cortical infarct with cavity formation in the occipital lobe.
Fig. 3 A ruptured microaneurysma in the brain perfused with contrast medium and Berlin Blue. ×400.
Fig. 4 An infarct (Inf) with occluded arterioles (Oa) and a microaneurysma (An) with an increased permeability in the surroundings (bottom). Perfused preparation, ×40.

Intracerebral hemorrhages varied in size from small slit hemorrhages to massive hemorrhages and were seen in most cases in the cerebral cortex and subcortical white matter. Rarely were they found in the basal ganglia. This fact differs from humans. In massive hemorrhagic focus, a thin-walled small artery was observed. Angiographically, these dilated arteries proved to be microaneurysmas (Fig. 3). Not only ruptured aneurysma existed but often several unruptured ones as well were observed in the surroundings of a hemorrhagic focus. Small hemorrhagic foci showed a tendency to fuse with each other. Arterioles and small arteries in the hemorrhagic focus revealed findings of fibrinoid necrosis and hyaline change.

From these findings, it appears that sodium chloride and perhaps cholesterol accelerate hypertensive vascular changes as in the case of renal arteries as shown in a separate paper [2]. In microscopical preparations of the perfused brain, permeated pigment existed in the surroundings of the aneurysma as shown in Fig. 4. It has been reported that dilated arteries show an increased permeability [1, 4]. The present experiment did not determine whether or not this increased permeability plays an important role in hemorrhage.

There was no definite difference in features of pathological changes between the NaCl and the Fat-Chol.-NaCl groups of animals.

New and old infarcts were also found mainly in the cerebral cortex and subcortical white matter. They occurred rarely in the basal ganglia. The predirection sites of infarct correspond to the borders between the medial and anterior or posterior cerebral arteries. Angiographically arteries in the subcortical white matter proved to be poorly distributed, making it appear as if ischemic changes occur here rather easily, while the basal ganglia showed a rich vascularization (Fig. 5). These angiographical findings may, to some extent, explain the difference of predirection sites of infarct between human cases and rats.

Though some infarcts took the form of hemorrhagic infarcts, some were in a combined form of infarct and hemorrhage. Hemorrhagic focus and infarct were rather sharply separated in the same preparation.

In the foci of infarcts arterioles and small arteries showed various changes. Some pial arteries showed cellular hyperplasia with narrowed lumina (Fig. 6). Lumina of the intracerebral arterioles and small arteries were also narrowed due to fibrinoid necrosis and hyalin deposition and also a slight increase of cells in number in the walls (Fig. 7). Some of them were completely occluded by thrombi (Fig. 4, 8) which was confirmed angiographically. Eosinophilic exsudate was often observed around affected arteries.

In untreated SHR the incidence of cerebral vascular diseases is less than 10 % and

Table Incidences of cerebrovascular diseases.

		NaCl			Fat-Chol.-NaCl			
		A	B_2	N	A	P_2	C	N
	Total cases	23	17	20	67	29	24	30
Infarct+intracerebral	Cases	22	6	0	53	10	14	0
hemorrhage	(%)	(79)	(35)	(0)	(79)	(34)	(58)	(0)
Infarct	Cases	20	7	0	45	10	11	0
	(%)	(71)	(41)	(0)	(67)	(34)	(42)	(0)
Intracerebral hemorrhage	Cases	4	0	0	18	2	3	0
	(%)	(14)	(0)	(0)	(27)	(7)	(13)	(0)
Subarachnoidal hemorrhage	Cases	1	1	2	2	2	3	1
	(%)	(3)	(6)	(10)	(3)	(7)	(13)	(3)
Fibrinoid necrosis	Cases	9	4	0	9	4	2	0
	(%)	(14)	(14)	(0)	(13)	(14)	(8)	(0)

N: normal Wistar rats

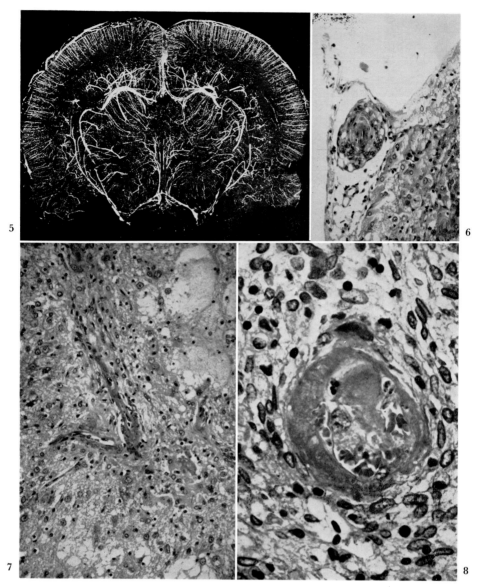

Fig. 5   Angiograph of the brain of normal rat. Subcortical white matter shows poor vasculari-
         zation, while the basal ganglia rich vascularization.
Fig. 6   Cellular hyperplasia of a pial artery. H.E., ×100.
Fig. 7   Fibrinoid necrosis of arterioles in a focus of infarct. H.E., × 100.
Fig. 8   Thrombosis in a focus of infarct. H.E., ×400.

occurred later than 200 days of age. As shown in Table 1, animals of both the NaCl and
the Fat-Chol.-NaCl groups showed extremely high incidence of cerebrovascular diseases.
Almost 80 % of the animals which belonged to substrain A developed infarct and or massive hemorrhage in both groups. Among these, small slit hemorrhages were omitted in
order to exclude agonal hemorrhage. No definite differences in the incidence of cerebrovascular diseases between the NaCl and the Fat-Chol.-NaCl groups could be found, while
there were definite differences among the three substrains. Incidence of cerebrovascular

diseases in substrain A was more than twice as high as that in substrain B_2. This fact indicates that heredity is an important factor in developing cerebrovascular diseases in addition to dietary factors such as sodium choloride and fatty substances.

SUMMARY

SHR given 1 % saline for drinking in place of tap water with and without a special high fat diet which contained cholesterol, developed with a high incidence cerebrovascular diseases, infarcts and hemorrhages.

There were definite differences in the incidences of cerebrovascular diseases among substrains A, B_2 and C.

REFERENCES

1. GIESE, J. (1964): Acta Pathol Microbiol Scand, **62**, 497.
2. HAZAMA, F., TANAKA, T., OOSHIMA, A., HAEBARA, H., AMANO, T., YAMAZAKI, Y. and OKAMOTO, K. (1972): *In* "Spontaneous Hypertension" (K. OKAMOTO ed.), p. 134, Igaku Shoin Ltd., Tokyo.
3. OKAMOTO, K., YAMORI, Y., OOSHIMA, A., PARK, C. HAEBARA, H., MATSUMOTO, M., TANAKA, T., OKUDA, T., HAZAMA, F. and KYOGOKU, M. (1972): *In* "Spontaneous Hypertension" (K. OKAMOTO, ed.), p. 1, Igaku Shoin Ltd., Tokyo.
4. OLSEN, F. (1969): Acta Pathol Microbiol Scand, **75**, 527.

DIETARY EFFECTS ON CARDIOVASCULAR LESIONS IN SPONTANEOUSLY HYPERTENSIVE RATS*

F. HAZAMA**, T. TANAKA**, A. OOSHIMA**, H. HAEBARA**,
S. AMANO**, Y. YAMAZAKI** and K. OKAMOTO**

In preliminary experiments dietary effects especially neutral fats, cholesterol, sodium chloride and their combinations were studied in relation to cardiovascular lesions in SHR. Feeding conditions and main pathological changes are shown in Table 1. Groups 2 and 5 developed considerable vascular changes and also sequential pathological changes in the brain, kidneys and heart within a short period. For this reason, the present experiments deal with detailed studies on dietary conditions.

Table 1 Feeding plans and main pathological changes in the preliminary experiments.

	1 Untreated		2 NaCl		3 Chol.-NaCl		4 Fat-Chol.		5 Fat-Chol.-NaCl	
	SHR	Cont.	SHR	Cont.	SHR	Cont.	SHR	Cont.	SHR	Cont.
Experimental periods	2–12 Mo.		2–3 Mo.		2–3 Mo.		6–12 Mo.		2–3 Mo.	
Cerebral vascular lesions	+	−	⧺	−	⫼		⧺	−	⧺	−
Kidney fibrinoid necrosis	+	−	⧺	−	⧺	−	⧺	−	⧺	−
Heart fibrinoid necrosis	+	−	⧺	−	⧺	−	+	−	⧺	−
Atherosclerosis	−∼±	−	−	−	⧺∼⫼	−	+∼⧺	−	⧺∼⫼	−

SHRs used were 2 to 4 months of age, of both sexes, and allotted into 3 groups, the first being the control. The control animals were fed on normal stock chow with ordinary drinking water. To the second group, 1 % saline was supplied for drinking (NaCl group). To the third, a high fat diet containing cholesterol and 1 % saline were supplied ad libitum (Fat-Chol.-NaCl group). The high fat diet consisted of 20 % tempura oil, 5 % cholesterol, 2 % bile powder (crude sodium cholate), and 73 % stock chow (Nihon Clea Co.).

Three groups of normal Wistar rats were maintained on identical diets as the SHR.

After various dietary feedings, some animals were sacrificed by decapitation, and materials for histopathology and electron microscopy were taken from various organs. Other animals which died spontaneously were also histologically studied.

As mentioned by OKAMOTO et al. [5] SHR can be divided into A, B and C substrains from the standpoint of breeding, biochemical characteristics and vulnerability of cerebral blood vessels.

SHR in both the NaCl and the Fat-Chol.-NaCl groups developed severe pathological changes in the kidneys within a short period, while control Wistar rats maintained on the same dietary conditions showed no remarkable changes. The surface of affected kid-

* This work was supported in part by a Grant-in-aid for Scientific Research from the Ministry of Education, Japan, and the Chiyoda Mutual Life's Subsidiary Fund for Social Welfare Works.
** Department of Pathology, Faculty of Medicine, Kyoto University, Kyoto, Japan

neys was fine granular, and basement membranes of the glomerular capillaries were, in general, thickened and partially necrotic. Arterioles and small arteries also revealed fibrinoid necrosis and cellular hyperplasia, most of which were accompanied by hemorrhages (Fig. 1). These findings correspond to those of malignant hypertension. The walls of medium-sized arteries were, in general, thickened and hyalinized. Kidneys of some animals which survived longer showed so-called thyroid-like change of the tubuli. In SHR of the Fat-Chol.-NaCl group, fat accumulation was observed in the glomeruli.

Table 2 Incidences of pathological changes in the kidneys and heart.

			NaCl			Fat-Chol.-NaCl			
			A	B_2	N	A	B_2	C	N
Kidney		Total Cases	26	17	20	63	29	23	17
	Fibrinoid necrosis	Cases	20	7	0	57	22	20	0
		(%)	(77)	(41)	(0)	(90)	(76)	(87)	(0)
	Hyperplastic arterio-, arteriolo-sclerosis	Cases	19	10	0	54	21	19	0
		(%)	(73)	(59)	(0)	(88)	(72)	(83)	(0)
	Fat accumulation in glomeruli	Cases	0	0	0	26	16	10	1
		(%)	(0)	(0)	(0)	(41)	(55)	(44)	(6)
	Tyroid-like change	Cases	8	2	0	15	10	7	0
		(%)	(31)	(12)	(0)	(24)	(39)	(31)	(0)
Heart		Total Cases	20	13	20	57	29	23	15
	Fibrinoid necrosis	Cases	9	1	0	28	6	11	0
		(%)	(45)	(8)	(0)	(49)	(21)	(48)	(0)
	Hyperplastic arterio-, arteriolo-sclerosis	Cases	6	2	0	22	5	13	0
		(%)	(30)	(15)	(0)	(39)	(17)	(57)	(0)
	Fibrosis	Cases	8	4	2	25	16	11	1
		(%)	(40)	(31)	(10)	(44)	(55)	(48)	(7)
	Diffuse	Cases	7	3	2	22	13	11	0
		(%)	(35)	(23)	(10)	(39)	(45)	(48)	(0)
	Perivascular	Cases	1	1	0	5	3	0	1
		(%)	(5)	(8)	(0)	(9)	(10)	(0)	(7)
	Scar or infarct	Cases	7	5	1	20	7	7	1
		(%)	(35)	(38)	(5)	(35)	(24)	(31)	(7)

N: normal Wistar rats

Significant pathological changes in the kidneys are summarized in Table 2. Incidence of fibrinoid necrosis and cellular hyperplasia of arterioles and small arteries in the NaCl and the Fat-Chol.-NaCl groups were very high in SHR, with the latter groups showing slightly higher incidence. It is a remarkable fact that in the Fat-Chol.-NaCl group about 90 % of animals of substrain A showed fibrinoid necrosis and cellular hyperplasia of the arteries. There were no findings of fibrinoid necrosis and cellular hyperplasia of the arteries in the kidneys of normal Wistar rats.

There was a definite difference in incidence of fibrinoid necrosis and cellular hyperplasia of the arteries between substrains A and B_2, especially in the NaCl group, the former being definitely higher than the latter.

In both groups of SHR, fibrinoid necrosis of the arterioles and small arteries in the kidneys occurred within a short period, mostly between 25 and 100 days after initiation of experimental feedings. In untreated SHR incidence of this change, occurring later than 200 days of age, was less than 10 %.

Macroscopically, the hearts of SHR in the Fat-Chol.-NaCl group were diffusely or locally whitish, especially at the perivascular areas, because of diffuse fat infiltration. In both the NaCl and the Fat-Chol.-NaCl groups, SHRs often revealed white nodules in the myocardium. These nodules correspond microscopically to the foci of cellular hyperplasia of the arterioles and small arteries with scar formation.

Findings of fibrinoid necrosis and hyperplastic arterio- and arteriolo-sclerosis in the heart were frequently observed among SHR of the NaCl and Fat-Chol.-NaCl groups (Fig. 2). In myocardium fibrosis, diffuse or perivascular, fresh as well as old infarcts were often observed (Fig. 3). Fat deposition was demonstrated with Sudan staining in the wall of coronary arteries in the Fat-Chol.-NaCl group of SHR (Fig. 4). In some cases fat infiltration was also observed in the heart muscles as well as in interstitial spaces.

In addition to these findings in the arterioles and small arteries, medium-sized intra-cardiac arteries showed various pathological changes in both the NaCl and the Fat-Chol.-NaCl groups. Many vacuoles were observed in arterial walls which were generally thickened and hyalinized. There was a variety in the size of the nuclei of arterial muscle cells. At hyalinization sites nuclei decreased in number.

Pathological changes in the heart are summarized in Table 2. Incidence of fibrinoid necrosis and cellular hyperplasia of intracardiac arterioles and small arteries in both the NaCl and the Fat-Chol.-NaCl groups was fairly high in SHR, the latter group showing slightly higher incidence. Among substrains A, B_2 and C there was a definite difference in the incidence of fibrinoid necrosis, and hyperplastic changes in arterioles and small arteries. Animals of substrains A and C showed definitely higher incidences of changes than those of substrain B_2. SHRs in both the NaCl and the Fat-Chol.-NaCl groups also showed high incidence of myocardial fibrosis, with incidence in the latter group being slightly higher.

Fibrinoid necrosis of intracardiac arterioles and small arteries occurred in the experimental SHR mostly between 30 and 100 days after initiation of specialized feeding, and 200 days in the untreated SHRs. Incidence of change was less than 10 %. There were also severe circulatory disturbances with high incidence occurring in the brain of SHR in both NaCl and Fat-Chol.-NaCl groups. These cerebral lesions have been reported in a separate paper [6].

In organs such as testes, pancreas, thyroid, adrenal and the wall of the intestinal tract, arterioles and small arteries showed frequent occurrence of cellular hyperplasia and fibrinoid necrosis.

In SHR of the Fat-Chol.-NaCl group, fat deposition was demonstrated in the wall of the aorta, common carotid arteries and renal arteries. Some differences in the fat deposition features between substrains A and B_2 were observed as reported in a separate paper [5]. In general, there was a greater deposition in substrain A. In substrain A, fat deposition was found not only in the intima where fatty substances existed mainly in the macrophages, but also in the medial layer of the above-mentioned arteries. In substrain B_2, fat deposition was localized in the subendothelial macrophages.

THANT [10] observed arteriosclerotic lesions in the common carotid arteries and peripheral arterial trees in SHR fed on a high fat diet; nevertheless the rats are regarded as being resistant to development of atherosclerosis. By comparison, it appears that NaCl loading in addition to a high fat diet accelerates development of atherosclerotic change.

Acceleration of dietary atherosclerosis has been reported in the case of renal hypertensive rats [2, 3, 4]. In these experiments, the process itself which causes hypertension may affect the cardiovascular system. SHR has the advantage that the process can be omitted.

The kidneys were observed electron microscopically in order to study the pathogenesis of extensive changes of the arterioles and small arteries.

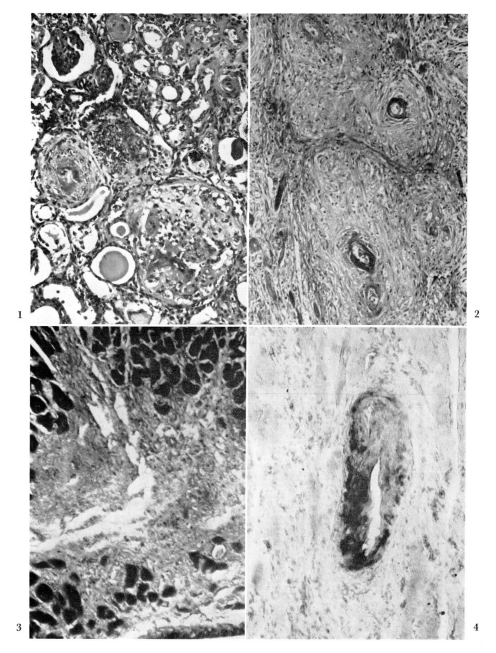

Fig. 1 Fibrinoid necrosis of the glomerular capillaries, arterioles and small arteries as well as cellular hyperplasia with hemorrhage in the kidney.   H.E., × 100.

Fig. 2 Cellular hyperplasia of arterioles and small arteries with fibrinoid necrosis in the heart. Mallory-Azan, × 100.

Fig. 3 An infarct in the heart.   Mallory-Azan, × 100.

Fig. 4 Fat deposition in the wall of coronary artery in the Fat-Chol.-NaCl group of SHR. Sudan III, × 100.

In the control SHR, endothelia of arterioles and small arteries had many small processes, pinocytotic vesicles and somewhat darker cytoplasma than normal rats (Fig. 5).
These findings may suggest that an uptake or transport of substances existing in the blood
is activated in the arterial endothelia. Smooth muscle cells of the arterioles and small
arteries showed occurrence of proliferation (Fig. 6) in 80 days old animals. The proliferated immature muscle cells revealed scanty myofibrils and an increased amount of
organellae, some of them degenerative. The degenerated muscle cells also contained vacuoles and sometimes lamellar structures (Figs. 7, 8). In an advanced stage, some of them
became macrophage-like cells, and others contained electron-dense homogeneous materials and lost their normal cytoplasmic structures. At the site of prominent proliferation
of muscle cells, a mass of immature cells protruded into the arterial lumen, destroying
the normal structure of the internal elastic lamina which splits into several finer elastic
laminae. Subendothelial and intercellular spaces were widened, basement-membrane-
like materials were found deposited. Adventitial fibrocytes increased in number and
contained dilated, rough surfaced endoplasmic reticula with amorphous substances.

In the NaCl group of SHR, similar pathological changes of the arterioles and small
arteries were observed but to a greater extent, with some renal arterioles completely
obstructed (Fig. 9). In the electron-dense, amorphous or granular substances, which
obstructed the arteriolar lumen, degenerated organellae and myofibrils could be recognized. Here cell borders were obscured, and it was impossible to differentiate intercellular
spaces from smooth muscle cells. Less degeneration was seen in neighboring immature
muscle cells.

From these findings, it can be presumed that an excessive uptake of sodium chloride,
conditioned by the hypertensive state or congenital abnormality of the endothelia, results
in toxic effects to the endothelia and newly proliferated muscle cells which appear to be
more susceptible than mature cells. Penetration of plasmal substances from the blood into
the arterial wall as well as destruction of muscle cells could be further accelarated. Consequently, deposition of amorphous substances, probably hyaline, takes place.

SHR fed on a Fat-Chol.-NaCl diet also developed extensive changes in the arterial
walls. Remarkable changes in these animals included proliferation of the smooth muscle
cells as well as adventitial cells, and general widening of the subendothelial and intercellular spaces with fine deposited vesicular or amorphous substances. Smooth muscle
cells showed a variation of cell size, with some greatly affected and often containing electron-dense bodies. Extensively proliferated adventitial cells consisted of fibroblasts and
macrophages with many fat droplets. In cases of fibrinoid necrosis, deposition of fibrin
crystals and cholesterol clefts were observed in the smooth muscle cells. In these cells
normal structure was completely destroyed (Fig. 10). Endothelia of the arterial wall also
showed various degenerative changes.

From the above mentioned findings, it can be presumed that due to abnormalities of
endothelia attributed to the hypertensive state and sodium chloride, the uptake or penetration of fatty substances as well as sodium chloride from the blood into the arterial wall
is accelerated. BELLIVEAU and MARSH [1] reported the fact that incidence of myocardial
and renal infarcts and the degree of fatty deposition in the aortas of rats on a high fat,
atherogenic diet were significantly increased when these rats were given 1 %– 2 % saline
to drink in place of tap water. It is reported by STEPANOVICH and GORE [9] that cholesterol feeding itself also caused an increased permeability of the aortic wall in rabbits.

Penetration of fatty substances seems to depend on proliferation of muscle cells and
sequential destruction of the normal arterial wall structure. This was confirmed by fat
and vital stainings. In the Sudan III preparations fatty substances were demonstrated in

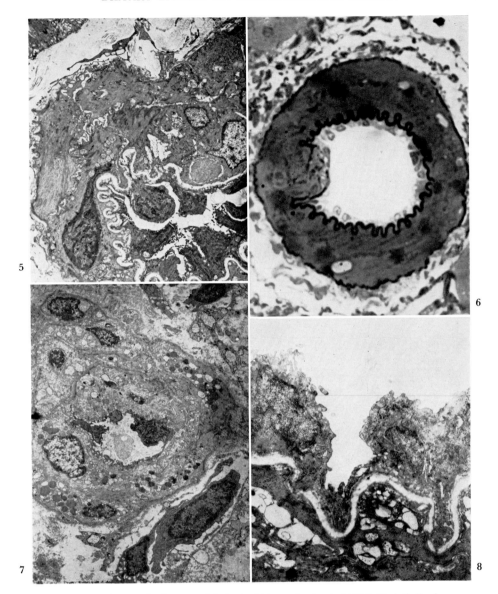

Fig. 5   Electron micrograph of an arteriole in the kidney of untreated SHR. Endothelia show many
         small processes, somewhat darker cytoplasma. Intercellular spaces are widened. × 2,000.
Fig. 6   Proliferation of medial smooth muscle cells of a renal arteriole in an untreated SHR.
         Toluidin blue, × 400.
Fig. 7   Electron micrograph of proliferated immature muscle cells with an increased amount of
         organellas of a renal arteriole in an untreated SHR. × 2,000.
Fig. 8   Electron micrograph of degenerated smooth muscle cells containing vacuoles and lamellar
         structures in a renal arteriole in an untreated SHR. × 5,700.

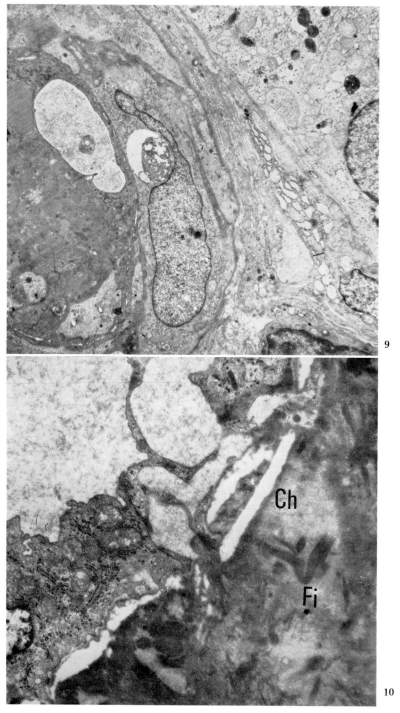

Fig. 9 Electron micrograph of completely occluded arteriole with electron dense amorphous substances which contain degenerated organellas in the kidney of NaCl group of SHR. × 4,000.

Fig. 10 Electron micrograph of cholesterol clefts (Ch) and deposition of fibrin crystals (Fi) in the
wall of renal small artery in an animal in the Fat-Chol.-NaCl group. × 10,000.

the intercellular spaces at the site of muscular proliferation. For the purpose of angiography, animals were perfused with a contrast medium mixed with Berlin Blue. The pigment was observed in the intercellular spaces also at the site of proliferation in the microscopical preparations. It has been reported that there is a close relationship between the destruction of internal elastic lamina and the increased permeability of plasmal substances [7, 8]. The question of whether or not increased penetration of plasmal substances can be attributed to destruction of the elastic lamina remains unclarified

SUMMARY

A test group of SHR given 1 % saline for drinking and another fed on a special high fat diet containing cholesterol plus 1 % salt in their drinking water developed high incidence of fibrinoid necrosis and cellular hyperplasia of the arterioles and small arteries. Extensive changes were observed in the kidneys, hearts, brains, etc.

Definite differences in the incidence of these pathological changes among substrains A, B_2 and C were observed.

Pathogenesis of vascular changes was discussed in light of electron microscopical studies.

REFERENCES

1. BELLIVEAU, R. and MARSH, M. E. (1961): A M A Arch Pathol, **71**, 559.
2. DEMING, Q. B., MORSHACK, E. H., BEVANS, M., DALY, M. M., ABELL, L. L., MARTIN, E., BRUN, L. M., HALPERN, E. and KAPLAN, R. (1958): J exp Med, **109**, 581.
3. EEDES, C. H. Jr., PHILLIPS, G. E., BALUSTEIN, A., HSU, I. C. and SOLBERG, V. B. (1965): Angiologia, **2**, 61.
4. KOLETSKY, S., CAROLYN, R. and RIVERAVELEZ, J. M. (1968): Exp Mol Pathol, **9**, 322.
5. OKAMOTO, K., YAMORI, Y., OOSHIMA, A., PARK, C., HAEBARA, H., MATSUMOTO, M., TANAKA, T., OKUDA, T., HAZAMA, F. and KYOGOKU, M. (1972): *In* "Spontaneous Hypertension" (K. OKAMOTO, ed.), p. 1, Igaku Shoin Ltd., Tokyo.
6. OKAMOTO, K., HAZAMA, F., HAEBARA, H., AMANO, S., TANAKA, T. and OOSHIMA, A. (1972): *In* "Spontaneous Hypertension" (K. OKAMOTO, ed.), p. 129, Igaku Shoin Ltd., Tokyo.
7. OLSEN, F. (1969): Acta Pathol Microbiol Scand, **75**, 527.
8. OONEDA, G., OOYAMA, Y., MATSUYAMA, K., TAKATAMA, M., YOSHIDA, Y., SEKIGUCHI, M. and ARAI, I. (1965): Angiology, **16**, 8.
9. STEFANOVICH, V. and GORE, I. (1971): Exp Mol Pathol, **14**, 20.
10. THANT, M. (1970): Jap Circ J. **34**, 83.

HISTOPATHOLOGICAL STUDY OF LESIONS IN THE CEREBROVASCULAR WALLS OF THE SPONTANEOUSLY HYPERTENSIVE RAT

Y. UMEHARA*, A. SASAKI*, Y. KUDO*
and T. MORI*

A Spontaneously Hypertensive Rat (SHR) was produced by Dr. Okamoto and Aoki [3, 4, 8], and studied seriously by their group.

From the histopathological point of view, a study of the lesion of the vessel wall in the central nervous system, heart, kidney and mesenterium of SHR, will enable us to observe the origin of so-called arteriosclerosis, and to investigate the pathogenesis of cerebrovascular diseases.

There are numerous reports by many researchers on arteriosclerosis and hypertention, which have a close relationship with cerebrovascular diseases.

However, no real cause or process of these pathological changes has yet been clarified.

It is evident that the use of SHR in arteriosclerosis research is very suitable and also more advantageous than the use of autopsy materials for studying vascular changes.

However, the relationship between the changes in the walls of vessels in SHR and arteriosclerosis in man may have to be discussed as a separate subject.

The purpose of this study is to clarify morphologically, the pathological changes and the process of serial changes in the walls of small arteries in the brain, heart, kidney and other organs of SHR, to examine the similarity or dissimilarity of these changes to arteriosclerosis, and to prove the initial changes of so-called arteriosclerosis by histochemical and histopathological method.

MATERIALS AND METHOD

An attempt was made to investigate whether various arteriosclerotic changes like atherosclerosis of peripheral arteries or arterioles, especially of the arteries in the brain, heart and kidney may be produced in SHR by feeding them on 1) a high-fat diet which contained 8 g lard oil (Yuki) in 20 g of stock chow diet (Oriental) for a period of 189 days, 2) a high-glucose diet which contained 18 g of glucose in 20 g of stock chow diet for a period of 123–138 days, 3) a high-fat diet and high-glucose diet which contained 4 g lard oil and 9 g glucose in 20 g of stock chow diet for a period of 123 days and 4) a high-NaCl diet which contained 0.4 g NaCl in 20 g of stock chow diet for a period of 40–50 days.

Histological preparations of semi-ultrathin section [10–13] were stained by a tri-basic or other staining methods to preserve the functional state of the blood vessels.

The experimental rats were divided into three groups; those in the prehypertensive or transitional stage (40 to 50 days old), those in the initial stage (4 to 6 months old) of hypertension, and those in the advanced stage (over one year old).

* Department of Pathology, Institute of Cerebrovascular Diseases, Hirosaki University School of Medicine, Hirosaki, Japan

RESULT

The following detailed pathological changes were observed in the vascular walls of nontreated SHR in the advanced stage of hypertension.

In the advanced stage [9], we noted endothelial cells that degenerated and came off easily with the deformation of these cell bodies, pycnosis, and pathologic changes of the organellas.

The borders among the homogeneous and amorphous layers of the subendothelial layer, basement membrane, and intima became indistinct, the layers themselves became thin and atrophic, and fibrils were observed here.

The most remarkable pathologic change in the vessel walls of peripheral small arteries and arterioles was an inward swelling of a portion of the vessel wall. This pathologic change was observed in the vessel walls of cerebral basilar arteries and central retinal arteries. On account of this swelling, the endothelial cells covering the inside of the walls were pushed into the lumen and then exfoliated.

The histopathologic findings in the swollen vascular walls were disorder, dispersion and disruption of the elastic fiber layers. We observed the abnormal protrusion of the lesions in the walls of these vessels.

In the swollen portions of vessel walls, the conjunction between the intima and media disappeared, and the elastic fibers migrated and colonized in the swollen tissue (Figs. 1, 2).

These lesions of pathologic swelling in vascular walls are called PN (Periarteritis nodosa). In the walls of the mesenteric arteries the following pathologic changes were also found: dispersion, disorder and the removal of the internal elastic fibers, various degeneration, fibrinoid degeneration, atrophy and exfoliation of endothelial cells in the endothelial layer, and collagenization, hyalinisation and fibrous thickening in the basement membrane and subendothelial layers which were sometimes edematous or infiltrated with inflammatory cells.

In particular, various pathologic changes were predominant in the medial muscle cell layer. We are convinced that the changes in the medial cells of arteries are of prime importance in the pathogenesis of arteriosclerosis and various degenerative lesions, and that these cells in the arterial media are the unique type of cells which are probably responsible for the production of collagen, elastin, myofibrils and for the thickning of basement membrane which contains acid muco-polysaccharide.

The vascular walls of the SHR fed on various diets showed the following pathological changes.

1) The effect on SHR of a high-fat diet. Degenerative lesions in the peripheral arteries or arteriosclerotic changes, especially in the arteries of the brain, heart and kidney were produced in SHR fed on a high-fat diet which contained 8 g lard oil in 20 g of stock chow diet for a period of 189 days.

Total cholesterol in the blood of SHR was elevated to 360 mg/dl and average blood sugar to 200 /mg/dl.

Microscopic findings: The appearance of lipid granules in endothelial cells, edematous thickening of vascular walls with many small faci of lipid granules, and the increase of intercellular spaces were found. But neither foamy cells nor atheromatous faci were observed.

In the medial layer, a few lipid ganules were seen, but in the adventitia these deposits were not found.

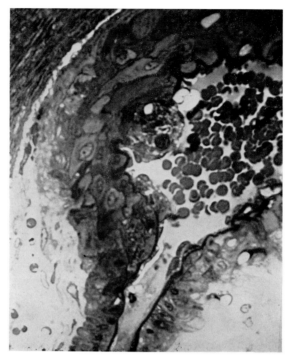

Fig. 1 A portion of the anterior cerebral artery of SHR. Inward swelling o elastic fiber and intimal layer. (Tribasic stain, × 100)

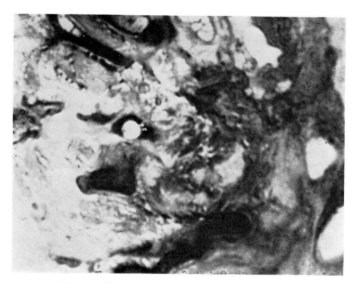

Fig. 2 Higher magnification of the same portion.
Disappearance of normal conjunction of intima and media in inwardly swollen wall. Elastic fibers migrate into swollen tissue. (Tribasic stain, × 1000)

2) The effect on SHR of a high-glucose diet. The necrotic or necrobiotic degenerative changes due to blood plasma infiltration, especially in the peripheral arteriolar wall of the brain, heart and kidney of SHR were produced by feeding them a high-glucose diet which contained 18 g cane sugar in 20 g of stock chow diet for a period of 123–138 days.

Total cholesterol in the blood of SHR in this series averaged 100 mg/dl, and blood sugar averaged 130 mg/dl.

Microscopic findings: In the vessel wall with nodular swelling, all cells of the arterial wall became swollen, turbid and cloudy, and tortuous beading was found in the internal elastic lamellae. The medial smooth muscle cells also become swollen and cloudy without lipid granules.

3) The effect on SHR of a high-fat and high-glucose mixed diet. Total cholesterol in the blood in this series was highest of all, reaching 380 mg/dl. The average blood sugar was 120 mg/dl.

The degenerative changes in peripheral vessel walls were the most severe.

Microscopic findings: The endothelial cells showed considerable degeneration, atrophy and exfoliation, and intimal cells showed a deposition of lipid granules and a cloudy swelling.

The severe pathological changes in internal elastic fibers and medial smooth muscle cells indicated the destruction of the histologic structure of the peripheral vessel walls.

4) The effect on SHR of a high-NaCl diet. The SHR fed on a high-NaCl diet which contained 0.4 g NaCl in 20 g of stock chow diet for a period of 45 to 50 days showed many disturbances such as encephalomalacia and intracerebral bleeding.

Microscopic findings: In the focus of the encephalomalacia in the SHR many small venous bleeding and necrotic foci were found like those in the encephalomalacia of human patients, and so-called fibrinoid degeneration was observed in the arterial walls. The arterial walls become thick and swollen, and showed colliquative necrosis to such a great degree that the lumen of the arteries became narrow and obstructed by thrombi or emboli.

In the surrounding area, many dilated arteries and veins were present, and the phenomenon of venous stagnation was observed.

The cerebral parenchyma consisted of a fine reticular structure with many degenerative nervous cells and phagocytes containing hemosiderin.

These findings suggested that the lesions of colliquative degeneration might have occurred on the bases of old bleeding.

DISCUSSION

We are attempting to examine pathologically the genesis of cerebrovascular disease (so-called cerebral apoplexy), on the basis of the disturbance of blood circulation in the central nervous system.

Compound abnormal phenomena, which are separately and collectively connected with some factors of the blood, the vessels, and blood circulation, have generally been observed as the main subject of this disease.

Some diseases related to this cerebral stroke are hypertension, arteriosclerosis, diabetes mellitus and the other diseases of the heart and kidney.

Basis to these diseases are lesions in the walls of small arteries and arterioles.

In order to obtain accurate finding regarding lesions in vascular walls in the cerebral parenchyma, fresh materials and semi-ultrathin sections prepared from them and stained by spesial stainings are necessary and useful.

We firmly believe that the best experimental animal for this purpose is the SHR (OKAMOTO and AOKI).

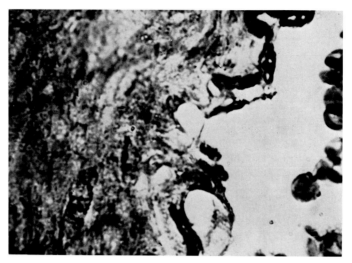

Fig. 3　The other portion of the same case.
Degeration, atrophy and exfoliation of endothelial cells, destruction and disappearance of internal elastic lamellae, and severe degeneration of medial smooth
muscle layer. (Azan stain, × 1000)

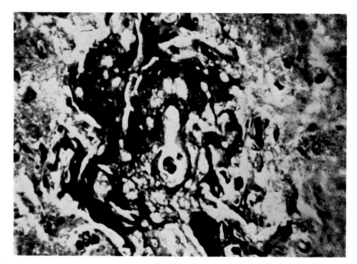

Fig. 4　In the surrounding area, many dilated arteries and vein are present.
The cerebral parenchyma consists of a fine reticular structure with many degenerative nervous cells and phagocytes containing hemosidirine. The swollen and
fibrinoid necrotic arterial wall in the encephalomalacic focus of cerebral parenchyma of SHR. (Luxol fast blue stain, × 400)

Spontaneous hypertension in SHR is similar to essential hypertension in human beings,
but many difficult problems of hormonal functions, catecholamine, and others must be
studied. Therefore, we can not state positively that the experimental results obtained from
SHR are exactly like the vascular lesions in human beings.

The lesions in arterial walls in the 3 stages—the pre-hypertensive, the initial, and the
advanced—seem most likely to be produced under the influence of hypertension.

We studied histopathologically the pathogenesis of the swelling of arterial walls in the advanced stage and obtained the following conclusions:

It is evident that each layer of the vascular wall is affected by much mechanical change in blood circulation and a rise in blood pressure for a long time after birth. The influences of alteration in circulation and biochemical components of blood on medial smooth muscle layer and internal elastic lamellae have been regarded as important factors by many researchers.

It seems that together with the regressive and progressive lesions in the medial smooth muscle cells the various thickening or swelling of intima occur to strengthen the affected arterial wall. However, it is our opinion that the injury to the intima caused by the un-usual blood quality or flow, and the abnormal permeation or deposition of blood plasma are not the initial cause of the vascular lesions.

The mechanical effect on the medial smooth muscle layer of the changes in blood flow and the rise in blood pressure should be the gradual thickening and swelling of the vascular walls. The gradual increase in permeability of the wall may play an important role in the lesions in vascular walls in the later stage.

The increased permeability makes unusual blood components, such as excessive fat and triglyseride permiate easily into the wall and accumulate there.

As to the adaptive behaviour of medial smooth muscle cells, WISSLER [14], POOLE [9] and ONEDA [6] observed it and stated that the muscle cells might play an important role in the pathogenesis of cerebrovascular disease and other arterial lesions.

As to the genesis of the experimental encephalomalacic focus in SHR fed with a high-NaCl diet [2, 5], we examined the details, and obtained the histopathological findings of the focus; the bleeding focus primarily occurs in the small arteries and arterioles, and this nectoric focus becomes gradually enlarged into encephalomalacia, which is brought about by the subsequent ischemia due to the obstruction of the more proximal arteries. The resultant ischemia is the cause of experimental encephalomalacia.

The bleeding focus in the cerebral parenchyma at an advanced stage in the dietary treatment may be due to the unusual blood flow that is occasioned by the occlusion of the vascular lumen because of the thickening and swelling of vascular walls, and red infarc-tion may be seen in the case of venous bleeding.

Investigation concerning the lesions in cerebral circulation is very important. They may be related to the etiological influence of hypertension, to diabetes mellitus and hyper-glycemia or to abnormal saccharide metabolism.

When a pathological examination of cerebrovascular diseases is made, the importance of hypertension and abnormal saccharide metabolism should be kept in mind.

SUMMARY

We observed vascular lesions in SHR in relation to aging and 3 stages of hypertension (the pre-hypertensive, initial, and advance stages) and then noted the following findings which seem to have resulted from the influence of rising blood pressure.

1) The swelling and edematous thickening of blood vessel walls, the homogeneous and uniform structure of subendothelial layers, including the basement membrane of endothe-lial cells, and an increase in quantity or an alteration in comporment of the fluid in the intercellular apace.

2) The nodular swelling of blood vessel walls, the dispersion, dissolution and dis-appearance of internal elastic lamellae and, the degeneration, atrophy, migration and proliferation of medial smooth muscle cells.

The experimental studies on the vascular walls of SHR fed on a high-fat diet, a high-glucose diet, and two metabolic mixed diets indicated that the pathological changes were similar to atherosclerosis and angionecrosis.

The findings obtained from the NaCl-diet experiment very much resemble the encephalomalacia accompanying cerebral hemorrhage in human beings. This cerebral hemorrhage in SHR indicates that the hemorrhage took place because of cerebroangionecrosis and a break in the vascular walls.

But we can not definitely regard some experimental effects of these nutritive factors as the pathogenesis of cerebrovascular diseases in human beings, and we are unable to negate absolutely the relation between many pathogenic conditions of human cerebral stroke and the encephalomalacic lesions in SHR.

REFERENCES

1. OKAMOTO, K. and AOKI, K. (1963): Jap Circ J, **27**, 282.
2. TAKEDA, T. TABEI, R., HASHIMOTO, Y., NOSAKA, S., FUKUSHIMA, M., YAMABE, H., MAMORI, Y., ICHISHIMA, K., HAEBARA, H., MATSUMOTO, M., MARUYAMA, T., SUZUKI, Y. and TAMEGAI, M. (1966): Saishin-Igaku, **21**, 1881 (in Japanese).
3. OKAMOTO, K., AOKI, K., NOSAKA, S. and FUKUSHIMA, M. (1964): Jap Circ J, **28**, 943.
4. UMEHARA, Y., KIMURA, T. and MORI, T. (1970): Blood and Vessel, **1**, 1233.
5. UMEHARA, Y. and MORI, T. (1969): Jap J Const Med, **32**, 73.
6. UMEHARA, Y. and MORI, T. (1970): Jap J Const Med, **33**, 20.
7. UMEHARA, Y. and MORI, T. (1971): Jap J Const Med, **34**, 55.
8. WISSLER, R. W. (1968): J Atheroscler Res, **8.**, 201.
9. POOLE, J. C. F., CROMWELL, S. B. and BENDITT, E. P. (1971): Am J Pathol, **62**, 391.
10. JELLINEK, H. (1970): Angiology, **21**, 636.
11. ONEDA, G., YOSHIDA, Y. and SUZUKI, K. (1971): J Jap College Angiology, **11**, 197.
12. OKAMOTO, K. TANAKA, T., BOKU, S. and HAZAMA, M. (1971): Jap J Const Med, **34**, 57
13. UMEHARA, Y. (1970): Geriatr Med, **8**, 201.
14. KOBAYASHI, I. (1971): Jap J Geriatr, **8**, 158.

LIFE-SPAN, HEMATOLOGICAL ABNORMALITIES, THROMBOSIS AND OTHER MACROSCOPICAL LESIONS IN THE SPONTANEOUSLY HYPERTENSIVE RATS

A. NAGAOKA*, K. KIKUCHI*, H. KAWAJI*
T. MATSUO* and Y. ARAMAKI*

Previously it was reported that the male spontaneously hypertensive rats (SHR) maintained on a standard diet for a long term died a spontaneous death from cardiovascular decompensation manifested by systemic edema, hydrothorax, ascites, and thrombus formation in the hepatic veins, mesenteric arteries and left atrium [8]. However, no abnormality in blood coagulation or viscosity was demonstrated in this strain of rats at any stage of development [10]. The appearance of an abnormal glycoprotein in the plasma of SHR at advanced ages was found to correlate roughly with the progression of hypertension [7]. Moreover, in the hepatic vein, which is the preferential site of the thrombus formation, the histopathological observation by means of a scanning electronmicroscope demonstrated a process of platelet aggregation on the wall of the vessels before the completion of the thrombus formation. In this process of observation a number of platelet adhesions, aggregation of platelets with other cellular elements such as erythrocytes and leucocytes, and a severe occlusive deposition of blood cells in the lumen of small branches of the hepatic veins followed by the thrombus formation at the orifices were observed. Electron microscopic study of the hepatic vein indicated swelling of the endothelial cells, loosening of the cellular junctions, and dilatation of subendothelial space, with proliferation of collagen fibers, all of which are considered to be precursory lesions of the thrombus formation [3].

The present report deals with more detailed observations of life-span and pathological changes in the SHR of both sexes, and the effect of cholesterol feeding on the formation of thrombus.

METHODS

Macroscopical abnormalities in relation to the advance of hypertension. The SHR of F_{20} and F_{21} as well as their original strain, the normotensive Wistar rats, all weaned at the age of 4 weeks and reared under the specific pathogen free (SPF) condition, were used. Five to 7 rats kept in a metal mesh cage were allowed free access to the commercial diet (Niphon CLEA, CE-2) and drinking water previously vapor-sterilized. Though the animals exhibited no abnormality in general conditions until 10 months of age, thereafter systemic edema, respiratory difficulty, and marked decrease in body weight occurred. Many of the moribund animals were laparotomized under anesthesia with ether and the blood sample was taken from the abdominal aorta with a syringe containing a minute amount of heparin for biochemical examinations. The severity of abnormalities at autopsy was assessed macroscopically and described as a grade from zero to 3.

Feeding with high cholesterol diet. The 20 SHR and 20 normotensive Wistar rats at the age of 2 months were divided into treated and control groups respectively. The treated

* Biological Research Laboratories, Research and Development Division, Takeda Chemical Industries, Ltd. Osaka, Japan

groups consisting of 12 rats of each strain were maintained on a cholesterol diet (diet A) containing 2 % cholesterol, 0.5 % cholic acid, 0.15 % propylthiouracil and 97.35 % standard diet, and another cholesterol diet (diet B) which differed from the former in lacking propylthiouracil. These 2 kinds of diets were alternately administered at intervals of 1 to 2 months for 14 months, while, the control groups of both strains, each consisting of 8 rats, were fed only on the standard diet. Three animals in each cholesterol-fed group, and 2 in each control group were sacrificed 6 months after the start of the experiment in order to determine the progression of pathological changes, and the remaining animals were sacrificed at the end of 14 feeding months. The blood pressure of the tail artery was measured by a microphonic method [9] 2 to 3 days before every exchange in diet and the blood sampled from the tail vein by tail-end clipping was used for the estimation of lipids. Total cholesterol in the plasma was measured following the method of ABELL et al. [4] and triglycerides were measured by use of the specific kit (WAKO). The body weight and food-intake for 24 hours were measured once a week.

   Disk electrophoresis of plasma protein and quantitative analysis of plasma albumin. Following the method of DAVIS [2], plasma in volume of 4 μl was submitted to electrophoresis for 2 hours at 2 mA/tube in 7.5 % polyacrylamide gel at pH 8.3 and the protein fractions thus obtained were stained with Amido Black 10B. The total protein and the albumin in the plasma were measured following the methods of LOWRY et al. [6] and CHEN and SHARTON [1], respectively. The amounts of the abnormal protein present in the plasma of SHR were scored, according to the size and the density of the electrophoretic band, into 5 grades. Since this protein is located after the albumin band, it is referred to as post-albumin in this text.

RESULTS

1. Life-span and macroscopical pathological changes

   The spontaneous death and moribund condition in the SHR occurred at 10 months of age and after. As shown in Fig. 1, the mortality rate of the SHR until 15 months of

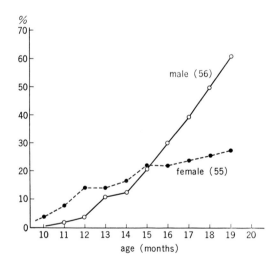

Fig. 1 Mortality rate in the SHR fed on standard diet for a long term under the specific pathogen free condition. The control Wistar rats showed no death during the same observation period. Numerals in parentheses refer to number of rats studied.

age was slightly higher in the females than in the males. However, the number of males showing systemic edema and respiratory difficulty from hydrothorax increased progressively thereafter. Consequently, in the SHR the mortality rate in the males increased more markedly than in the females, while none of the 35 female and 73 male normotensive Wistar rats died during the same observation period.

The incidence of pathological abnormalities in 43 male SHR that died or were sacrificed within 18 months of age was as follows. Cardiac hypertrophy or dilatation was observed in all SHR, and whitish or dark necrotic lesions were present on the pericardial surface of the ventricles in 30 % of these animals. The nephrosclerosis with uneven surface was present in 95 % of the rats. The bead-like aneurysma (94 %) in the mesenteric arteries with thrombi seemed to progress from the peripheral site to the central site, and most of these thrombi were organized. The incidence of thrombus formation in other sites was 68 % in the left atrium, 61 % in the hepatic vein and 80 % in one of these sites. Many of these thrombi were whitish in color, but red thrombi were also frequently observed. The thrombosis in the cardiovascular system was accompanied with systemic edema (68 %), hydrothorax (82 %), ascites (58 %), and congestion in the liver (83 %). On the other hand, in the case of the female SHR, 22 of the 26 SHR died suddenly without showing any sign of cardiovascular decompensation such as systemic edema, hydrothorax and respiratory embarrassment, but the remaining 4 animals showed such decompensation signs. Moreover, severe hemorrhage in the thoracic or peritoneal cavity and also at the subcutaneous site of the thorax was observed in many of the females which died suddenly. These hemorrhages were not observed in the male SHR. The localized bleeding in the corpus callosum and the subcortical structures of the brain was present in 3 of the 32 males and in one of the 8 females examined.

Since the lethal course was somewhat different in the male and female SHR as mentioned above, the pathological abnormalities in both sexes were macroscopically compared at various ages. The incidence of the cardiovascular lesions was slightly more frequent in the males than in the females at the age of 7 months, but in the higher age it was of equal frequency in both sexes. In contrast with these vascular lesions, the incidence of edema and thrombus formation in the hepatic vein, left atrium or mesenteric arteries was higher in the males than in the females at all ages from 7 to 22 months.

2. Effects of the cholesterol feeding on the thrombus formation

The feeding of animals with the cholesterol diet A containing propylthiouracil caused a reduction in both body weight and blood pressure in both SHR and normotensive Wistar rats. However feeding with diet B restored the reduced weight and blood pressure to their control level. The maintenance of both strains on the cholesterol diets also retarded the progression of hypertension, although the blood pressure of the SHR treated with cholesterol diets was in the range from 170 to 190 mm Hg after 7 months. The range was markedly higher than the 110 to 130 mm Hg of the treated or untreated Wistar rats.

As shown in Fig. 2, though the plasma cholesterol level in the SHR and Wistar rats fed with the control diet rose gradually with aging, the level in the SHR was always lower than that in the Wistar rats. The feeding on diet A markedly and consistently elevated the cholesterol level in both strains, but the elevated level fell again as a result of diet B. The plasma triglyceride level in control groups of both strains showed no differences until the 10th month of the feeding period, but the level of SHR only rose markedly thereafter. However, though the triglyceride level in both strains treated with the cholesterol diets was slightly decreased by diet A and restored by diet B, the elevation of the level observed in control SHR was prevented by the treatment.

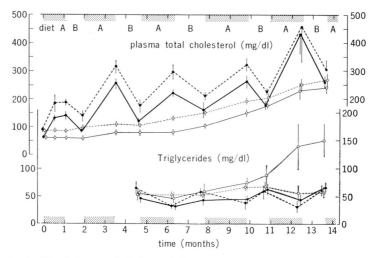

Fig. 2 The influence of cholesterol diets on plasma total cholesterol and tri-glycerides of the SHR and normotensive Wistar rats. Two kinds of cholesterol diets (A and B) were alternately administered for 14 months. The solid and dotted lines show the values for the SHR and Wistar rats, and the thick and thin lines show the values for the rats treated with cholesterol and standard diets, respectively. Results are mean ± standard deviations.

In 3 of the 6 SHR fed with the control diet, whose plasma triglyceride level rose at a later period, systemic edema and thrombus formation developed (Table 1). Quite un-expectedly, however, no systemic edema or thrombus formation were found in the groups fed with the cholesterol diets. The other cardiovascular changes were also retarded slightly in the treated SHR group. In the normotensive Wistar rats no cardiovascular changes or thrombus formation were observed. Other findings at autopsy in the animals of both strains of rats sacrificed at 6 and 14 months after the start of the experiment were hypertrophy of the thyroid glands and fatty deposition in the liver.

Table 1 Macroscopical autopsy findings in the SHR fed with cholesterol and standard diets for 14 months.

Kind of diet	SHR fed with cholesterol diets									SHR fed with standard diet					
Rat No.	1	2	3	4	5	6	7	8	9	1	2	3	4	5	6
Cardiac hypertrophy	+	+	+	+	++	+	+	+	++	++	++	++	+	++	++
Nephrosclerosis	+	−	−	−	++	++	+	−	+	++	++	+	+	+	+
Bead-like changes in mesenteric arteries	−	++	+	+	+++	++	+++	+	++	+	+++	+++	+	+	+
Thrombosis in left atrium	−	−	−	−	−	−	−	−	−	+++	−	+	−	−	+++
Thrombosis in hepatic vein	−	−	−	−	−	−	−	−	−	+++	−	+	−	−	+++
Systemic edema	−	−	−	−	−	−	−	−	−	+++	−	+++	−	−	+++
Hydrothorax	−	−	−	−	−	−	−	−	−	+++	−	+++	−	−	+
Ascites	−	−	−	−	−	−	−	−	−	+++	−	+	−	−	+
Congestion in liver	−	−	−	−	−	−	−	−	−	++	+	+++	−	−	+

−: no lesion, +: slight, ++: mild, +++: severe

3. Relationship between post-albumin content and pathological changes

The post-albumin appeared markedly in the plasma of the SHR of either sex at 10 months of age and after. Its contents were found to be correlated positively with the severity of nephrosclerosis and bead-like changes in the mesenteric arteries, and negatively with the ratio of albumin/globulin in the plasma. Though the post-albumin in the plasma was present in all of the 23 SHR with vascular thrombosis, the contents of the post-albumin did not correlate with the extent of the thrombosis. The post-albumin was also detected in some of the SHR without the thrombosis.

DISCUSSION

Even under the SPF environment the life-span of SHR was significantly shorter than that of the normotensive Wistar rats. The male SHR succumbed mainly to the thrombosis in the cardiovascular system but the female SHR died suddenly from extensive capillary hemorrhage in the thoracic or peritoneal cavity. These differences in reaction in the sexes can not be explained clearly from the results of the present experiment, because the progression of the hypertension and the feeding conditions were not significantly different between the male and female SHR. One possible explanation is that since in our behavioral studies [12] on the SHR the sensitivity in response, such as escape or vocalization, to external stimuli was higher in the females than in the males, a variety of stress stimuli seems to activate the endocrine functions more strongly in the females than in the males, and finally leads to adrenal dysfunction and sudden death with hemorrhage. Another is that the susceptibility of the males to thrombosis as well as to stress stimuli is different from that of the females, since the preferential occurrence of thrombosis in the male animals has been reported by WILSON et al. [13] and RENAUD [11] as being induced by the dietary factor.

It has been indicated by KOLETSKY et al. [5] and other many investigators that the feeding of experimental hypertensive rats with high cholesterol or fat diet facilitates the development of atherosclerosis. In the present experiment we could not demonstrate any acceleration of the thrombus formation in the SHR fed with high cholesterol diets. Though the cholesterol level in the plasma was not so high in this experiment, the level in the SHR fed with the cholesterol diets was higher than that in the animals fed with the standard diet. So, as far as the present studies are concerned, it is concluded that the plasma cholesterol in the SHR was not involved in the progression of hypertension nor in the occurrence of the thrombus formation. However, the maintenance of the male SHR on the standard diet produced a rather abrupt and progressive rise in plasma level of triglycerides at a later stage. Therefore, this increased level of triglycerides might be a contributing cause to the thrombus formation. Moreover, these facts seem to suggest that abnormal lipid metabolism occurs in the SHR at advanced ages.

The enlargement of the thyroid glands probably reflecting the effect of propylthiouracil contained in cholesterol diet A was demonstrated by the present study. The depression of the thyroid activity by propylthiouracil is quite likely to produce the retardation of the adrenal and cardiovascular decompensation, since the presence of hyperthyroidism in the SHR has already been reported by YAMABE [14]. Therefore, the pathological significance of the post-albumin in plasma as well as the mechanism of thrombus formation and platelet aggregation in the SHR sould also be studied in relation to the thyroid function.

SUMMARY

The purpose of this paper was to investigate the life-span and pathological changes in the SHR of both sexes in more detail, and the effects of cholesterol feeding on the thrombus formation.

The life-span of the SHR was significantly shorter than that of the control Wistar rats even under the specific pathogen free condition. The mortality rate of SHR at 18 months of age was 50 % in 56 males and 25 % in 55 females, while control Wistar rats showed no death during the same observation period. Autopsy of these male SHR disclosed the following incidence of pathological abnormalities: cardiac hypertrophy (100 %), nephrosclerosis (95 %), bead-like changes in mesenteric arteries (94 %), systemic edema (68 %), and thrombosis in the hepatic vein (61 %) and the left atrium (68 %). Most of the female SHR died suddenly mainly of intraperitoneal or intrathoracic hemorrhage.

The SHR fed on cholesterol diets for 14 months did not show systemic edema, thrombosis or death, but in 50 % of the SHR fed on a control diet thrombosis was detected. This finding suggests that the plasma cholesterol in the SHR is not involved in the progression of hypertension nor in the occurrence of thrombus formation, and that the depression of thyroid activity by propylthiouracil contained in the cholesterol diet is likely to produce retardation of the cardiovascular decompensation manifested by systemic edema and thrombus formation.

REFERENCES

1. CHEN, H. P. and SHARTON, H. (1963): Am J Clin Pathol, **40**, 651.
2. DAVIS, B. J. (1964): Ann N Y Acad Sci, **121**, 404.
3. KAWAJI, H., NAGAOKA, A., TSUKUDA, R., MIURA, I. and FUKUI, H. (1971): Jap J Constitut Med, **34**, 59.
4. ABELL, L. L., LEVY, B. B., BRODIE, B. B. and KENDALL, F. H. (1952): J Biol Chem, **195**, 357.
5. KOLETSKY, S., ROLAND, C. and RIVERA-VELEZ, J. M. (1968): Exp Mol Pathol, **9**, 322.
6. LOWRY, O. H., ROSEBROUGH, N. J., FARR, A. L. and RANDALL, R. J. (1951): J Biol Chem, **193**, 265.
7. MATSUO, T., NAGAOKA, A., MORISHITA, K. and SUZUOKI, Z. (1971): Jap J Constitut Med, **34**, 44.
8. NAGAOKA, A., KAWAJI, H., IMAI, Y. and FUKUI, H. (1970): Jap J Pharmacol, **20**, 509.
9. NAGAOKA, A., KIKUCHI, K. and ARAMAKI, Y. (1970): Jap Circ J, **34**, 489.
10. NAGAOKA, A., SUDO, K., ORITA, S., KIKUCHI, K. and ARAMAKI, Y. (1971): Jap Circ J, **35**, 1379.
11. RENAUD, S. (1965): J Atheroscler Res, **5**, 43.
12. SHIMAMOTO, K. and NAGAOKA, A. (1972): *In* "Spontaneous Hypertension" (K. OKAMOTO, ed.), p. 86, Igaku Shoin Ltd., Tokyo.
13. WILSON, J. L., ASHBURN, A. D. and WILLIAMS, W. L. (1971): Anat Rec, **168**, 331.
14. YAMABE, S. (1970): Jap Circ J, **34**, 233.

FURTHER STUDIES ON THE CARDIOVASCULAR SYSTEM IN SPONTANEOUSLY HYPERTENSIVE RAT

M. KYOGOKU*a), H. HAEBARA*, A. OOSHIMA*, Y. YAMORI*, S. IKEHARA*, T. OHTA**, T. OKUDA* and K. OKAMOTO*

It was reported by us [3, 6, 12] that not only morphological but also chemical or functional abnormalities could be found in the vascular system of SHR during the course of hypertensive state. We are going to present, here, the several further observations about the vascular abnormalities of spontaneously hypertensive rats (SHR).

Reactivity of the cerebral basilar artery of SHR against barium chloride.

SHR and Wistar-Kyoto (WK) as a control around 4–8 months of age were mostly used for the experiments. Under Nembutal (pentobarbital) anesthesia, (40 mg/kg i.p.), cerebral basilar artery and some of their branches were exposed and 2.5% barium chloride dropped on the vascular wall.

Usually, prompt narrowing of the arteries occurred, and after washing out the barium chloride, two phases of dilatation followed, the early transient type and the delayed rather continuous type.

The grade of narrowing of the basilar artery was around 34–35% of the original width in Wistar-Kyoto (WK) and 44–47% in SHR.

About the vasodilatation (V.D.), in WK 44% of the animals showed the early V.D. mostly in their branches, and 27% of the WK showed late V.D. mostly in their basilar arterial stems. However, in SHR, *only one* animal showed delayed V.D. and *none* showed the early transient type of V.D. Comparing the grade of these two kinds of vascular reactivity of SHR with that of WK, *either* of the reactions, contraction and dilatation, are *weaker* in SHR. In other words, the wall of the basilar artery of the spontaneously hypertensive rat does not function as much as that of the normotensive rat, Wistar-Kyoto.

By such a gross observation, no remarkable changes were observed in the wall of the basilar artery at this age. However, histopathologically already some muscular hypertrophy and partial fibrosis of the media were seen in the basilar artery.

Histometrical examination of cardiovascular system of SHR

Heart weight, cross-sectional luminar area of the aorta, thickness of aortic wall were measured.

The heart weight is significantly greater in SHR even on the 40th day after birth, and increases more with age.

It was revealed that the thickening of the aortic wall was more severe in the proximal part of the aorta, and the dilatation also started from the proximal part of aorta and these thickenings already started at an early age.

As was reported previously [3], the mean and minimal luminal diameter of the jejunal small arteries and arterioles in SHR were significantly smaller than WK in the range of 70–85% of the control diameters.

* Department of Pathology, Faculty of Medicine, Kyoto University, Kyoto, Japan.
  Present address:
*a)Department of Pathology, Kobe University School of Medicine, Kobe, Japan.
** Department of Neurosurgery, Osaka City University Medical School, Osaka, Japan.

When the ratio of the jejunal arterial diameter to the aortic luminal area was taken, the ratio was always lower in SHR than WK and the rate of decrease with age was greater in SHR. This might be one of the morphological evidences that the peripheral vascular flow resistance is greater in SHR even in their early stage of hypertension.

Enzymatic activity in the vascular wall of SHR [10, 11]

The activity of five kinds of enzyme, alkaline phosphatase [1], acid phosphatase [1], lactic dehydrogenase [2], malic dehydrogenase [5] and glucose-6-phosphate (G-6-P) dehydrogenase [4] were examined in the saline extract of the mesenteric arteries, aorta and heart of SHR at various ages.

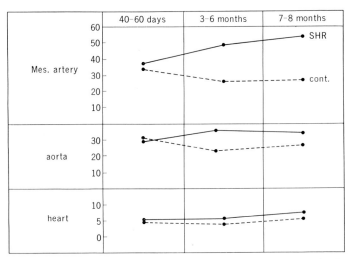

Fig. 1 Alkaline phosphatase activity of the cardiovascular system in SHR. Activity is expressed as μM of the product per mg of protein per hour (BESSEY et al.'s method [1]).

Among them, the most remarkable phenomenon was observed in the activity of alkaline phosphatase (ALP). On the basis of activity per unit protein, the ALP in mesenteric arteries of WK *decreased* (gradually) with age; on the contrary, that of SHR *increased* with age. Those were very high contrasts. The same tendency to a lesser degree was seen in the aorta (Fig. 1). Acid phosphatase in mesenteric as well as aortic arterial walls was higher in SHR but the tendency to decrease with age was almost the same as WK. The G-6-P dehydrogenase activity in the aorta and lactic dehydrogenase in the heart was significantly higher in SHR.

Alkaline phosphatase which may be related to the metabolism of active phosphorous compounds including ATP, and acid phosphatase, a lysosome enzyme, may have some relation to the activity of cyclic AMP, both having a close relation to the activity of muscle cells or some receptors in the vascular wall.

As was mentioned before, in F_{23}–F_{25} generations, SHR of 40 days after birth are not *pre*hypertensive, but are already early hypertensive, showing around 140 mm Hg of blood pressure. Thus, all of those phenomena seemed to start at the early development of hypertension.

YAMORI and OKAMOTO did find congenital abnormalities in the isozyme pattern of esterase in the kidney and liver of SHR [13]. The co-dominant transmission of this isozyme was clearly demonstrated in the hybrid F_1 and F_2. About the esterase activity of the vascular bed, four esterase isozymes were demonstrated in the saline extract of the mesenteric artery and the aorta. The two bands of slow electrophoretic movability of vascular extract from SHR, always moved much slower than those from WK.

And in our preliminary experiments, the saline extract of the mesenteric arteries of the F_1 hybrid obtained between SHR and WK, demonstrated those 4 bands, two of each from both parental strains, on the starch. It may imply the existence of some genetic enzymatic abnormalities in the vasculature of SHR, as a basis of morphological or functional alterations of blood vessels.

Vascular changes and the disc electrophoresis pattern of serum

Twelve to fifteen discs were detectable on the polyacrylamide gel electrophoretic patterns of rat serum. The disc pattern of the serum of SHR was roughly the same as that of WK. However, in some line of SHR, we call it substrain A, α_1-1 globulin or socalled postalbumine was quite dark even in their early hypertensive (40-days-old) stage. This component was strongly PAS positive and weakly alcian blue positive, and the amount of this component increased more and more with age.

Besides, when some treatment on the body of SHR was applied, such as cholesterol feeding, high sodium dieting and sensitization with antigen, this α_1-1 component in any SHR substrain increased more even in their early stage of life (Fig. 2). We checked the correlation between plasma cholesterol level and the amount of α_1-1 globulin but failed to find the correlation. "The saline alone" group sometimes showed a very high level of α_1-1 globulin. Perhaps "sodium" might be more important to the increment of α_1-1 globulin.

When we checked the tissue changes of the animals showing high α_1-1 globulin contents, we noticed the high percentage of vascular fibrosis, granulation, diffuse fibrosis, basophilic degeneration, and thrombi in the heart as well as in the kidney. The grade of

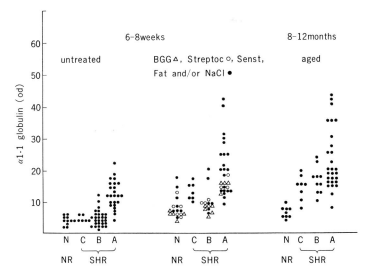

Fig. 2 Serum α_1-1 globulin in SHR substrains. Effect of aging, dietary conditions (high fat-cholestral diet and/or 1% sodium chloride in drinking water) and sensitization with antigens (bovine gamma globulin (BGG) or Streptococcus type A6).

such histologic changes was rated from grade 1 to 3, and these ratings were summed for each animal and plotted with α_1-1 globulin content on the chart. Very high correlations existed between α_1-1 globuline content and tissue fibrosis. Here again, "A" substrain had higher α_1-1 globulin and more fibrosis than "B" or other groups (Fig. 3). But there was no correlation between α_1-1 globulin contents and the angionecrosis or bleeding.

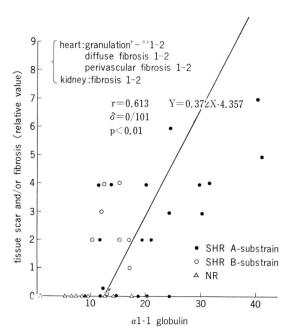

Fig. 3 Correlation between serum α_1-1 globulin level and the grade of tissue scar and/or fibrosis. Ordinate shows the sum of the grades of the findings in the heart and kidney of individual rats.

SUMMARY

Several further observations about the vascular abnormalities of SHR were presented. Reactivity of the cerebral basilar artery of SHR against barium chloride was less than that of Wistar-Kyoto. Histometrical examination of cardiovascular system of SHR revealed that the peripheral vascular flow resistance was greater in SHR even in their early stage of hypertension.

Alkaline phosphatase activity in the mesenteric artery and aorta was always higher in SHR than Wistar-Kyoto, and besides, in SHR it increased with age where that of Wistar-Kyoto decreased. The activities of acid phosphatase, G-6-P dehydrogenase, and lactic dehydrogenase were higher in SHR by case. The isozyme pattern of esterase of the saline extract from mesenteric artery and aorta in SHR was congenitally different from that of control rat Wistar-Kyoto. The amount of α_1-1 globulin or post albumin component of the serum in SHR had a high correlation with the grade of fibrosis or tissue damage around the vasculature. Substrain A of SHR showed the highest amount of this component.

REFERENCES

1. BESSEY, O. A., LOWRY, O. H. and BROCK, M. J. (1946): J Biol Chem, **164**, 321.
2. HILL, B. R. (1956): Cancer Res, **16**, 460.
3. ICHIJIMA, K. (1969): Jap Circ J, **33**, 785.
4. KORNBERG, A. and HORECKER, B. L. (1955): *In* "Methods in Enzymology" (COLOWICK, S. P. and KAPLAN, N. O. eds.), Vol 1, p. 323, Academic Press, New York.
5. NEILANDS, J. B. (1955): *In* "Methods in Enzymology" (COLOWICK, S. P. and KAPLAN, N. O. eds.), Vol. 1 p 449 Academic Press, New York.
6. NOSAKA, S., YAMORI, Y., OHTA, T. and OKAMOTO, K. (1972): *In* " Spontaneous Hypertension" (OKAMOTO, K ed.), p. 67 Igaku Shoin Ltd., Tokyo.
7. OHTA, T., NISHIMURA, S. and OKAMOTO, K. (1972): Jap J Const Med, **36**, in press.
8. OKAMOTO, K. (1969): *In* "International Review of Pathology" (G. W. RICHTER and M. A. EPSTEIN, eds.), Vol. 7, p. 227, Academic Press, New York.
9. OKAMOTO, K., AOKI, K., NOSAKA, S. and FUKUSHIMA, M. (1964): Jap Circ J, **28**, 943.
10. OOSHIMA, A. (1972): Jap Circ J. **36**, in press.
11. OOSHIMA, A, YAMORI, Y., OKUDA, M. and OKAMOTO K. (1972): Jap J Const Med, **36**, in press.
12. TABEI, R. (1966): Jap Circ J, **30**, 717.
13. YAMORI, Y. and OKAMOTO, K. (1970): Lab Invest, **22**, 206.

ON THE FUNDUS OF SPONTANEOUSLY HYPERTENSIVE RATS

S. TAKAHASHI*

The essential changes of the ocular fundus in hypertension have been reported by many researchers [1, 2, 4, 5, 8, 11].

In spontaneously hypertensive rats, which are generally regarded to resemble human patients with essential hypertension [7], the fundus changes have been sequentially observed in the 14th through 18th generations. Also, the histological studies [3] of retinal arterioles, sometimes with the aids of the trypsin digestion method [9] and the electron microscope [10], were performed especially in relation to cerebral hemorrhage. The present report deals with the results of my experiments up to date.

EXPERIMENTAL METHOD

The fundus was observed by an ophthalmoscope, without anesthetising the animal, with the pupil dilated by mydrin P (Tropicamide + Phenylephrine hydrochloride). After this observation the animal was killed and the organs were subjected to the following histopathological examinations. Eyes and other organs were extracted and fixed in 10 per cent formalin. Most eyes were embedded in paraffin but some eyes were digested by trypsin according to the Kuwabara-Cogan's method [6]. The paraffin-embedded specimens were sectioned (5 microns in thickness) and the stained with H. E., Elastica van Gieson and PAS.

RESULTS OF EXPERIMENTS

The ratio of the caliber of retinal arterioles and their accompanying veins was 1:3 to 2:3 at the prehypertensive stage in SHR, while it was 1:3 to 1:4 in the hypertensive stage. During the period of progressive blood pressure elevation, the blood vessels sometimes exhibited an alternating appearance of wide and narrow portions. When the blood pressure was stabilized, a narrowing of retinal arterioles was commonly seen and the variation of the blood vessel calibers also. As the elevation of blood pressure continued, the caliber showed irregularities (Fig. 1; 1), changing into an aneurysm (Fig. 1; 2–3) and assuming the form of a rosary (rosary-like artery) (Figs. 4–6). Those aneurysm which assumed an appearance of a rosary-like artery were mostly found 1 to 3 mm from the edge of the optic disc, but sometimes were found in the peripheral part of the vessel. Figure 2 shows a rosary-like artery of the sixth type.

How soon did the aneurysm or rosary-like artery appear after the onset of hypertension? In F_{14} they appeared after 7 to 11 weeks, in F_{15} and F_{16} they appeared in the earlier weeks and in F_{18} they appeared mostly after 1 to 2 weeks. There was little difference in the time of appearance, except that in the later generations they tended to appear earlier.

The course of retinal arterioles was straight in the early stage of hypertension. In the late stage of hypertension, however, the blood vessels showed tortuosity and irregular dilatation; sometimes tortuosity was seen even in the early stage.

* Department of Ophthalmology, Hirosaki University School of Medicine, Hirosaki, Japan

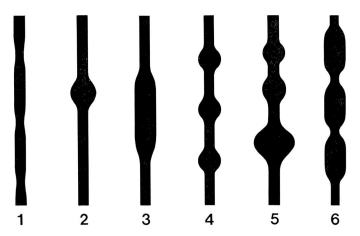

Fig. 1 Types of caliber- irregularities in retinal arterioles.

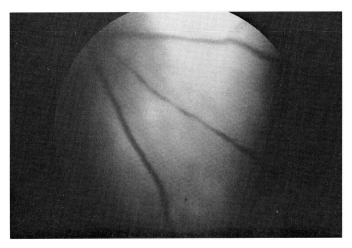

Fig. 2

Similarly, in other types of hypertension such as DCA hypertension and adrenal regeneration hypertension, such tortuosity of retinal arterioles was seen in many cases. In other words, in other hypertensive rats tortuosity was frequently observed while in SHR straightening appeared first and then tortuosity and irregular dilatation followed. This is a characteristic difference between SHR and the other experimental hypertensive rats.

When the elevation of blood pressure was sustained for a long time, venules showed a slight swelling, too. Some of them showed tortuosity in a spiral form and the others a partial swelling.

Sustained elevation of blood pressure from around 12 weeks after birth resulted in a lot of preretinal hemorrhages starting after 19 weeks. The hemorrhage appeared in various forms; punctiform and fleck-shaped in the fundus of SHR.

In the late stage of hypertension some SHR showed retinal opacity and papilledema. Retinal opacity was seen around the optic disc and blood vessels, resembling scattered patches of raw cotton wool of various sizes and shapes.

The above are the findings obtained mainly in the blood vessels of the retina by means of a ophthalmoscope. What histopathological changes underlay them?

In this regard the result from the trypsin digestion method is mentioned first. By means of the trypsin digestion method the retinal tissues were digested except for the blood vessels so that the latter could clearly be observed. As shown in Figure 3, some SHR showed caliber irregularity of retinal arterioles in the same way as in the ophthalmoscopic examination.

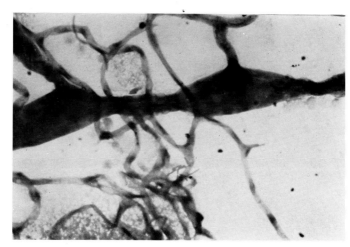

Fig. 3

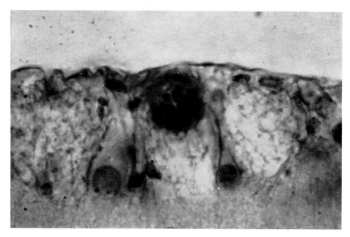

Fig. 4

The capillaries were swollen and tortuous, finally taking the appearence of a ball.

Figure 4 shows narrowed retinal arterioles and their rosary like change. Around the wall of retinal arterioles some edematous swelling was noticed. In the longituidinal section narrowing and dilatation corresponding with the caliber irregularity was recognized in the lumens of the blood vessels.

As mentioned before, the ophthalmoscopic examination revealed a sort of venous swelling. However, no considerable change could be detected histologically in the venous wall but only that the vein protruded into the vitreous body.

In the cases in which retinal opacity and papilledema were seen by the ophthalmo-scopic examination, some round-form PAS positive substance was present in the nerve fiber layer. This was consisered a socalled cytoid body.

It was noteworthy that we encountered cerebral hemorrhages at a high incidence at the autopsy. In some cases the hemorrhage, such as the ventricular hemorrhage, was easily recognized with a naked eye but some other hemorrhages could be first recognized with the aid of histological examinations.

Cerebral hemorrhages were found in 34 out of 99 SHR with no difference between sexes. The incidence of the cerebral hemorrhage in each generation was as follows. Cerebral hemorrhage was encountered at the highest incidence in F_{15} in which about half the animals were affected, while it was at the lowest incidence in F_{16} in which one fifth were affected. The incidences in the other generations were within these extremities and showed no significant differences between them to one another.

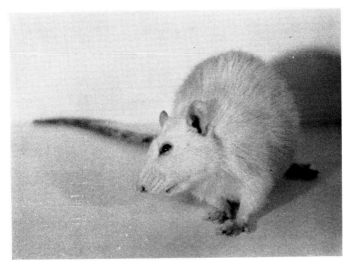

Fig. 5

Figure 5 is a photograph showing an hemorrhage-attacked SHR with an extraordinary position of its head. Such a rat was considered as paralysed. At the autopsy cerebral hemorrhage was assured. Therefore, this might correspond with so-called hemiplegia in man. Such symptoms were manifest in 15 out of 34 SHR with cerebral hemorrhage.

In addition, the relationship between the incidence of cerebral hemorrhage and blood pressure level was investigated in SHR. The blood pressures of 29 out of 34 SHR with cerebral hemorrhage exceeded 200 mm Hg. Since the cerebral hemorrhage occurred often at the peak of blood pressure, the intimate relationship seems to be obvious. The blood pressures of 14 out of 15 SHR with hemiplegia were higher than 200 mm Hg.

A relation of the fundus findings to cerebral hemorrhage could be noticed. The nar-rowing of retinal arterioles was seen in all 99 SHR: 73 per cent of these SHR showed moderate narrowing, 13 per cent severe, and the other 14 per cent slight. Moreover moderate narrowing was observed in 70 per cent of SHR with cerebral hemorrhage. Slight narrowing appeared in 15 per cent, and severe narrowing in another 15 per cent.

In the 15 SHR with hemiplegia moderate narrowing in the retinal arterioles was seen in 60 per cent and severe narrowing in 20 per cent.

Generally, the caliber irregularity of the retinal arterioles could be divided into three groups: a rosary-like artery, a mixed form of rosary appearance and indentation, and pure indentation. Pure indentation was seen in the largest number while the mixed form was seen in the smallest number. The incidence of the caliber irregularity in SHR with cerebral hemorrhage was the same as that in SHR as a whole.

Statistical data concerning the course of retinal arterioles were as follows. In SHR retinal arterioles showed for the most part the tendency of straightening, but tortuosity was seen very rarely. Cerebral hemorrhage attacked 21 out of 70 SHR with straightening of retinal aterioles while 9 out of 16 SHR with the tortuosity were attacked by the cerebral hemorrhage. In other words, when the retinal aretrioles show tortuosity in SHR, there is a more than 50 % probability of the presence of cerebral hemorrhage. In addition, 8 out of 21 SHR with cerebral hemorrhage and retinal arteriolar straightening and 5 out of 9 SHR with cerebral hemorrhage and retinal arteriolar tortuosity showed hemiplegia. Eight out of 70 SHR with retinal arteriolar straightening and 5 out of 16 SHR with retinal arteriolar tortuosity were affected by hemiplegia.

Finally, the relationship between cerebral hemorrhages and the changes of the retina and the optic disc is given below. About 50 per cent of the total SHR showed retinal opacity, white patches or papilledema, whereas retinal hemorrhages were seen in only 4 SHR. These changes were encountered in the animals with cerebral hemorrhages at an incidence less than half of the above. On the other hand, cerebral hemorrhages were observed in 3 out of 4 SHR with the retinal hemorrhages. In addition, SHR with retinal hemorrhages showed hemiplegia. Retinal opacity, white patches and papilledema were found in 11 out of 15 SHR with hemiplegia. These facts suggest that in the case where a change is noticed in the retina and optic disc the development of hemiplegia and the presence of cerebral hemorrhage are highly suspicious.

CONCLUSION

Sequential ophthalmoscopic and histopathological observations of the ocular fundus of SHR, F_{14} through F_{18}, yielded the following results.

1) Hypertension was observed in all the cases.

2) The fundus changes are as follows:

   a) Narrowing of retinal arterioles was the first change related to the elevation of blood pressure.

   b) Caliber irregularity appeared next.

   c) The caliber irregularity could be classified into socalled 'caliber irregularity type', 'aneurysm type' and 'rosary-like artery type'. Some of the aneurysm types changed into a rosary-like artery type. In the late stage of hypertension, indentation was added to the rosary-like artery type.

   d) The rosary-like artery tended to appear earlier and earlier as the generation proceeded from F_{14} to F_{18}. A genetic factor is likely involved in the development of this change.

   e) In the late stage of hypertension, hemorrhage, white patches, opacity and papilledema were seen in the fundus of some cases.

3) The histopathological studies revealed edematous swelling in the wall of retinal arterioles in some cases, but most cases did not show so remarkable a change as was expected from the ophthalmoscopic findings. In the cases with retinal opacity and papilledema a round PAS positive substance was found in the nerve fiber layer. This was considered identical with a so-called cytoid body.

4)   Autopsy and histological examinations revealed cerebral hemorrhage in 34 out of 99 SHR studied. Fifteen out of these 34, when alive, showed an extraordinary positioning of the head with a close similarity to that of so-called human hemiplegia.

REFERENCES

1.   ABT, K. and BRÜCKNER, R. (1950):   Ophthalmologica, **119**, 17.
2.   BYROM, F. B. (1963):   Lancet, **7280**, 516.
3.   IRINODA, K., TAKAHASHI, S. and YAMANOBE, R. (1968): Jap J Const Med, **31**, 234.
4.   KEYES, J. E. L. and GOLDBLATT, H. (1937):   Arch Ophthalmol, **17**, 1040
5.   KEYES, J. E. L. and GOLDBLATT, H. (1938):   Arch Ophthalmol, **20**, 812.
6.   KUWABAHA, T. and COGAN, D. G. (1960):   Arch Ophthalmol, **64**, 904.
7.   OKAMOTO, K. and AOKI, K. (1963):   Jap Circ J, **27**, 282.
8.   TAKAHASHI, S. (1964):   Acta Soc Ophthalmol Jap, **68**, 870.
9.   TAKAHASHI, S. and WATANABE, J. (1969):   Acta Soc Ophthalmol Jap, **73**, 1429.
10. WATANABE, J. (1970):   Acta Soc Ophthalmol Jap, **74**, 999.
11. UYAMA, M. (1963):   Acta Soc Ophthalmol Jap, **67**, 1377.

CARDIAC HYPERTROPHY IN SPONTANEOUSLY HYPERTENSIVE RATS

T. TAKATSU* and C. KASHII*

There have been many experimental investigations on various aspects of cardiac hypertrophy [7], such as morphology, including ultrastructure of the myocardial cells [1, 14], hemodynamics [5, 15], protein synthesis [8, 18], energetics [2, 3] and so forth, but the results seem to be contradictory.

In most of the investigations animals with experimentally induced pulmonic [1, 2, 5, 15] or aortic stenosis [7, 8, 18] and in some cases those with Goldblatt hypertension [14] were used as materials. Spontaneously hypertensive rats (SHR) develop a gradual elevation of the blood pressure in 100% [13], which must induce cardiac hypertrophy gradually. They are, therefore, considered to be the best subjects for the study of cardiac hypertrophy. The present paper resports an investigation of the development of cardiac hypertrophy in SHR by light- and electron microscopy and by histochemistry of enzymes related to energy metabolism of the myocardium.

MATERIALS AND METHODS

In 1966 SHR were obtained from the Department of Pathology, Kyoto University, through the courtesy of Prof. OKAMOTO, and now they are in generations F_{19-21}. In the present study a total of 83 SHR were used with 67 control animals of the Wistar strain supplied by the Animal Center Laboratory, Faculty of Medicine, Kyoto University.

The systolic blood pressure was measured indirectly by the tail-water plethysmographic method from the 7th week after birth, and the heart was removed immediately after decapitation every other week from the 5th to the 21st week. The body and heart were weighed, and the ratio heart weight/body weight was determined. The free wall of the left ventricle near the apex was observed morphologically by light- and electron microscopy. The diameter of myocardial cells was determined by light microscopy and the ratio of the area occupied by myofibrils to that occupied by mitochondria was determined by electron microscopy.

The activity of the following enzymes in the myocardium was determined histochemically: Glucose-6-phosphate dehydrogenase (G6PDH) [11] and lactic dehydrogenase (LDH) [10] as representative enzymes in glycolysis, β-hydroxybutyrate dehydrogenase (β-HBDH) [10] related to lipid metabolism, succinic dehydrogenase (SDH) [9] and isocitric dehydrogenase (IDH) [11] in the Krebs cycle, ATPase [16] to form high energy phosphate bond, and monoamine oxidase (MAO) [6] in catecholamine metabolism (Fig. 1).

In a comparative study cardiac hypertrophy was induced by aortic constriction in a total of 20 rats of the Wistar strain each weighing 120–150 g. The ascending aorta was constricted by a tight ligature around it and a No. 19 guage injection needle placed adjacent to it. This needle was subsequently removed. The heart was observed for 12 weeks after the constriction.

---

* The Third Division, Department of Internal Medicine, Osaka Medical College, Takatsuki, Osaka, Japan

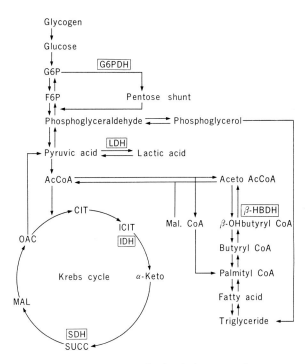

Fig. 1 Energy production in heart muscle.

RESULTS

The blood pressure in SHR rose gradually from the 7th week after birth to reach 184 mm Hg in the 19th week, while that in control rats was below 140 mm throughout the experimental period (Fig. 2).

The body weight as well as the heart weight progressively increased with age, though the increase in the heart was more prominent in SHR (Fig. 2). The ratio heart weight/ body weight was significantly larger from the 13th week in SHR than in control animals (Fig. 3). The diameter of myocardial cells of the left ventricle increased progressively to about 20μ in SHR and 15μ in controls by the 19th week (Fig. 3).

With respect to the ultrastructure of the myocardial cells, there seemed to be no significant changes in myofibrils during the experimental period, whereas there were changes in other organelles. In an early stage, for instance, in the 9th week there was an increase in the area of sarcoplasm especially in the perinuclear region and in glycogen granules (Fig. 4). During the 15th week marked changes appeared in the mitochondria, which were increased in number and different in size; some of them showed degenerative changes (Fig. 5). The sarcoplasmic reticuli were also increased in number, and some were dilated, as was the tubular system. These findings were even more pronounced in the 21st week. The ratio of the area occupied by myofibrils to that occupied by mitochondria became smaller from the 15th week on (Fig. 3).

In regard to enzyme activity (Table 1) the reaction to LDH and SDH indicated an increase of activity in the myocardium in the early stages. However, the activity of other enzymes was not increased significantly except for β-hydroxybutyrate dehydrogenase which was increased noticeably throughout the experimental period, and especially

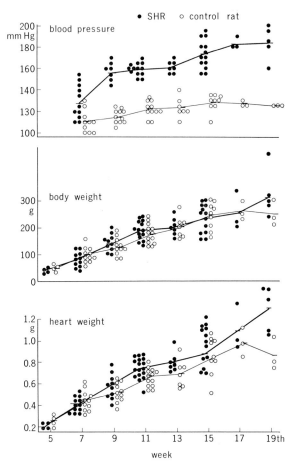

Fig. 2 Blood pressure, body weight and heart weight in SHR.

during the progressive elevation of blood pressure (Fig. 6, 7). The activity of MAO was increased later, when significant hypertension developed.

In animals with aortic constriction the ratio heart weight/body weight showed a bifid curve and the diameter of myocardial cells of the left ventricle was increased markedly in the late stages. Their ultrastructural appearance was different from that of SHR. Although the myofibrils revealed no significant changes like those of SHR, the changes in mitochondria and sarcoplasmic reticulum were marked in the early stages. The great increase in the activity of β-hydroxybutyrate dehydrogenase found in SHR was not observed in the rats with aortic constriction.

DISCUSSION

It is evident from these results that myocardial cells of the left ventricle were hyper-trophied in SHR as well as in rats with aortic constriction. However, in the former the morphological changes of myocardial cells appeared gradually and were marked in late stages, while in the latter the changes were prominent in early stages. These differences might be due to the difference in effect of slow or sudden induction of afterload on the heart.

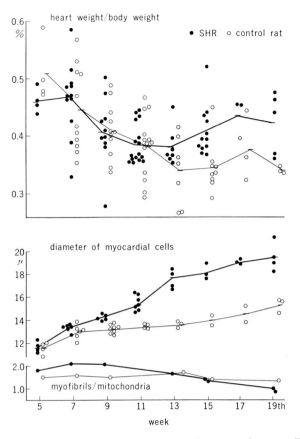

Fig. 3 The ratio heart weight/body weight, diameter of myocardial cells
and the ratio myofibrils/mitochondria in SHR.

Table 1 Activity of enzymes in the myocardium of SHR.

week\nenzyme	5	6	7	9	11	13	15	17	21
G6PDH	→	→	↑	↑	→	→	↑	↑	→
LDH	↑	↑	↑	↑	↑	↑	↑	↑	↑
β–HBDH	↑↑	↑↑	↑↑	↑↑	↑↑	↑↑	↑↑	↑↑	↑
SDH	↑	↑	↑	↑	↑	↑	↑	↑	→
IDH	↓	↓	↓	↓	↑	→	→	↑	↓
ATPase	→\n(?)	→	→	→	→	→	→	→	→
MAO	→	→	→	↑	↑	↑↑	↑↑	↑↑	↑↑

notes :
→ normal, ↑ slightly increased, ↑ moderately increased, ↑↑ markedly
increased, ↑↑ much markedly increased, ↓ slightly decreased.

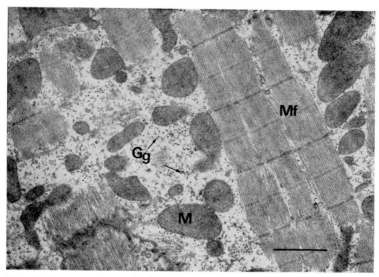

Fig. 4 Electron micrograph of the myocardial cell in SHR in the 9th week after birth. Myofibrils (Mf) and mitochondria (M) show no significant changes; the area of sarcoplasm and glycogen granules (Gg) are increased. × 26,000.

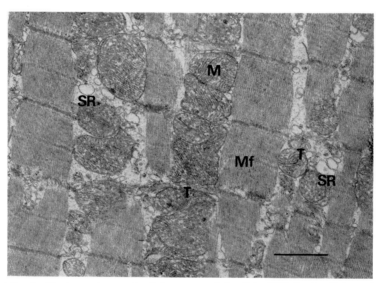

Fig. 5 Electron micrograph of the myocardial cell in SHR in the 15th week after birth. Mitochondria (M) show difference in size and some degenerative changes; sarcoplasmic reticuli (SR) as well as tubular system (T) are increased in number and dilated. × 26,000.

One of the purposes of this investigation was to answer the question as to whether hyperplasia of myocardial cells or increase in the number of myofibrils plays the greater role in cardiac hypertrophy. There were no abnormalities in the morphology of the myofibrils, such as widening or duplication of the Z-band [1]. The ratio of the area of myofibrils/mitochondria decreased in later stages, whereas the area of sarcoplasm increased. However, the data obtained so far fail to give any clue to the solution of this problem.

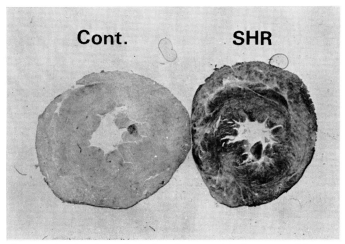

Fig. 6   Histochemistry of β-hydroxybutyrate dehydrogenase of the myocardium in SHR and control rat in the 5th week after birth.

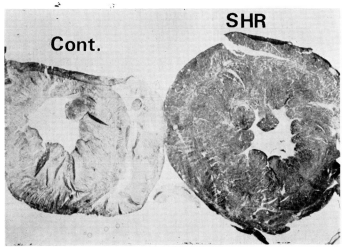

Fig. 7   Histochemistry of β-hydroxybutyrate dehydrogenase of the myocardium in SHR and control rat in the 9th week after birth.

   Cardiac hypertrophy is a morphological representation of enhanced protein synthesis
in myocardial cells, for which much energy must be used. Up to the present time it has
not been decided whether the heart preferably derives its energy from carbohydrates or
lipids, although the latter are considered by BING et al. [4] as a major source of energy in
the myocardium. And in cardiac hypertrophy WITTELS et al. [17] reported a decrease of
lipid metabolism accompanied by an increase of carbohydrate metabolism, while NEELY
et al. [12] observed the opposite results. In SHR the activity of β-hydroxybutyrate dehydrogenase was markedly increased throughout the experimental period, especially as
the blood pressure rose, whereas it was not prominent in animals with aortic stenosis.
Although the activity of lactic dehydrogenase was increased in SHR, that of glucose-6-
phosphate dehydrogenase rose only minimally. These results suggest that lipid metabolism

increased much more than carbohydrate metabolism in SHR. Therefore, it might mean that in SHR much of the energy necessary for cardiac hypertrophy is derived more economically from lipids than from carbohydrates, and that there are some genetic abnormalities in metabolism in SHR.

SUMMARY

1. Cardiac hypertrophy in SHR was observed by light- and electron microscopy, and compared with that in rats with induced aortic constriction.

2. The gradual development of cardiac hypertrophy as the blood pressure rose was proved by the ratio heart weight/body weight and the diameter of myocardial cells.

3. There were marked changes in mitochondria and sarcoplasmic reticulum in the late stages, when the ratio between myofibrils and mitochondria was definitely decreased.

4. Most of the enzymes related to energy metabolism in the myocardium showed increased activity, especially β-hydroxybutyrate dehydrogenase. The latter finding might indicate some genetic factors in energy metabolism in SHR.

REFERENCES

1. BISHOP, S. P. and COLE, C. R. (1969): Lab Invest, **20**, 219.
2. FEINSTEIN, M. B. (1962): Circ Res, **10**, 333.
3. FOX, A. C., WIKLER, N. S. and REED, G. E. (1965): J Clin Invest, **44**, 202.
4. DANFORTH, W. H., BALLARD, F. B., KAKO, K., CHOUDHURY, J. D. and BING, R. J. (1960): Circulation, **21**, 112.
5. GEHA, A. S., DUFFY, J. P. and SWAN, H. J. C. (1966): Circ Res, **19**, 255.
6. GLENNER, G. G., BURTNER, H. J. and BROWN, G. W., JR. (1958): J Histochem Cytochem, **6**, 389.
7. MEERSON, F. Z. (1969): Circ Res, Suppl II, **25**, 1.
8. MOROZ, L. A. (1967): Circ Res, **21**, 449.
9. NACHLAS, M. M., TSOU, K. C., DE SOUZA, E., CHENG, C-S. and SELIGMAN, A. M. (1957): J Histochem Cytol, **5**, 420.
10. NACHLAS, M. M., WALKER, D. G. and SELIGMAN, A. M. (1958); J Biophys Biochem Cytol, **4**, 29.
11. NACHLAS, M. M., WALKER, D. G., and SELIGMAN, A. H. (1958): J Biophys Biochem Cytol, **4**, 467.
12. NEELY, J. R., BOWMAN, R. H. and MORGAN, H. E. (1969): Am J Physiol, **216**, 804.
13. OKAMOTO, K., TABEI, R., FUKUSHIMA, M., NOSAKA, S., YAMORI, Y., ICHIJIMA, K., HAEBARA, H., MATSUMOTO, M., MARUYAMA, T., SUZUKI, Y. and TAMEGAI, M. (1966): Jap Circ J, **30**, 703.
14. POCHE, R., DE MELLO MATTOS, C. M., REMBARZ, H. W. and STOEPEL, K. (1968): Virchows Arch Pathol Anat, **344**, 100.
15. SPANN, J. F., JR. (1969): Am J Cardiol, **23**, 504.
16. WACHSTEIN, M, and MEISEL, E. (1957): Am J Clin Pathol, **27**, 13.
17. WITTELS, B. and SPANN, J. F., JR. (1968); J Clin Invest, **47**, 1787.
18. ZAK, R. and FISCHMAN, D. A. (1971): *In* "Cardiac Hypertrophy" (ALPERT, N. R. ed.), p. 273, Academic Press, New York & London.

CARDIAC MYOFIBRILLAR ADENOSINE TRIPHOSPHATASE ACTIVITY AND CALCIUM BINDING OF MICROSOME IN THE SPONTANEOUSLY HYPERTENSIVE RAT*

K. AOKI**, N. IKEDA** and K. HOTTA***

To understand the nature of hypertension from contractile properties of the cardiac muscle and the vascular smooth muscle, the ATPase activities of isolated myofibrils and fragmented sarcoplasmic reticulum were measured on the materials obtained from the heart of the spontaneously hypertensive rat (Okamoto-Aoki) (SHR) at the various stages of hypertension and compared with those of the normotensive Wistar rat (NR). The calcium uptake ability of the sarcoplasmic reticulum which may indicate the relaxing activity of the muscle was also measured.

EXPERIMENTAL PROCEDURES

Materials. Spontaneously hypertensive rats [5] and normotensive Wistar rats were fed on a commercial stock diet (Nippon Clea) and given tap water to drink. Blood pressures were determined by the tail water plethysmographic method [5]. For the preparation of myofibrils [1], rat hearts were quickly removed and immersed in a tris-HCl buffer, pH 7.5, at 2°C. To obtain relaxed myofibrils, rat hearts were perfused with calcium-free Ringer solution and then transferred into the tris-HCl buffer. Connective tissue was removed and the muscle was cut into small pieces and homogenized. Myofibrils were extracted by homogenization and centrifugation. Sarcoplasmic reticulum [3, 4] was prepared from the homogenate of the hearts by water extraction, and purified by differential centrifugation on a sucrose gradient.

Assay for ATPase activity [1]. Basal or calcium-dependent ATPase activity of cardiac myofibriles was measured in a tris-HCl buffer, pH 7.5 containing Mg and ATP in the absence and the presence of calcium, respectively. The ATPase activity of fragmented sarcoplasmic reticulum was measured in a medium containing KCl and Mg in the absence and the presence of calcium. The ATPase activity was measured by determining the liberated inorganic phosphate according to the Fiske and Subbarow method [2]. Protein concentration was determined spectrophotometrically by a modification of the Biuret method.

Calcium Binding Capacity. The calcium uptake of sarcoplasmic reticulum was measured by incubating the samples with various concentrations of calcium containing ^{45}Ca by separating them by ultracentrifugation.

RESULTS

Blood Pressure. Blood pressure in SHR continuously increased at a much greater rate than these of the normotensive rats. SHR began to develop hypertension at six weeks of age. The blood pressures of SHR were approximately 150 mm Hg, 180 mm Hg, and 200 mm Hg at 6, 10, and 20 weeks of age, respectively. However, the control normotensive

* This work was supported in part by U. S. Public Health Service Grant HE-11878-01 National Heart Institute and Grant 7062 from the Ministry of Education, Japan.
** Department of Internal Medicine and *** Department of Physiology, Nagoya City University School of Medicine, Nagoya, Japan

Wistar rats usually maintained a blood pressure of 120 to 140 mm Hg.

Heart weight. The ratio of heart to body weights increased in SHR. The cardiac hypertrophy was recognized by at least eight weeks of age.

Myofibrillar fragments. In myofibrils obtained by homogenization without the perfusion, a high concentration of sodium azide inhibited the mitochondrial ATPase activity. This azide-inhibited fraction of myofibrillar ATPase activity corresponded to about 40 % of the total ATPase activity. The relaxed myofibrils, obtained by perfusion with calcium free Ringer, contained only a minimum amount of mitochondria and other materials. The inhibition of ATPase activity of relaxed myofibrils by sodium azide was less than 15 %.

ATPase Activity. The ATPase activity of cardiac myofibrils from the hearts of rats aged 8 to 55 weeks, showed no significant differences between the NR and SHR. But the total ATPase activity per heart significantly increased in SHR, because of the cardiac hypertrophy observed in SHR. The basal and the calcium dependent ATPase activity of relaxed myofibrils were measured in the hearts of rats aged 30 to 45 weeks. The Basal ATPase activity was 0.063 and 0.072 μM per protein per minute in NR and SHR respectively. The calcium dependent ATPase activity was 0.072 and 0.053 μM per mg protein per minute in NR and in SHR, respectively. Thus, an increase in basal ATPase activity and a decrease of calcium dependent ATPase activity of relaxed myofibrils were noticed in SHR. However, the total ATPase activity per protein showed no significant difference because of cardiac hypertrophy in SHR.

Sarcoplasmic Reticulum. The ATPase activity of fragmented sarcoplasmic reticulum, obtained from the hearts of rats aged 20 to 25 weeks, was measured. The basal ATPase activity was 0.145 and 0.148 μM per mg protein per minute in NR and SHR, respectively. The calcium dependent ATPase activity was 0.100 and 0.174 μM per mg protein per minute in NR and in SHR, respectively. The basal ATPase activity was about the same in both NR and SHR. But, it was clear that the calcium dependent ATPase activity of sarcoplasmic reticulum in SHR considerably increased.

Calcium Binding Capacity. The number of maximum binding sites and binding constants of sarcoplasmic reticulum were calculated from the double reciprocal plotts of bound and free calcium in the medium. No difference in maximum binding site and low values of binding constant were observed in SHR. But, the values obtained here were considerably lower than those obtained in skeletal muscle.

DISCUSSION

The specific ATPase activity of cardiac myofibrils from SHR was not significantly different from that of NR. The rate of energy release in the heart per unit protein may be the same in the hearts of normotensive and hypertensive rats. However, since hypertensive rats showed cardiac hypertrophy, the release of chemical energy per heart increased in SHR. This increase in myocardial energy production in hypertension may be used by the heart to perform extra work brought about by high blood pressure. It appears that ventricular hypertrophy due to hypertension may prevent heart failure. Accordingly, the function of a hypertrophied heart in hypertension is characterized by an absolute increase in external work.

The calcium binding capacity of sarcoplasmic reticulum obtained from SHR heart was lower than that from NR. This fact indicates that the relaxing ability of SHR heart muscle may be reduced. The high value of Ca-ATPase activity in the sarcoplasmic reticulum of SHR heart may mean that it requires more ATP hydrolysis for the uptake of unit amount of calcium than that of a normal heart, although the role of ATPase in calcium binding is not clear.

SUMMARY

1. SHR began to develop hypertension within six weeks after birth. Hypertrophy of the heart was observed after eight weeks of age in SHR.

2. The cardiac myofibrillar ATPase activity of SHR showed no significant difference from that of normotensive rats of the same age. However, myofibrils from SHR showed little low in calcium dependent ATPase activity. The total ATPase activity per heart significantly increased because of cardiac hypertrophy. The requirement of extra energy for hypertension in the heart may be supplied by the increased heart mass, namely cardiac hypertrophy.

3. In the sarcoplasmic reticulum, high calcium dependent ATPase activity and low calcium binding capacity were noticed in SHR. The relation of ATPase activity with the calcium uptake of the sarcoplasmic reticulum has not yet been clarified, but in myogenic skeletal muscle disease, it was reported that the sarcoplasmic reticulum showed high calcium dependent ATPase activity and low calcium-binding capacity which may represent the hypofunction of a relaxing factor. Therefore, the findings in SHR, suggest that the relaxing ability may be reduced in the heart muscle and possibly in other vascular smooth muscle.

REFERENCES

1. AOKI, K., IKEDA, N. and HOTTA, K. (1971): Jap Circ J, **35**, 329.
2. FISKE, C. H. and SUBBAROW, Y. (1925): J Biol Chem, **66**, 375.
3. KATZ, A. M. and REPKE, D. I. (1967): Circ Res, **21**, 767.
4. MEAD, R. J., PETERSON, M. B. and WELTY, J. D. (1971): Circ Res, **24**, 14.
5. OKAMOTO, K. and AOKI, K. (1963): Jap Circ J, **27**, 282.

Chapter VI

ENDOCRINE FACTORS

PATHOLOGY OF THE ADRENAL CORTEX IN SPONTANEOUSLY HYPERTENSIVE RATS

H. TSUCHIYAMA*, H. SUGIHARA* and K. KAWAI*

In previous studies it has been noted that hypertension is often associated with endocrine disorders in man and experimental animals [12, 13]. AOKI [1] first studied the endocrine organs in spontaneously hypertensive rats (SHR) and detected some histological changes in them even in the prehypertensive stage. Moreover, he demonstrated that removal of the pituitary, adrenals or thyroid in the prehypertensive stage prevents the development of hypertension.

A review of the literature on the adrenal cortex in SHR [1, 14, 15] has shown the following: (1) The area of the glomerular zone and the summed areas of the fascicular and reticular zones are increased in SHR. The hypertrophy and increase in lipid content of the glomerular and fascicular zones are detectable even in the prehypertensive stage. (2) With the persistence of hypertension these changes become more marked; and increase in weight of adrenals, irregularity of cell cords of the fascicular zone, and decrease in width of the reticular zone are noted. (3) Glucose-6-phosphate dehydrogenase and triphosphopyridine nucleotide disphorase activity increase in the adrenal cortex in SHR.

The purpose of this paper is to examine critically the histochemical and ultrastructual alterations of the adrenal cortex of SHR in relation to the functional state.

MATERIALS AND METHODS

Forty-four spontaneously hypertensive male rats (SHR) F15–16 that had been produced by OKAMOTO and AOKI [11], ranging from 40 days to 16 months, were prepared for this study. Another 138 Wistar strain rats of the same age distribution supplied by the Animal Center Laboratory of Kyoto University were used as the control animals. They were kept in a room with a temperature range of $18°$ to $20°C$ and were fed Oriental stock chow diet (MF and NMF, Oriental Yeast Co., Japan).

Unfixed frozen sections were obtained by cryostat from the left adrenal of 26 SHR and 90 control rats. These were treated by HARDONK's method for the demonstration of secondary alcohol dehydrogenase (SAD) activity using isopropanol as the substrate (HARDONK, 1965); and by LEVY's method for 3β-hydroxysteroid dehydrogenase (3βHSD) activity using dehydroepiandrosterone as the substrate. The other gland was fixed in formalin, and frozen sections 10μ thick were cut and stained with oli red 0 for lipids. The remainder of the formalin-fixed adrenal was embedded in paraffin and cut in 5μ thick

* Department of Pathology, Nagasaki University School of Medicine, Nagasaki, Japan

sections. The sections were stained with hematoxyline-eosin and Gomori's silver staining method.

The adrenal glands were obtained from 18 SHR and 48 control rats for ultrastructural observation. Using the perfusion method under Nembutal anesthesia small pieces of the adrenal cortex were fixed in 0.1 M phosphate-buffered 1.0 per cent glutaraldehyde followed by 1.3 per cent osmium tetraoxide. After dehydration in acetone, the material was embedded in Epon 812 according to the method of Luft. Thick sections (1μ) stained with toluidine blue were examined with the light microscope in order to identify and select areas for more detailed study. Adjacent thin sections were double stained with a saturated aqueous solution of uranil acetate followed by lead citrate. Micrographs were taken with a JEM 7A electron microscope.

RESULTS

1. Histochemical Findings

In the control rats 40–60 days old, the SAD activity of many adrenals was characterized by a weakly positive stain in the zona glomerulosa without clear demarcation from the zona fasciculata. The activity ranged from moderate to high in the outer and middle fasciculata, and was high in the inner fasciculata and reticularis. On the other hand, SHR of the same age showed a slight decrease of SAD activity in the inner zona fasciculata. The control animals revealed a marked intensity of 3βHSD activity in the zona glomerulosa. The fascicular and reticular zones, in contrast, were comparatively inactive for this enzyme. There was no detectable difference of 3βHSD activity between SHR and the control rats at this age.

In the control rats aged 4–6 months, the zona glomerulosa exhibited a weakly positive reaction for SAD activity, and it was distinctly demarcated from the outermost portion of the zona fasciculata which showed a high SAD activity. This enzyme activity was intensely positive in the outer-to-middle fascicular zone. Lipid droplets in these portions were coarse and were present in a moderate to large amount. In the inner fascicular zone, the SAD activity ranged from positive to negative and there was a minimal or almost negative stain for lipid. The zona reticularis revealed a positive SAD activity which was more intense toward the inside. The SAD activity in SHR of the same age was reduced in the middle-to-inner fasciculata, but the outer fasciculata showed less pronounced changes. In the zona golmerulosa, the SAD activity showed no difference from that in the controls. The most conspicuous change in 3βHSD activity in SHR was seen in the zona fasciculata and here the activity was moderately increased in the middle-to-inner portions.

In the control rats aged 12–16 months, the distribution of SAD activity was similar to that in rats of 4–6 months of age, but the activity was further increased in the reticularis, which is composed of large cells with a moderate accumulation of fine lipid droplets. The SAD activity of SHR in the same age group was reduced in the inner zona fasciculata. The zona glomerulosa had minimum change in SAD activity. The distribution of 3βHSD activity in both the control animals and SHR was almost the same as in the 4–5 months old group. Although nodularity of the zona fasciculata was also present in the control group, it appeared to be more abundant in SHR. These nodules showed a tendency to exhibit strong SAD activity and abundant coarse lipid droplets.

2. Ultrastructural Findings

In SHR aged 40–60 days, the Golgi complex of the cells of the zona glomerulosa was moderately enlarged, and the amount of smooth-surfaced endoplasmic reticulum was slightly increased in some areas. The Golgi complex was occasionally composed of distended cisternae surrounded by vesicles. Also, there was much more variation in the shape of the mitochondria and the appearance of their cristae. The lamellae of enlarged mitochondria ran a straight course parallel to each other and their limiting membranes were thicker than that of the typical intramitochondrial cristae (Figs. 1 and 2). At this stage, on the other hand, the cell organelles of the fascicular and reticular zones in SHR did not so differ from their counterparts in the control animals.

In the zona glomerulosa cells of SHR aged 4–6 months, Golgi complexes with somewhat dilated cisternae and dense bodies were well developed (Figs. 3 and 4). Near the Golgi complex, elongated mitochondria containing lamellae oriented in several directions were often observed (Fig. 5). Some mitochondria contained amorphous deposits within their matrix. These intramitochondrial deposits varied considerably in size and number. These findings were more prominent in the zona glomerulosa cells of SHR than in those of the control group. In the zona fasciculata of SHR, particularly in the inner portion, smooth-surfaced endoplasmic reticulum was increased and dilated. Marked concentration of the mitochondria containing vesicular elements was also noted (Figs. 6 and 7).

In most SHR aged 12–16 months, fine zonal structure changes were similar to those observed in SHR at 4–6 months of age. The cells of the zona glomerulosa showed a prominent Golgi complex adjacent to the nucleus. The dense bodies could be found not only in the Golgi area, but scattered throughout the cytoplasm. Large droplets which had round profiles and were delimited from the adjacent cytoplasm by a single membrane, were occasionally seen in the zona glomerulosa. The contents of the droplets were either homogenous and of high electron opacity, or fine granular particles (Fig. 8). The cells of the zona fasciculata were characterized by a greater concentration of mitochondria and well developed smooth-surfaced endoplasmic reticulum. The mitochondria were usually spherical and the cristae were short tubular infoldings of the inner membrane. The smooth-surfaced endoplasmic reticulum showed a tendency to tubular dilatation in some areas. An increased number of dense bodies and lysosomes including lipofuscin pigment were noted in the inner fascicular and reticular zones. When the cells forming the cortical nodule were examined by electron microscopy, the most prominent changes consisted of numerous mitochondria with circular cristae, large intramitochondrial deposits, lamellar arrangement of the smooth-surfaced endoplasmic reticulum and a few giant lipid droplets (Figs. 9 and 10). These features clearly differed from those in the surrounding cortical tissue.

DISCUSSION

In this study of the adrenal cortex in SHR, we have pointed out a few characteristic histochemical and ultrastructural changes in various stages of the development of hypertension.

In the initial stage of hypertension, 3βHSD activity was increased in the zona fasciculata, while SAD activity was decreased in the middle and inner parts of the zona fasciculata. In regards to fine structure, the Golgi complex was well developed in the zona glomerulosa, to mitochondria often possessed arrays of tubules parallel to the long axis of the mitochondria, intramitochondrial deposits were found; and in the zona fasciculata an increase in the amount of smooth-surfaced endoplasmic reticulum and of mitochondria with vesicular cristae was seen.

Many studies of the Golgi complex in steroid-producing cells have reported that this organelle is significantly larger in actively secreting cells [5]. Recent biochemical investi-

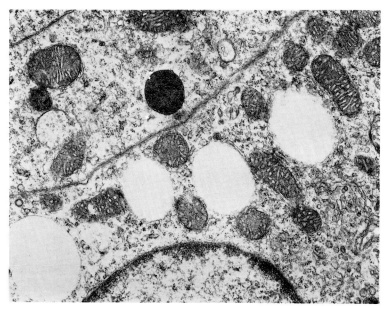

Fig. 1 This shows the fine structure of the zona glomerulosa of a control rat aged 40 days. × 15,800.

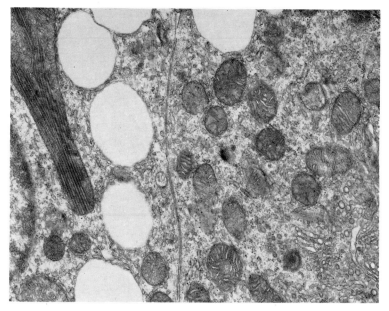

Fig. 2 In SHR of the same age, the Golgi complex of the zona glomerulosa is already enlarged. Note a giant mitochondria with characteristic parallel arrays of tubules (left corner). × 15,800.

gations have emphasized the importance of steroid conjugates, particularly sulfates, in biosynthetic reactions [2]. Long [9] suggested that this conjugation of steroid hormones occurs in the Golgi complex of adrenocortical cells and that the product secreted is the more water-soluble sulfate or glucuronide.

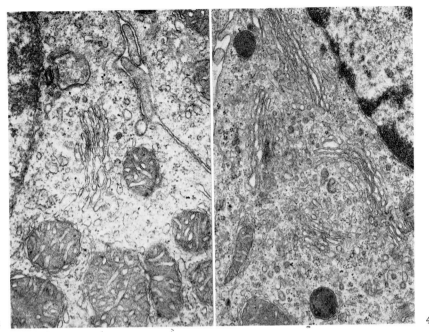

Fig. 3 This shows the fine structure of the zona glomerulosa of a control rat aged 4 months. × 21,000

Fig. 4 In the zona glomerulosa in SHR of the same age, the Golgi complex is moderately enlarged, and dense bodies are abundant. × 21,000.

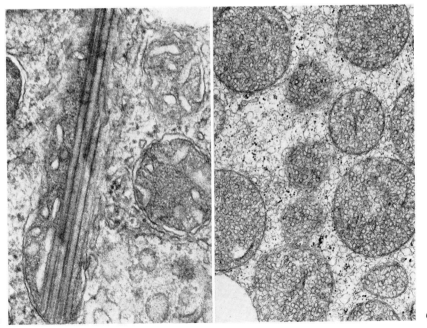

Fig. 5 Note the characteristic appearance of the mitochondria containing parallel arrays of tubules oriented in several directions. × 35,000.

Fig. 6 This shows the fine structure of the zona fasciculata of a control rat aged 4 months. × 24,500.

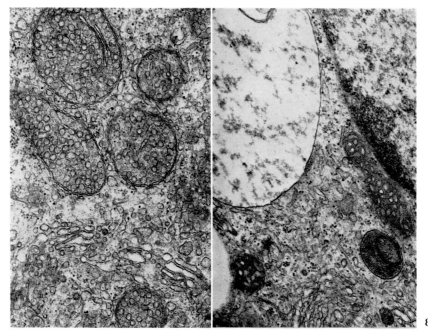

Fig. 7 In the zona fasciculata in SHR of the same age, smooth-surfaced endoplasmic reticulum is increased and somewhat dilated. Moderate concentration of mitochondria containing vesicular cristae is also found. × 24,500.

Fig. 8 In an electron micrograph of SHR in the advanced stage of hypertension, the zona glomerulosa cell contains a cytoplasmic droplet showing a degenerative appearance. ×21,000.

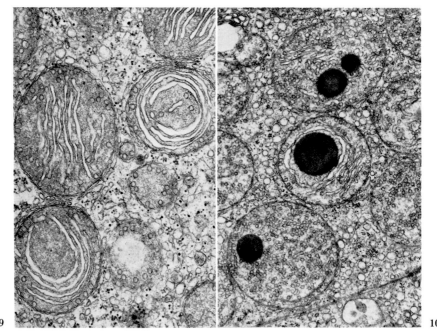

Fig. 9 An electron micrograph from a cortical nodule of the zona fasciculata in SHR. Numerous mitochondria are often characterized with circulating cristae. × 24,500.

Fig. 10 Similar to Fig. 9. Large intramitochondrial deposits and lamellar arrangement of the smooth-surfaced endoplasmic reticulum are seen. × 14,000.

Mitochondria containing parallel arrays of tubules and intramitochondrial deposits in the zona glomerulosa have been observed in sodium depleted animals [7]. Some workers have regarded these mitochondrial alterations as intermediated corticosterone and 18-hydroxycorticosterone and the final product aldosterone [6].

CHRISTENSEN [3] summarized the evidence and suggested that the amount of smooth-surfaced endoplasmic reticulum in different species was directly proportional to the amount of precursor cholesterol synthesized in the cells. On the other hand, LONG and JONES suggested tentatively that the amount of smooth-surfaced endoplasmic reticulum may be related to the type of hormone synthesized and its rate of production. Certain steps in the transformation of cholesterol to adrenocortical hormones are mediated by enzymes including 3β-hydroxysteroid dehydrogenase and 21 hydroxylase thought to be localized in the microsomal fraction of homogenized cortical cells. Moreover, it is assumed that the smooth-surfaced endoplasmic reticulum comprises the major portion of the microsomal fraction [10]. According to HARDONK [8], secondary alcohol dehydrogenase seemed to be related to the dehydrogenase activity in the transofrmation from 20α-22R-dihydroxycholesterol to pregnenolone, which does not have to occur in the same cells of a steroid-producing tissue as the oxidation of the 3β-ol group. It is known that this primary degradation of the cholesterol side chain to form pregnenolone by enzyme occurs in the mitochondrial fraction.

From the results reported in many papers, it may be expected that in increased of secretory activity of the zona glomerulosa and fasciculata in SHR plays a significant role in the initial stage of hypertension.

During the development of hypertension, there were progressive changes in the morphology of organelles and in the histoenzymatic activity of the adrenal cortical cells. The activity of SAD was decreased irregularly in the zona fasciculata and an increase of 3β-HSD activity was seen in the same zone. Increased amount of the Golgi complex and a smooth-surfaced endoplasmic reticulum in the glomerular and/or fascicular zones were predominant features in the advanced stage of hypertension. In addition to these alterations there was a gradual increase in the number of cytoplasmic droplets and dense bodies including lipofuscin pigments. The electron density and contours of cytoplasmic droplets resemble those of degenerative lipid vacuoles. In the inner fascicular and reticular zones, there were numerous lysosomes and lipofuscin pigment granules. The histochemical and ultrastructural findings of the cortical nodules varied slightly from nodule to nodule. However, most of the nodules in SHR could be distinguished from the surrounding cortex in terms of their SAD activity, lipid content and dramatic appearance of fine structures. These findings in the nodules suggest that many nodules play a role in the storage of steroid precursors but not in such an active secretion of corticosteroids.

From the above-mentioned evidence it may be concluded that the adrenal cortex of SHR in the advanced stage still reveals hyperactive changes on one hand, but tends to approach of exhaustion on the other hand.

At the prehypertensive stage of SHR, there existed ultrastructural changes in the cells of the zona glomerulosa. The Golgi complex of the zona glomerulosa was enlarged in SHR and by accepted cytological criteria appeared to be active. It has been shown that the active Golgi complex is more dispersed and the cisternae appear shorter and often distended. Moreover, the cells of the zona glomerulosa occasionally contained mitochondria with characteristic lamellae and a well developed endoplasmic reticulum. The distribution of SAD activity was similar to that in SHR aged 4–6 months. It is therefore assumed that active steroid biosynthesis of the glomerular and fascicular cells in SHR is already present in the prehypertensive stage.

Thus, our investigations have established that the morphological changes of the adrenal cortex in SHR occur even in the prehypertensive stage and they become more obvious during the processes of development of hypertension. However, it can not be determined whether these changes of the adrenal cortex play a primary etiologic role in the development and maintenance of hypertension or whether they act as secondary factors controlled by the vasomotor center of the brain and the autonomic nervous system.

SUMMARY

The structural alterations of the adrenal cortex in spontaneously hypertensive rats have been studied by light and electron microscopy. In the initial stage of hypertension, 3β-hydroxysteroid dehydrogenase activity is increased in the zona fasciculata, and secondary alcohol dehydrogenase activity is decreased in the middle and inner parts of the zona fasciculata. In fine structure studies, the Golgi complexes are well developed in the zona glomerulosa and there is an increase in the amount of smooth-surfaced endoplasmic reticulum and of mitochondria with vesicular cristae in the zona fasciculata. During the development of hypertension, there are progressive changes of the adrenocortical morphology in spontaneously hypertensive rats. In addition to the above alterations there is an increase in the number of cytoplasmic droplets, and dense bodies, including lipofuscin pigment granules, are also observed. In the prehypertensive stage, the Golgi complex of the zona glomerulosa is moderately enlarged and dilated in some areas. Also, there is more variation in the shape of the mitochondria and the appearance of their cristae. These observations are discussed in relation to the functional state of the adrenal cortex in various stages of hypertension.

REFERENCES

1. Aoki, K. (1963): Jap Heart J, **4**, 426.
2. Calvin, H. I., Vande Wiele, R. L. and Lieberman, S. (1963): Biochem, **2**, 648.
3. Christensen, A. K. (1965): J Cell Biol, **26**, 911.
4. Crisp, T. M., and Browning, H. C. (1968): Am J Anat, **122**, 169.
5. Fawcett, D. W. (1966): "An Atlas of Fine Structure. The Cell. Its Organelles and Inclusions." W. B. Saunders Co., Philadelphia.
6. Giacomellei, F., Wiener, J. and Spiro, D. (1965): J Cell Biol, **26**, 499.
7. Gordon, G. B., Miller, L. R. and Bensch, K. G. (1964): Lab Invest, **13**, 152.
8. Hardonk, M. J. (1965): Histochemie, **5**, 235.
9. Long, J. A. and Jones, A. L. (1967): Am J Anat, **120**, 463.
10. Long, J. A. and Jones, A. L. (1970): Anat Rec, **166**, 1.
11. Okamoto, K. and Aoki, K. (1963): Jap Circ J, **27**, 282.
12. Rather, L. J. (1951): Am J Pathol, **27**, 717.
13. Shamma, A. H., Goddard, J. W. and Sommers, S. C. (1958): J Chronic Dis, **8**, 588.
14. Tabei, R. (1966): Jap Circ J, **30**, 717.
15. Tsuchiyama, H., Sugihara, H. and Kawai, K. (1971); Jap J Const Med, **34**, 35.

MORPHOLOGICAL STUDIES ON ENDOCRINE ORGANS IN SPONTANEOUSLY HYPERTENSIVE RATS

R. TABEI*, T. MARUYAMA*, M. KUMADA* and K. OKAMOTO*

It has been reported that the endocrine system, as well as the autonomic nervous system, also plays an important role in the pathogenesis of hypertension in spontaneously hypertensive rats [10] (SHR hereafter). The results obtained by the morphological studies on endocrine organs of SHR was demonstrated comparing them to those of the control animal.

1. Adenohypophysis

It has been reported by AOKI and others [1] that an increase in the percentage of basophils in that of SHR starts from the prehypertensive stage, and that these changes were exaggerated as hypertension persisted. Moreover, the hypertrophy and the change similar to hyaline substance were observed in basophils [1]. By electron microscopy, these basophils are morphologically differentiated into four kinds of cells, that is ACTH, TSH, FSH and LH producing cells [5].

Fig. 1 (a) is the adrenocorticotropic hormone (ACTH) producing cell of the adult control rat. In the cytoplasm, secretory granules which are haloed granules unique to ACTH producing cells (as shown in this photograph), endoplasmic reticulum (ER) and mitochondria were observed [5]. Fig. 1 (b) is the picture of the ACTH producing cell of adult SHR. There were less granules in the cytoplasm compared to that of the control. Mitochondria showed a mild tendency to enlargement. In addition, in the cytoplasm of ACTH producing cell of SHR, the tendency of higher density of the cytoplasmic matrix was observed and also the growth of the membrane structure was pronounced. These findings seem to suggest that there is less retention of the product in the cell of SHR due to the enhancement of secretory activity.

There is the other kind of basophile, that is, the thyroid stimulating hormone (TSH) producing cell in the anterior pituitary.

Fig. 2 (a) shows TSH producing cell of the adult control rat [5]. There were a few granules around the cytoplasm. Fig. 2 (b) is the picture of TSH producing cell of an adult SHR and it contains much less granules and it seems to have the same tendency as that of ACTH producing cell of SHR.

From these findings it may be considered that there is much less retention of the product and TSH producing or secretory activity of the cell may be accelerated in SHR. No relevant change was observed in the other types of cells in the adenohypophysis.

2. Neurohypophysis

Fig. 3 (a) is the picture of the secretory nerve terminal of the neurohypophysis of the adult control rat. Many granules and less vesicles could be observed. Fig. 3 (b) is the secretory nerve terminal of the neurohypophysis of adult SHR [4]. Granules were decreased in number. On the contrary, there were observed many vesicles. From these findings it may be considered that retention of pituitrin, probably vasopressin is less, and the secretory activity is increased in SHR. When the percentage ratio of the number of neurosecretory granules and vesicles were calculated in unit area of the neurohypophysis

---

* Department of Pathology, Faculty of Medicine, Kyoto University, Kyoto, Japan

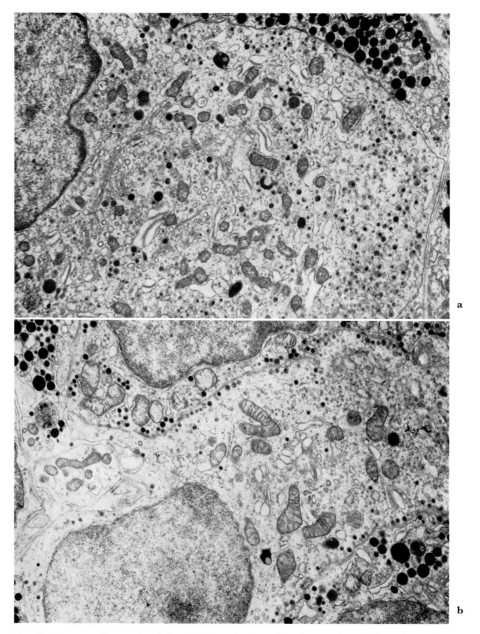

Fig. 1 Electron micrographs of the ACTH producing cell in the anterior pituitary. ($\times$ 5,000)
a. Control rat (7 months of age). In the cytoplasm, quite a few haloed granules are observed.
b. SHR (7 months of age). There are fewer granules in the cytoplasm.

on the electron micrographs, the number of vesicles of SHR was about twice that of the control [4]. On the other hand, the number of granules was slightly decreased compared to the control [4]. From these figures it may be considered that there exists the hyper-secretory state of pituitrin, probably vasopressin, in the neurohypophysis of SHR.

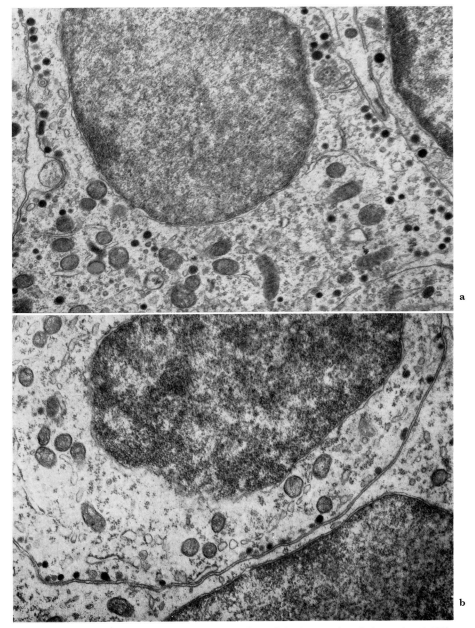

Fig. 2 Electron micrographs of the TSH producing cell in the anterior pituitary. ($\times$ 10,000)
a. Control rat (7 months of age). There are a few granules around the cytoplasm.
b. SHR (7 months of age). There are fewer granules in the cytoplasm.

3. Adrenal cortex

It has been reported that there exists the hypertrophy and an increase in lipid content of the fascicular zone in SHR from the prehypertensive stage [1]. Histometrically, the fascicular zone was significantly larger in adult SHR [1]. Histochemical results also suggested that this zone in SHR is in hyperfunctional state from the prehypertensive stage [14].

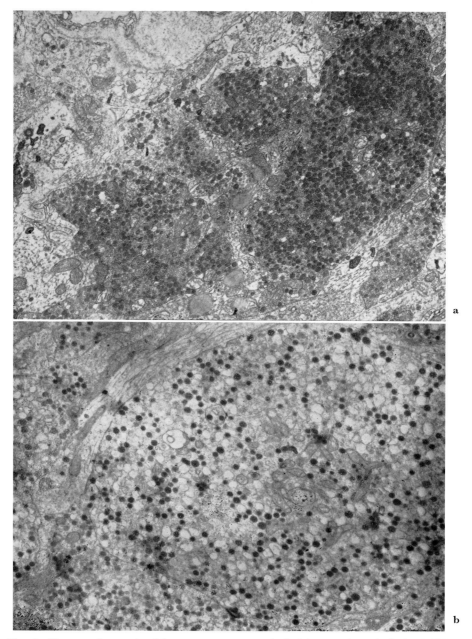

Fig. 3 Electron micrographs of the secretory nerve terminal of the neurohypophysis. ($\times$ 5,000)
a. Control rat (8 months of age). Many granules and less vesicles are observed.
b. SHR (8 months of age). Number of granules is decreased and many vesicles appear.

Fig. 4 (a) is the electron micrograph of the cell in the fascicular zone of the young control rat. Mitochondria, ribosomes and lysosomes are observed. Fig. 4 (b) is that of young SHR. Increase in the number of ribosomes, lysosomes, distention and increase in number of smooth surfaced endoplasmic reticulum and vacuolization of mitochondria were observed [6]. These findings closely resembled the finding obtained from the adrenal

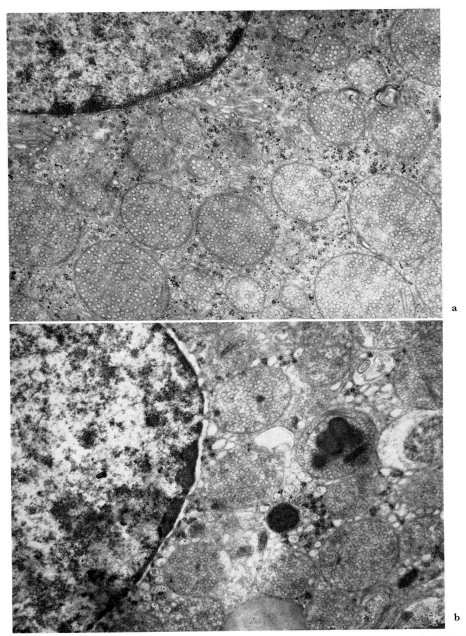

Fig. 4 Electron micrographs of the epithelial cell of the fascicular zone of the adrenal cortex. ($\times$ 10,000)
a. Control rat (55 days old). Mitochondria and ribosomes are observed.
b. SHR (57 days old). Increase in number of ribosomes and lysosomes, distention and increase in number of smooth surfaced endoplasmic reticulum, and vacuolization of mitochondria are observed.

cortex with continuous administration of ACTH for a certain period [13]. These findings seem to suggest that there exists the hyperfunction of the fascicular zone of the adrenal cortex of SHR, and it may correspond to the finding of the basophils in the adenohypophysis suggestive of hyperfunction.

4. Adrenal medulla

Histometrical results have demonstrated that the area of the noradrenaline storing cell islets of SHR was about twice the size of that of the control from eighteen days after birth [7, 14].

Fig. 5 (a) is an electron micrograph of osmophilic noradrenaline storing cells of the adrenal medulla of the control rat of 14 months of age. The noradrenaline granules and vesicles in the cytoplasm of the noradrenaline storing cell can be observed. Fig. 5 (b) is the picture of the same in SHR at the same age. In that of SHR, the noradrenaline storing granules were increased in number, and moreover the size and shape were irregular [6]. Vesicles were also increased in number [6].

According to the results from the calculation of the noradrenaline storing granules and vesicles in adrenal medullary cytoplasm on the electron micrographs [6], both granules and vesicles were increased in SHR through all three, *i.e.* pre-, initial and advanced hypertensive stages. The number of vesicles was increased starting from the prehypertensive stage, and it was about 1.4–2.6 times that of the control. The number of granules was also about 1.3 times that of the control. These results correspond well to those obtained by quantitative analysis that the amount of noradrenaline in the adrenal gland of SHR was twice of that of the control from the prehypertensive stage, and that rate of synthesis of noradrenaline and the enzyme activity was increased in SHR [8, 11, 12]. These results may be considered as peripheral indication of the central sympathetic overactivity in SHR [10, 14].

5. Thyroid

It was also reported that histometrical results such as areas of follicle, follicle cells, lumen of follicle, follicle cell height and the number of follicle cells were significantly increased in SHR starting from the prehypertensive stage [1]. Histochemically, increase in the activity of acid phosphatase of the follicle cells was detected in SHR from the prehypertensive stage [14]. From these and other results from the studies on the thyroid activity [10, 15], it has been considered that the thyroid of SHR is in a hypersecretory state from the prehypertensive stage.

Fig. 6 (a) is an electron micrograph of the follicular cell of the thyroid of the adult control rat. The endoplasmic reticulum is rather dilated. Fig. 6 (b) is a picture of that of adult SHR. Middle-sized colloid droplets which appeared in the cytoplasm were demonstrated remarkably in the thyroid of SHR [10]. These droplets may be considered to be colloid droplets reabsorbed from the follicle. Dense bodies are also observed in the thyroid of SHR.

The origin or nature of these dense bodies may be presumed to be lysosome or degenerated substance coming from reabsorbed colloid droplets. Moreover, in the follicular cells of the thyroid of SHR, tendency of the proliferation of the endoplasmic reticulum and also the enlargement of Golgi area, and tendency of elongation and of slight increase in number of pseudopods in apical zones were observed [10]. These results are similar to the finding in the thyroid of the normal rat treated with TSH for a certain period [2].

From these findings, it may be considered that there is an increase in the secretory activity of the thyroid of SHR, and this finding corresponds to that of TSH secreting cells in the anterior pituitary which may also indicate the hypersecretory state.

6. Hypothalamus

Moreover, studies on the nerve cells of the hypothalamus of SHR performed by the morphological techniques [3, 9, 10] such as histometry, enzyme histochemistry and

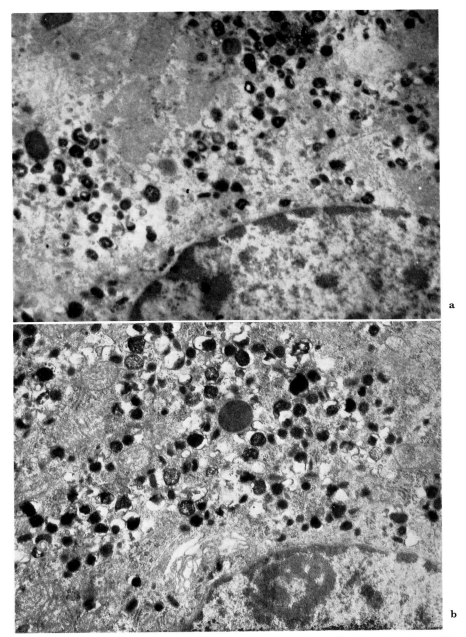

Fig. 5 Electron micrographs of the osmophilic noradrenaline storing cell of the adrenal medulla.
  (× 10,000)
a. Control rat (14 months of age). Noradrenaline granules and vesicles in the cytoplasm.
b. SHR (14 months of age). Increase in number of large and small sizes, and moreover irregular
  noradrenaline storing granules and vesicles are observed.

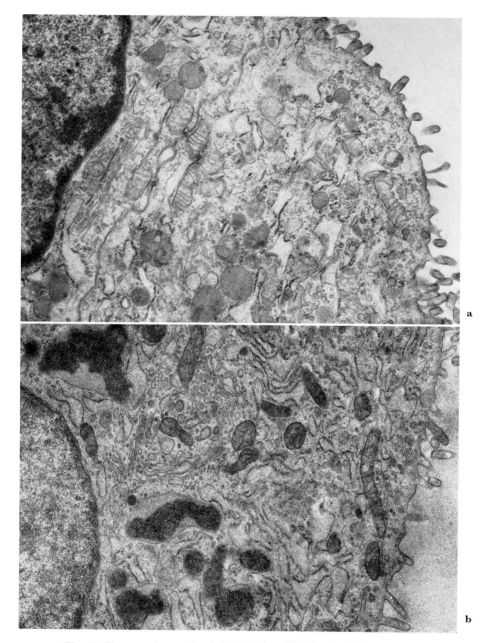

Fig. 6   Electron micrographs of the follicular cell of the thyroid. ($\times$ 5,000)
a. Control rat (7 months of age). The endoplasmic reticulum is rather dilated.
b. SHR (7 months of age). Colloid droplets and dense bodies are remarkable, and the enlargement
of Golgi area are observed.

fluorescence microscopy on noradrenaline, has demonstrated the following:

(i) It was indicated that the hypothalamus of SHR showed the finding similar to that under the hypersecretory state of both ACTH and TSH.

(ii) The finding obtained was suggestive of augmented activity of secretion of vasopressin and oxytocin.

7. Summary

All these results so far seem to indicate the following. In the endocrine system of SHR, there exists hyperfunction in both the adenohypophyseo-adrenocortical and the adenohypophyseo-thyroidal systems, the hypersecretory state of pituitrin, probably vasopressin and the sympathetic overactivity. Thus in conclusion, these changes in the endocrine system of SHR possibly participate in the pathogenesis of hypertension in SHR.

REFERENCES

1. Aoki, K., Tankawa, H., Fujinami, T., Miyazaki, A. and Hashimoto, Y. (1963): Jap Heart J, **4**, 426.
2. Ekholm, R. and Smeds, S. (1966): J Ultrastruct Res, **16**, 71.
3. Haebara, H., Ichijima, K., Motoyoshi, T. and Okamoto, K. (1968): Jap Circ J, **32**, 1391.
4. Kumada, M. (1972): Jap Circ J, **36**, in press.
5. Kurosumi, K. (1968): Arch Histrol Jap, **29**, 329.
6. Maruyama, T. (1969): Jap Circ J, **33**, 1271.
7. Morisawa, T. (1968): Jap Circ J, **32**, 161.
8. Nagatsu, T., Mizutani, K., Nagatsu, I., Umezawa, H., Matsuzaki, M. and Takeuchi, T. (1971): Jap J Const Med, **34**, 34.
9. Okamoto, K., Tabei, R., Nosaka, S. Fukushima, M., Yamori, Y., Matsumoto, M., Yamabe, H., Morisawa, T., Suzuki, Y. and Tamegai, M. (1966): Jap Circ J, **30**, 1483.
10. Okamoto, K. (1969): *In* "International Review of Experimental Pathology" (G. W. Richter and M. A. Epstein, eds.), Vol 7, p. 227. Academic Press, New York.
11. Ozaki, M., Suzuki, Y., Yamori, Y. and Okamoto, K. (1968): Jap Circ J **32**, 1367.
12. Ozaki, M. (1971): Jap J Const Med, **34**, 33.
13. Sakamoto, S. (1959): Folia Endocrinol Jap, **35**, 723 (in Japanese).
14. Tabei, R. (1966): Jap Circ J, **30**, 717.
15. Yamabe, H. (1970): Jap Circ J, **34**, 233.

NEW TYPE OF SPONTANEOUSLY HYPERTENSIVE RATS WITH HYPERLIPEMIA AND ENDOCRINE GLAND DEFECTS

S. KOLETSKY*

In the course of breeding spontaneously hypertensive rats of the Okamoto-Aoki strain in our laboratory, there appeared among the litters, apparently as genetic mutants, rats which developed marked obesity, hyperlipemia, and endocrine gland disturbances. The latter appeared to involve the adrenals, pancreas, gonads and also possibly the pituitary. These animals have been tentatively designated as 'obese' spontaneously hypertensive rats.

This report describes the preliminary observations that were made on 12 such animals. At present breeding procedures are being employed to preserve the unusual genetic traits of these rats. Additional animals are needed to characterize the hyperlipemia more completely, to elucidate the nature of the endocrine gland disturbances, and to provide adequate histologic studies of the pathological lesions present in various tissues and organs.

GENETIC BACKGROUND

The injurious gene responsible for the obese SHR is apparently recessive since its characteristic effect is not evident when it is paired with its allele. The harmful phenotype occurs in both sexes and represents a homozygous recessive trait which can be inherited only when the parents are heterozygous and each carries the same recessive allele.

In this situation as shown in Table 1 the probability is that about 50% of the offspring

Table 1 Genetic status of obese SHR.

	Harmful trait is homozygous recessive Both parents must be heterozygous - each carries same recessive allele Ff x Ff		
Offspring	FF 1/4 homozygous dominant	2 Ft 1/2 heterozygous & carry recessive allele	ff 1/4 homozygous recessive- abnormal genotype

would be heterozygous carriers (Ff) of the recessive allele like the parents and would be of normal phenotype, 25% would be heterozygous for the normal or dominant allele (FF) and of normal phenotype while the remaining 25% would be homozygous for the recessive gene ff) and represent the deleterious phenotype.

So far heterozygous parents which must be mated to yield the affected phenotype have been identified only by the fact that their litters contain the abnormal offspring.

ABNORMALITIES OF OBESE SHR

As shown in Table 2 the abnormal changes in SHR comprising the injurious pheno-

---

* Case Western Reserve University Medical School, Department of Pathology, Cleveland, Ohio U.S.A.

Table 2 Abnormalities of obese SHR.

Obesity
Hypertension
Hyperlipemia
Endocrine dysfunction
        adrenal—plasma corticosterone elevated
                    cortical hyperplasia of adrenals
        Pancreas—glycosuria, hyperglycemia
                    hyperplasia islets of Langerhans
        gonads—infertility
        pituitary - ? ACTH elevated

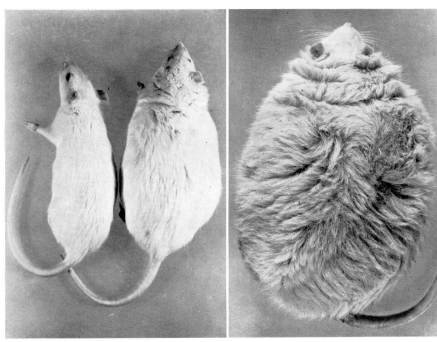

Fig. 1 Obese SHR and SHR of usual pheno-   **Fig. 2** Obese SHR 9 months of age.
type, both 2 months old.

type included the development of marked obesity which was associated with hyperlipemia, hypertension and endocrine gland dysfunction.

At about 4–6 weeks of age both male and female rats showed a rounded or bulging contour of the body especially involving the lower portion of the trunk. This distingui- shed the pathological animals from the usual type of SHR (Fig. 1). Thereafter the animals became progressively more obese and developed bulging deposits of fat around the shoul- ders, thighs, abdomen and buttocks. The fore and hind limbs as well as the face were not involved. By 6 months of age the body shape was rounded (Fig. 2). The development of obesity was associated with hyperphagia which was especially evident between 6 weeks and 4 months of age.

After 3 or 4 months the fur of the animals became ruffed and underwent progressive discoloration. The latter may have been related to the marked and persistent proteinuria which these rats exhibited.

Only sketchy data on the levels of blood pressure in these abnormal rats is available at present although it was determined that hypertensive levels, *i.e.* in the vicinity of 180 mm Hg, were present uniformly in animals 6–8 months old.

An interesting facet of the abnormal SHR was the presence of hyperlipemia. Serum lipids were already elevated in animals only 6 weeks old and thereafter continued to rise progressively with increasing age.

Table 3   Serum lipids.

Obese SHR		
6 weeks–4 months.	cholesterol	95–185 mg%
	triglycerides	130–285
5–9 months.	cholesterol	200–885 mg%
	triglycerides	650–3600
SHR-usual type		
6 weeks–9 months.	cholesterol	55–100 mg%
	triglycerides	30–75

Table 3 shows the range of serum cholesterol and triglycerides during the first 9 months of life and also the corresponding control values for SHR with usual phenotype. Although determinations in the latter are limited in number, no significant change in either serum cholesterol or triglycerides has been noted so far in relation to age.

The elevation in serum triglycerides in the obese SHR occurred earlier and was more pronounced than the rise in serum cholestrol.   Moreover subsequently the triglcyerides rose more rapidly and were relatively higher than were the cholesterol values.   At 5–9 months of age serum triglycerides ranged from 650 to 3600 mg% and the serum was often milky to creamy in consistency.   Serum cholesterol was within normal limits or only slightly elevated at first, *i.e.* at 6 weeks of age, and then also underwent progressive elevation, reaching levels of 200–885 mg% when the animals were 5–9 months old.

The hyperlipemia was in all probability endogenous in origin since the animals were on standard Purina chow which has only a 5% content of fat. Evidently most of the food eaten by these rats is converted to fatty acids.

Table 4   Plasma corticosterone.

Rat	Age (months.)	Corticosterone (μg%)	
		Mean	Range
Obese SHR	2–4	43	34–56
	5–9	26	10–40
SHR (usual type)	2–9	23	19–27
Sprague-Dawley	2–9	16	14–20

Plasma corticosterone levels were determined by the method of HYDE and DAIGNEAULT [1]. Table 4 shows that the mean plasma corticosterone in obese SHR 2–4 months old was distinctly higher than the corresponding levels for the usual SHR and for Sprague-Dawley rats. The determinations in both control groups were made on animals 2–9 months old and the levels over this period were in the same general range. On the other hand the plasma corticosterone of the obese SHR appeared to decline gradually after the fifth month so that the levels in animals 5–9 months old approached those of SHR with usual phenotype (Table 4). The significance of this change is not clear. The few adrenals of obese SHR studied morphologically so far were enlarged and showed cortical hyperplasia.

Involvement of the pancreas of the abnormal SHR was indicated by the presence in some rats of glycosuria and hyperglycemia. The latter are unusual findings since in the rat more than 80% of the pancreas has to be eliminated experimentally in order to produce diabetes mellitus. The glycosuria and hyperglycemia probably represent adrenal rather than pancreatic diabetes and this is supported by the presence of giant hyperplasia of the islets of Langerhans in the few animals studied morphologically.

It has not been possible to successfully mate male or female obese SHR with each other or with SHR of usual phenotype. The animals appear to be sterile and thus the gonads participate in the endocrine gland abnormalities.

The function of the pituitary has not yet been determined. However we are entertaining the possibility that the obese SHR secrete excess amounts of ACTH and that perhaps this is responsible for the dysfunction noted in other endocrine glands.

SUMMARY

A mutation in the course of breeding spontaneously hypertensive rats resulted in an injurious phenotype which is inherited as a homozygous recessive trait from heterozygous parents each of which carries the same recessive allele. The harmful phenotype is characterized by obesity, hypertension, endogenous hyperlipemia and endocrine gland abnormalities. Such animals should constitute a valuable animal research model for various types of studies.

REFERENCE

1. HYDE, P. M. and DAIGNEAULT, E. A. (1968): Steroids, **11**, 721.

Chapter VII

RENAL FACTORS AND ELECTROLYTES

ABSENCE OF HYPERACTIVE RENAL HUMORAL PRESSOR SYSTEM IN SPONTANEOUSLY HYPTERTENSIVE RATS

S. KOLETSKY*, P. SHOOK* and J. RIVERA-VELEZ*

The pathogenesis of the high blood pressure in spontaneously hypertensive rats of the Okamoto-Aoki strain is not established. Genetic factors are evidently involved. AOKI [1] reported that removal of the pituitary, adrenals or thyroid of SHR in the prehypertensive stage prevented the development of subsequent hypertension while removal during hypertension caused a lowering of the blood pressure to normotensive levels. NOLA-PANADES and SMIRK [11] questioned the role of the adrenals on the ground that their genetically hypertensive rats subjected to adrenalectomy continued to have high blood pressure when the animals were maintained on 1% saline instead of tap water for drinking.

The renin-angiotensin system is not involved in the genesis of spontaneous hypertension according to SOKABE [12]. This author determined the total renin content of the kidney and also the pressor activity of renal venous blood by grafting the kidney onto a bilaterally nephrectomized recipient rat and noting the rise in blood pressure of the recipient. The renin activity of the kidneys of SHR in the early stage of hypertension was about the same as for normal rats, but later on decreased significantly in comparison with the controls.

The renin-angiotensin activity of SHR was also studied in our laboratory in order to explore further whether this sytem might contribute to the origin and/or maintenance of high blood pressure in SHR.

METHOD

Three parameters of the renal humoral pressor system were investigated, *i.e.* the juxtaglomerular index (JGI) of the kidneys [7], the vasopressor activity of renal venous blood as determined by bioassay, and renal vein plasma renin activity. These were previously studied in rats with unilateral renovascular hypertension which, in its incipient and early stages, shows some evidence for the etiologic participation of the renin-angiotensin system [8–10].

The JG indices were determined on a resected kidney or on a cylindrical biopsy of renal tissue about 5×3 mm which was removed from the kidney with a dermatome.

---

* Case Western Reserve University, Medical School, Department of Pathology, Cleveland, Ohio U.S.A.

Step serial sections of the biopsy provided 100 different glomeruli for counting. Renal vein plasma renin activity was measured by the method of GOULD and others [6] using 0.5 ml plasma obtained from the left renal vein by venipuncture. For vasopressor activity of renal venous blood, 0.5 ml blood was withdrawn from the left renal vein of SHR and injected immediately into the cannulated femoral vein of a recipient rat treated 30 minutes previously with pentolinium tartrate (4 mg/100 gm body weight subcutaneously) for ganglion blockade. The response was the rise in arterial pressure of the recipient as measured on a Hg manometer connected by catheter to the femoral artery. Each assay was controlled by injecting 0.5 ml renal venous blood from a normal animal into the same recipient. The increment (in mm Hg) in pressor response of the hypertensive over the normotensive blood represented the pressor activity of the hypertensive blood and an increment greater than 8 mm Hg was considered a positive assay.

The determinations were made in male and female SHR from 6 weeks to 12 months of age and whose blood pressure ranged from 130–210 mm Hg. About half the SHR were 6 weeks–6 months of age and half were 7–12 months old. Blood pressures were obtained under anesthesia by attaching a cannula in the femoral artery to a Hg manometer. In most instances the animals were tested at successive age intervals so that the results represented the prehypertensive, labile and established or chronic stages of the hypertension.

Negative and positive controls were used in establishing each parameter of renin-angiotensin activity in SHR. The negative control was a normal Sprague-Dawley rat about the same age as the SHR being tested. The positive control consisted of rats with unilateral renovascular hypertension whose high blood pressure was induced from 1 hour to 2 days before testing by constricting the aorta just above the ostium of the left renal artery while the contralateral kidney remained *in situ* [8]. The JG indices were obtained on the ischemic left kidney of these animals and the blood samples for renal vein plasma renin activity and for pressor activity were taken from the left renal vein.

RESULTS

The mean and range of the JGI for SHR, normal Sprague-Dawley rats, and acute renal hypertensive rats are shown in Table 1. The SHR index was lower than for the normotensive controls and the difference between the two groups was highly significant ($p < .001$), while the JGI of the acute renal hypertensive rats was substantially higher than for SHR and for the normotensive controls. The mean JGI of SHR 2–6 months of age was approximately the same as for animals 7–12 months old.

Table 1 Juxtaglomerular index.

Rat	JGI	
	Mean±SD	Range
SHR	24±4	10–35
Normotensive controls	33±6	22–44
Acute renal hypertensive	99±12	85–130

n=30 for each group

The renal vein plasma renin activity of the SHR was not significantly different from that of normal rats (Table 2). In contrast the activity of acute renal hypertensive rats was substantially higher than for SHR and for normal animals and the difference in comparison with each of the latter two groups was highly significant ($p < .001$).

The mean and standard deviation of renal vein plasma renin activity of SHR 2–6 months of age was 258 ± 102 as compared to 147 ± 101 when the animals were 7–12 months

Table 2 Plasma renin activity.

Rat	Renal vein PRA*	
	Mean±SD	Range
SHR	216±93	60–360
Normotensive controls	196±58	120–240
Acute renal hypertensive	942±390	480–1320

n=35 for each group
*Ng angiotensin II/ml plasma/16 hr. incub.

Table 3 Pressor activity of renal vein blood.

Rat	Bioassays		
	No.	% pos.*	% neg.
SHR	44	5	95
Acute renal hypertensive	42	86	14

* Response to hypertensive blood exceeded that to normotensive
by more than 8 mm Hg.

old. The difference between the younger and older age groups was statistically significant (p<.01).

Bioassays of renal venous blood from SHR were essentially negative for vasopressor activity as were assays made with blood from the normotensive control rats (Table 3). In contrast venous blood from the ischemic kidney of rats with acute unilateral renovascular hypertension caused a rise in blood pressure of the recipient, *i.e.* 6–24 mm Hg, which in the great majority of instances exceeded by more than 8 mm the rise produced in the same recipient by blood from the normotensive controls.

DISCUSSION

No evidence was obtained that the renal humoral pressor system of SHR was hyperactive at any time in the course of the high blood pressure. This seems to parallel the situation in human benign essential hypertension [2–5].

The juxtaglomerular indices of SHR were significantly lower than those of the normotensive controls. Renal venous blood from SHR was generally devoid of pressor activity as determined by bioassay. In fact SHR blood usually yielded a smaller response in the recipient than did blood from the normotensive animals. On the other hand the renal vein plasma renin activity was approximately the same in the two groups. Of interest is the observation that the mean renal vein plasma renin activity of SHR 2–6 months old was significantly greater than for SHR 7–12 months old. Perhaps this was due to long standing hypertension and/or to the development of nephrosclerosis.

SUMMARY

SHR had a significantly lower JG index than did normal rats. Bioassays of renal venous blood for a vasopressor agent were essentially negative including tests on animals 6–8 weeks old when the blood pressure was rising to hypertensive levels. Renal vein plasma renin activity was normal except for reduced activity in SHR with long standing high blood pressure. Hence the origin and maintenance of high blood pressure in SHR is probably not due to overactivity of the renal humoral pressor system. Moreover the lack of pressor activity of the renal venous blood of SHR excludes release by the kidney of a vasoconstrictor agent other than renin-angiotensin as the cause of the high blood pressure.

REFERENCES

1. AOKI, K. (1963): Jap Heart J, **4**, 443.
2. BARBOUR, B. H., HILL, J. and BARBOUR, A. M. (1966): Proc Soc Exp Biol Med, **121**, 124.
3. BROWN, J. J., DAVIES, D. L., LEVER, A. F. and ROBERTSON, J. I. S. (1964): Can Med Assoc J, **90**, 210.
4. FITZ, A. E. and ARMSTRONG, M. L. (1964): Circulation, **29**, 409.
5. GOORNO, W. E. and KAPLAN, N. M. (1965): Ann Intern Med, **63**, 745.
6. GOULD, A. B., SKEGGS, L. T. and KAHN, J. R. (1966): Lab Invest, **15**, 1802.
7. HARTROFT, P. M. and HARTROFT, W. S. (1953): J Exp Med, **97**, 415.
8. KOLETSKY, S., JACKSON, E. B., Jr., HESS, B. M., RIVERA-VELEZ, J. M. and PRITCHARD, W. H. (1966): Proc Soc Exp Biol Med, **122**, 941.
9. KOLETSKY, S., RIVERA-VELEZ, J. M., MARSH, D. G. and PRITCHARD, W. H. (1967): Proc Soc Exp Biol Med, **125**, 96.
10. KOLETSKY, S. and RIVERA-VELEZ, J. M. (1970): J Lab Clin Med, **76**, 54.
11. NOLA-PANADES, J. and SMIRK, F. H. (1964): Aust Ann Med, **13**, 320.
12. SOKABE, H. (1966): Jap J Physiol, **16**, 380.

THE ROLE OF SODIUM BALANCE AND THE PITUITARY-ADRENAL AXIS IN THE HYPERTENSION OF SPONTANEOUSLY HYPERTENSIVE RATS

L. BAER*, A. KNOWLTON* and J. H. LARAGH*

INTRODUCTION

The role of genetic determinants for the development of hypertension has been studied for several decades. These studies, in part, have been focused on three congenital forms of hypertension in rats developed by SMIRK, DAHL, OKAMOTO and AOKI [12, 3, 7]. Unlike DOCA-salt or Goldblatt models, these congenitally hypertensive rats require no drug treatment or surgical procedures to raise blood pressure. Thus, the spontaneous and sustained nature of the hypertension bears similarities to essential hypertension in man. Moreover, in spontaneously hypertensive rats (SHR) pathological changes—including vascular disease, cardiomegaly, myocardial infarction, nephrosclerosis and cerebral hemorrhage—have been described. SHR have also been shown to bear another resemblance to some human forms of hypertension. Adrenal cortical hyperplasia has been observed in SHR and in some patients with hypertension [8, 10]. In addition, earlier reports have suggested that SHR have low renal renin content and depressed juxtaglomerular cell granularity (13, 5). Altogether these results indicate similarities between the hypertensive process of SHR and some human forms of hypertension.

The studies reported herein further characterize the role of sodium metabolism and the adrenal gland in the hypertension of SHR.

In addition, we have carried out a number of studies of the renin-angiotensin system in control rats and SHR. Although these studies were internally consistent and in general agreement with previous reports, we have elected not to report these findings in detail at this time. This is because plasma renin concentration in SHR, measured by bioassay, was always very low in SHR when compared to that in control Wistar rats. We are now using a radioimmunoassay method to measure plasma renin activity. With this method, low renin values can be measured with much greater accuracy than with bioassay techniques. Our preliminary studies of renin in SHR using this technique confirm the results of our previous bioassay measurements that renin is not increased and may be below that in normal Wistar rats.

METHODS

The strain of SHR used in these studies were direct descendants of the original strain developed by OKAMOTO and AOKI. Normotensive Wistar rats matched for sex and weight were used as controls. Blood pressure was measured using the microphonic tail method [4]. For determination of plasma electrolytes, approximately 2 ml of blood were drawn from the jugular vein under ether anesthesia. Plasma sodium and potassium were measured on an Instrumentation Laboratories, Inc. flame photometer.

* Department of Medicine, Columbia University College of Physicians and Surgeons, New York, N. Y., U.S.A.

The normal sodium diets consisted of Purina rat chow containing 0.42% sodium. The low sodium diet consisted of a modified Hartroft low sodium diet (General Biochemicals).

Total adrenalectomy was performed under ether anesthesia through bilateral flank incisions. Following adrenalectomy, the adrenalectomized and nonadrenalectomized control and SHR groups were all placed on a high sodium intake by substituting 0.9% saline for their drinking water and continuing the normal sodium rat chow. In order to assess the adequacy of total adrenalectomy, all the animals were placed on a low sodium diet at the conclusion of the experiment. The adrenalectomized animals died within one week. Those animals that survived the period of sodium depletion after adrenalectomy were considered incompletely adrenalectomized and were excluded from the evaluation.

RESULTS

Figure 1, illustrates the effect of four weeks of sodium depletion on the blood pressure of a group of young control rats and young SHR. The mean blood pressure of the two

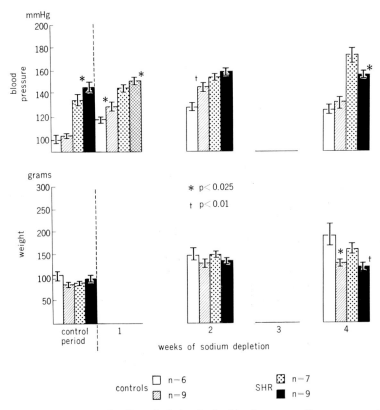

Fig. 1 Effect of 4 weeks of sodium depletion in the blood pressure of young normotensive Wistar rats and young SHR. The Wistar group (n=6) and the SHR group (n=7) maintained on normal sodium diets are indicated by the open bars and the dotted bars respectively. The sodium depleted Wistar group (n=9) and the SHR group (n=9) are indicated by the hatched bars and the black bars respectively. The control period refers to measurement while all groups were on a normal sodium diet prior to the start of sodium depletion.

groups of young SHR, 135 and 137 mm Hg, is already considerably higher than in the control groups, 102 and 104 mm Hg (p < 0.001). However, the blood pressure of these young SHR is still in the prehypertensive range when compared to older SHR. Four weeks of sodium depletion significantly slowed the characteristic rise of blood pressure in the sodium deprived SHR (156±3 mm Hg): p < 0.02. In both sodium deprived SHR and controls, body weight was significantly lower when compared to the groups fed the normal sodium diet. In contrast to the similar effects of sodium depletion on body weight in both groups, only in sodium deprived SHR was the blood pressure significantly altered. It should also be noted that the blood pressure of the sodium deprived SHR did not fall during the four week period of sodium depletion: 147±mm Hg vs. 156±3 mm Hg, and may even have increased.

Plasma potassium and sodium concentrations were measured in three groups of control rats (n=26) and SHR (n=26) while they were maintained on normal sodium diets. SHR consistently exhibited a lower mean plasma potassium concentration when compared to the control groups (p < 0.001). The mean difference between control and SHR in plasma potassium concentration in all of the three experiments was 0.5 mEq/l. Thus SHR have a mean depression of plasma potassium concentration of approximately 10%. In contrast to these differences in plasma potassium concentration in the two groups of rats, plasma sodium concentration was similar.

Figure 2, illustrates the effect of corticosterone (compound B) administration (1 mg/rat/day) in control rats and SHR. B was administered for 8 weeks to suppress the pituitary-adrenal axis. B had no significant effect on the blood pressure of control rats. In contrast, B treatment in SHR slowed the development of hypertension and this effect was maximal at 4–5 weeks. At this time the blood pressure of B-treated SHR was consistently 25–30 mm Hg lower than in the untreated group. However, with continued B treatment blood pressure rose progressively so that by the 8th week, blood pressure was similar in both B and untreated SHR groups (186±4 vs. 199±6 mm Hg).

Figure 3, illustrates the effect of total adrenalectomy (adx) on young control rats and SHR. The blood pressure of these SHR, while already higher than age-matched control animals, was considerably lower than older SHR with established hypertension. All groups were given 0.9% saline to drink. Four weeks after total adrenalectomy, the blood pressure of adx SHR rose from 146±3 to 160±2 mm Hg while the blood pressure of the non-adx SHR group rose to higher levels (135±5 to 174±6 mm Hg). Thus, despite adrenalectomy, blood pressure in adx SHR did not fall but rose although the increase in blood pressure in this group was less than in the unoperated SHR group (p < 0.02).

DISCUSSION

A number of considerations led to the study of the effect of the pituitary-adrenal axis on the suppressed renin and hypertension of SHR. Adrenal hyperplasia in SHR has been reported previously and we also observed these adrenal changes in our studies [8]. It has also been reported that aldosterone secretion is increased in SHR [9]. The lower plasma potassium concentration observed in our SHR also suggests the possibility of mineralo-corticoid excess. Accordingly, it appeared possible that an adrenal factor by producing sodium retention could lead to the hypertension of SHR. The corticosterone (compound B) experiments demonstrated that the rate of development of hypertension was slowed by the administration of B for 8 weeks. This result supports the view that an abnormal pituitary-

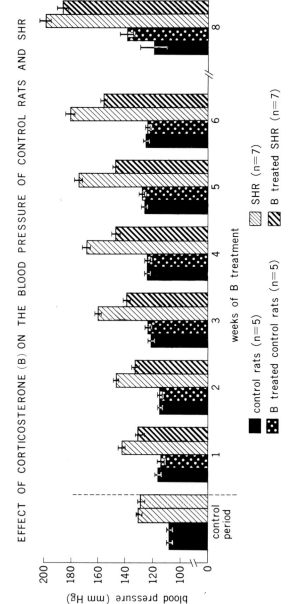

Fig. 2 Effect of corticosterone (compound B) on the blood pressure of control rats and SHR. The dose of corticosterone in these experiments was 1 mg/rat/day. The n of B-treated control rats was 5 and of B-treated SHR n=7. The black bars represent untreated control rats and the black and white dotted bars represent B-treated control rats. The black hatched bars represent untreated SHR and the white hatched bars represent B-treated SHR.

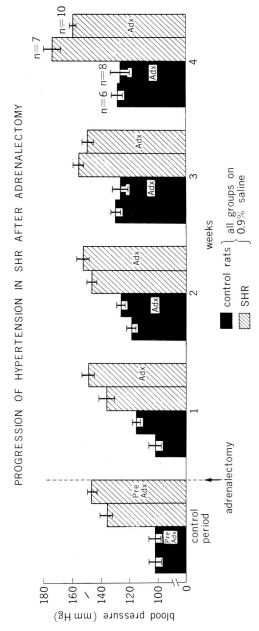

Fig. 3 Effect of total adrenalectomy (adx) on the hypertension of SHR. The n of non-adx control rats was 6 and of non-adx SHR n=7. The n of adx control rats was 8 and of adx SHR n=10. The black bars represent control rats and the hatched bars represent SHR. Adx identifies the totally adx groups.

adrenal axis is present in SHR [8]. However, SHR still became hypertensive despite B treatment. Moreover, B did not lower the blood pressure of SHR. These findings indicate that the pituitary-adrenal axis is not critically involved in the development or maintenance of the hypertension of SHR. These effects of B treatment in SHR are to be contrasted with the adrenal regeneration form of hypertension in which the same dose of B prevents the development of the hypertension in this other experimental model [11]. The experiments involving adrenalectomy (Fig. 3) also rule out the adrenal gland as a primary factor in the hypertension of SHR because total adrenalectomy in SHR failed to correct the hypertension and blood pressure even rose after adrenalectomy.

The experiments involving chronic sodium depletion demonstrated that the progressive rise of blood pressure of SHR could not be blocked by a low sodium diet. Chronic sodium depletion in our experiments delayed the development of the hypertension but it neither restored blood pressure to normal levels nor did it totally block the progressive rise of blood pressure in SHR with aging. This finding is similar to that reported by LOUIS et al [6]. Moreover, our results suggest that the effect of sodium depletion on the blood pressure of young SHR may be non-specifically related to their failure to thrive because the sodium deprived group failed to grow at a normal rate. Altogether these findings of the relationship of sodium to the hypertension of SHR indicate that sodium balance is not a critical factor in the disease process.

A number of the features of SHR described in the present study, bear a similarity to another hypertensive disorder that has recently been described in patients and has been termed pseudoprimary aldosteronism or idiopathic adrenal hyperplasia [1, 2]. SHR and patients with pseudoprimary aldosteronism exhibit mild hypokalemia and adrenal cortical hyperplasia. Total adrenalectomy in these patients, as in SHR, reverses the hypokalemia, but the hypertension is not fully corrected. Thus, in both SHR and patients with pseudoprimary aldosteronism, the hypertension is not primarily mediated by the adrenal gland, although in both situations, adrenal hyperplasia is present. Accordingly, SHR may share mechanisms in common with certain forms of hypertension in man and should prove to be a valuable tool in their study.

SUMMARY

The relationship of sodium balance and the pituitary-adrenal axis to the hypertension of spontaneously hypertensive rats (SHR) was studied. SHR exhibited adrenal hyperplasia and their plasma potassium levels were 10% lower than the control Wistar groups. Severe sodium depletion for 4 weeks in young SHR delayed the progression of hypertension but it did not reduce the blood pressure to normotensive levels. This effect of sodium depletion may be nonspecific and need not imply a critical role of dietary sodium in the mechanism of the hypertension of SHR because severe sodium depletion was also associated with retarded growth of the animals.

Suppression of the pituitary-adrenal axis with corticosterone (compound B) for 8 weeks delayed the development of severe hypertension in SHR, but it did not prevent or reverse the hypertensive process. Total adrenalectomy also did not cure the hypertension.

These results suggest that sodium balance and the adrenal cortex are not primarily involved in the hypertension of SHR. This animal model resembles at least one form of human hypertension with adrenal hyperplasia (pseudoprimary aldosteronism or idiopathic adrenal hyperplasia) because these patients also exhibit mild hypokalemia and are similarly not cured by adrenalectomy.

REFERENCES

1. BAER, L., SOMMERS, S. C., Krakoff, L. R., NEWTON, M. A. and Laragh, J. H. (1970): Circ Res, **26** and **27,** Suppl I, I–203.
2. BIGLIERI, E. G., SCHAMBELAN, M., SLATON, P. E. and STOCKIGT, J. R. (1970): Circ Res, **26** and **27,** Suppl I, I–195.
3. DAHL, L. K., HEINE, M. and TASSINARI, L. (1962): J Exp Med, **115,** 1173.
4. FRIEDMAN, M. and FREED, S. C. (1949): Proc Soc Exp Biol Med, **70,** 670.
5. HAGA, M., SOKABE, H. and OKAMOTO, K. (1966): Jap Circ J, **30,** 1479.
6. LOUIS, W. J., TABEI, R. and SPECTOR, S. (1971): Lancet, **2,** 1283.
7. OKAMOTO, K. and AOKI, K. (1963): Jap Circ J, **27,** 282.
8. OKAMOTO, K., AOKI, K., NOSAKA, S. and FUKUSHIMA, M. (1964): Jap Circ J, **28,** 943.
9. RAPP, J. P. and DAHL, L. K. (1971): Endocrinology, **88,** 50.
10. SHAMMA, A. H., GODDARD, J. W. and SOMMERS, S. C. (1958): J Chron Dis, **8,** 587.
11. SKELTON, F. S. (1958): Endocrinology, **62,** 365.
12. SMIRK, F. H. and HALL, W. H. (1958): Nature **182,** 727.
13. SOKABE, H. (1964): Jap J Physiol, **16,** 380.

RESPONSIVENESS OF SPONTANEOUSLY HYPERTENSIVE RATS TO A HYPERTENSION-INDUCING SUBSTANCE OF THE KIDNEY

K. OGINO*, J. KIRA* and M. MATSUNAGA*

Concerning renal or hormonal pressor substances, such as renin or catecholamines, extensive studies on acute pressor effects have contributed to explanations of the pressor mechanism. As to their role in sustaining clinical hypertension, however, evidence is lacking except for cases of hypertension with renal or endocrine disorders. This is particularly true in essential hypertension where these substances are not considered active participants in sustaining high blood pressure. Investigations have been carried out on resulting hypertension following the administration of pressor substances, especially angiotensin [1, 3, 4]. MASSON, et al. [5–8] reported that an experimental hypertension similar to renovascular hypertension was produced in the rat by repeated injections of endocrine kidney extract, crude renin, or semi-purified hog renin mixed with tissue extract, gelatin etc.

Recently, KIRA and colleagues [2] studied the relationship between renin content and hypertension-inducing potency of kidney extracts obtained from normal rats as well as rats undergoing various treatments. It was found that the hypertension-inducing potency of these extracts did not always parallel the renin content, and the extract from adrenalectomized rats had a high potency for inducing hypertension.

This implies a participation of a renal substance other than renin in inducing and sustaining hypertension.

The effects of kidney extracts from adrenalectomized rats on normal rats and SHR are compared in this study.

METHODS

Adrenalectomized rats were given water (I) or 1% saline (II), then these and non-treated rats (III) were sacrificed a week after by bleeding and kidney extracts were prepared. The extracts are referred to as Extract I, II and III respectively. Each extract was injected subcutaneously into the rat at noon and midnight each day. Blood pressure was measured 10 to 12 hrs. after injection by a tail plethysmographic method.

The incubation mixture for determination of renin concentration was at pH 6.5 and consisted of kidney extract, adequate renin substrate and angiotensinase inhibitors. The mixture was deproteinized by heating following incubation at 37°C, and pressor activity was bioassayed.

RESULTS

1) *Substantiation of a hypertension-inducing potency unrelated to renin content in the kidney extract.* The left kidneys of Wistar rats weighing approximately 100 gm were removed. In the first experiment, 0.5 ml of each extract was subcutaneously injected every twelve hrs. into the uninephrectomized rats six to seven days after nephrectomy. The course of blood pressure and body weight were followed for ten days; then, the rats were bled to death for histological examination.

---

* Department of Internal Medicine, Faculty of Medicine, Kyoto University, Kyoto, Japan

Blood pressure in each group began to rise approximately 4 days after the beginning of injection, and steadily increased. Blood pressure elevation was most marked in Extract I group, slightest in III and intermediate in II. Thus, animals of Extract I group developed manifest hypertension six to seven days after the beginning of injection. Increase in body weight was impaired most markedly in Extract I group and slightly in Group III. Animals in Extract I group were in poor condition, suggesting the presence of a toxic factor in the extract. Ratios of heart weight to body weight at termination time of the experiment were the highest in Extract I group and next in Group II.

Renin concentration was similar in Extract I and II, and slightly lower in Extract III.

In the second experiment, the amount of Extract I injection was reduced so that the injected renin content would be less than that of Extract III. Nevertheless, the blood pressure in Extract I group was much more elevated than in Group III and maintained the high level of 200 mm Hg 10 days after the beginning of injection. Increase in body weight was impaired in Extract I group, but less than in the former experiment.

The high ratio of heart weight to body weight in Extract I group at the termination time of the experiment indicated the influence of induced hypertension on the heart. These results suggested that Extract I contained a substance with a hypertension-inducing potency, not connected to renin activity.

2) *Comparison of effects of the kidney extract on normal rats and SHR.* Young SHR without manifest hypertension were used. Normal Wistar rats of approximately the same age and body weight were utilized as the control group. Extract I, that is the kidney extract from adrenalectomized rats which had been given water, was subcutaneously injected in the same manner as mentioned above into the SHR and control rats each weighing about 100 gm. This was done 2 to 4 days after left nephrectomy. Blood pressure and body weight were observed for seven days. Figure 1 shows changes in blood pressure; solid, broken and dotted lines correspond to the groups injected with 0.5 ml, 0.25 ml of Extract I and 0.5 ml of saline, respectively. Injection of Extract I elevated the blood pressure significantly in both SHR and control rats.

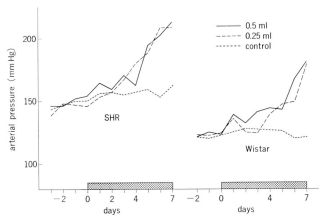

Fig. 1   Injection of extract of adrenalex. rat-kidney.

In this experiment, however, no difference in the responsiveness between SHR and control rats was observed. Next, a lesser amount of Extract I was injected into the younger SHR without manifest hypertension as well as the control rats, both types weighed about 60 gm.

Figure 2 shows that blood pressure rose significantly in both SHR and control rats injected with 0.1 ml of Extract I, as compared to the blood pressure of rats injected with 0.1 ml of saline. It appeared that SHR was more sensitive to Extract I than the control rats.

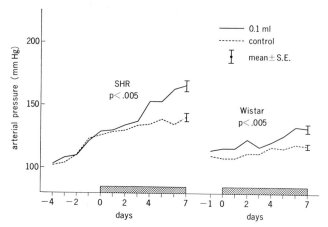

Fig. 2   Injection of extract of adrenalex. rat-kidney.

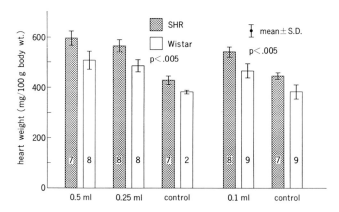

Fig. 3   Cardiac hypertrophy in treated rats.

Figure 3 is a histogram showing heart weight per 100 gm of body weight at termination of the experiment. Heart weight was significantly increased in SHR and control rats injected with Extract I. This indicates the influence of hypertension induced by Extract I.

CONCLUSION

1)   An experimental hypertension was produced in rats by subcutaneous injections twice daily of kidney extracts from the same strain. The kidney extract had a hypertension-inducing potency which was remarkable in the extract from the adrenalectomized rat given water and was not parallel with the renin content.

2)   It is suggested from these studies that the kidney extract possibly contains a substance with a hypertension-inducing potency, other than renin.

3)   SHR seemed to be hyper-responsive to the hypertension-inducing effect of the rat kidney extract.

ACKNOWLEDGEMENTS

The authors are grateful to Prof. Dr. Okamoto for provision of SHR and to M. Ohara for assistance with the manuscript.

REFERENCES

1. Dickinson, C. T. and Lawrence, J. R. (1963):   Lancet, **1**, 1354.
2. Kira, J., Onishi, K., Yamamoto, J., Konishi, N., Yamatori, K. and Kamiguchi, T. (1971): Jap Circ J, **35**, 1591.
3. Koletsky, S., Rivera-Velez, J. M. and Pritchard, V. H. (1966):   Arch Pathol, **82**, 99.
4. McCubbin, J. W., DeMoura, R. S., Page, I. H. and Olmsted, F. (1965):   Science, **149**, 1394.
5. Masson, G. M. C., Kashii, C., Panisset, J. C., Yagi, S. and Page, I. H. (1964): Circ Res, **14**, 150.
6. Masson, G. M. C., Kashii, C. Matsunaga, M. and Page, I. H. (1964):   Science, **145**, 178.
7. Masson, G. M. C., Kashii, C., Matsunaga, M. and Page, I. H. (1965):   Proc Soc Exp Biol Med, **120**, 640.
8. Masson, G. M. C., Kashii, C., Matsunaga, M. and Page, I. H. (1966):   Circ Res, **18**, 219.

EFFECT OF SPONTANEOUS AND RENAL HYPERTENSION ON A PARABIOTIC PARTNER IN RATS*

A. EBIHARA**

Although many papers have been published on the pathogenesis of hypertension in man and animals, it is still obscure whether it is mediated by a humoral principle or by neurogenic factor. In this study we investigated the transmissibility of the congenital and renal hypertension to the partner united in parabiosis in rats. Our results indicate that hypertension resulting from renal artery constriction and partial renal infarction is transmissible through the parabiotic junction, but that congenital hypertension is not transmissible. The observations were interpreted as indicating that both types of renal hypertension involve (a) humoral factor(s) and that in congenital hypertension, there is no transmissible humoral factor.

MATERIALS AND METHODS

In these studies, 4-week-old male spontaneoulsy hypertensive rats and Wistar rats of the same age were used. All animals were kept in mesh cages, fed Purina Laboratory Chow and tap water *ad libitum*. Systolic blood pressure was determined by the tail microphone method [1] without anesthesia after animals were warmed for 10 minutes in a heating box maintained at 39°C.

Parabiosis was performed under sodium pentobarbital anesthesia by suturing scapulae, muscles and skin, making a common peritoneal cavity. Uninephrectomy was performed on the adjoining side of each rat at the time of the parabiosis operation.

Renal artery constriction was performed by ligation of the renal artery using a guide wire having a diameter of 0.36 mm. Hemi-infarct of the kidney was produced by ligating the posterior branch of the renal artery [3].

In the studies involving renal artery constriction and hemi-infarct of the kidney, the second operation was performed 6 weeks after parabiosis operation.

RESULTS

Fig. 1 illustrates that when a normotensive uninephrectomized Wistar rats is joined in parabiosis with a normotensive uninephrectomized sham-operated one, the systolic blood pressure does not significantly change over a 12-week observation period.

Fig. 2 depicts the observation in 10 pairs of rats, in one of which renal artery stenosis was induced 6 weeks after parabiosis was established.

During the 1 week after partial ligation of the main renal artery, the rats showed a significant blood pressure increase. The blood pressures of the partner rats in parabiotic union were significantly elevated over the 12-week observation period.

Fig. 3 shows similar observations in 8 pairs of rats, one of which had a hemi-infarct of the kidney induced by ligation of a major renal artery branch.

Again, the uninephrectomized partner in parabiosis showed a significant increase in the blood pressure.

* This work was supported by Lilly Research Grant.
** Department of Internal Medicine, Faculty of Medicine, University of Tokyo, Tokyo, Japan

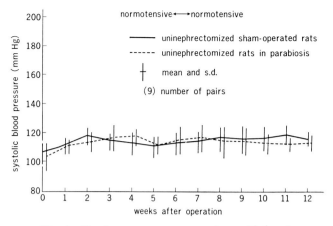

Fig. 1 Blood pressure measurement in parabiotic rats.

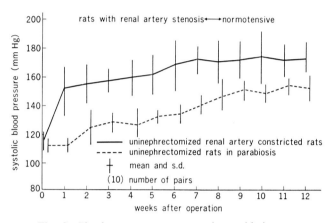

Fig. 2 Blood pressure measurement in parabiotic rats.

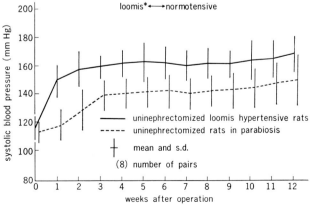

*Hemi-infarct induced by ligation of major renal artery branch

Fig. 3 Blood pressure measurement in parabiotic rats.

Fig. 4 gives results in 6 pairs of uninephrectomized spontaneously hypertensive rats joined with uninephrectomized normotensive Wistar rats.

The blood pressure observations over a period of 12 weeks indicates no increase of pressure in the normal rats and no interference with the normal progression of hypertension in the spontaneously hypertensive partners.

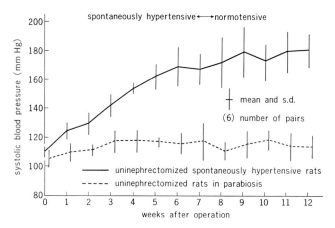

Fig. 4 Blood pressure measurement in parabiotic rats.

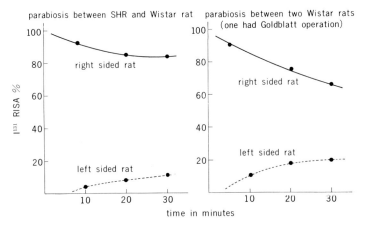

Fig. 5 Exchange between parabiotic partners. Appearance and disappearance of I^{131} RISA injected intravenously to the right sided rat.

Fig. 5 reveals the results of experiments of blood exchange rate between the two rats of parabiosis. As shown in this figure, both in the instance of the combination of a spontaneously hypertensive rat and a normal Wistar rat and in the parabiosis between a rat with renal artery constriction and a normotensive rat, a significant appearance of I^{131} tagged albumin was observed in the blood of the parabiotic partner in 30 minutes after intravenous injection.

DISCUSSION

These studies indicate that the hypertension in spontaneously hypertensive rats is not transferred to the parabiotic partner. It is, thus, interpreted that the hypertension in this strain is not mediated by a transmissible humoral factor.

SOKABE [4] reported that the spontaneously hypertensive rat did not show increased renin activity in the renal venous blood nor in the renal tissue as compared with the normotensive control rat. The results of our studies indicate that the hypertension resulting from main renal artery narrowing and from hemi-infarct of the kidney induced by ligation of a major renal artery branch is transmitted to a parabiotic partner. It is still obscure whether the chronic stage of these experimental models of hypertension is mediated by humoral factors *per se* or whether early influence of a humoral factor affects neurogenic control. Spontaneous hypertension in parabiotic rats was reported by HALL and HALL [2]. In our studies, such spontaneous hypertension was observed in approximately 25 per cent of parabionts between Wistar rats. The second operation (renal artery operation) was performed only in parabionts which did not show an elevation of blood pressure by the sixth postoperative week—based on our experience that such hypertension, if it develops, will be apparent by that time. In these studies, such spontaneous hypertension was not observed in any Wistar rat partner connected in parabiosis with a spontaneously hypertensive rat.

CONCLUSION

Parabiotic studies in rats have indicated that the hypertension following renal artery constriction as well as that associated with renal hemi-infarct results in hypertension in the parabiotic partner. When spontaneously hypertensive rats were united with normotensive rats, no transmission or amelioration of the blood pressure was noted.

ACKNOWLEDGMENT

The author gratefully thanks Dr. B. L. MARTZ for his encouragement and correction of the manuscript and Dr. M. IIO for his contribution in measuring the body fluid exchange rate with radioactive albumin.

REFERENCES

1. FRIEDMAN, M. and FREED, S. C. (1949): Proc Soc Exp Biol Med, **70**, 670.
2. HALL, C. E. and HALL, O. (1951): Am Med Assoc Pathol, **51**, 527.
3. LOOMIS, D. (1946): Arch Pathol, **41**, 231.
4. SOKABE, H. (1965): Nature, **205**, 90.

FLUID EXCHANGE BETWEEN PARABIOTIC RATS OF THE BROOKHAVEN STRAINS*

K. D. KNUDSEN**, L. K. DAHL**, J. IWAI** and M. HEINE**

In our laboratory we have developed two rat colonies with disparate predisposition to hypertensive disease. Their acronyms, R and S rats, indicate their relative resistance (R) or senstivity (S) to various manipulations used to produce experimental hypertension. Ancestors for both colonies were originally selected from the same batch of Sprague-Dawley rats on the basis of their reponse to salt (NaCl) intake [1].

By continued selective breeding the complementary traits have been improved so that R rats are tolerant to salt intake, while S rats given a diet containing 8% NaCl develop malignant hypertension and die within 5–12 weeks. Left to their own on a low sodium intake, both strains remain healthy although some of the S rats become mildly hypertensive. These colonies provide a valuable tool for controlled studies of experimental hypertension.

The two strains have retained a high degree of tissue compatibility. Organs may be transplanted between R and S rats, and we have united them in parabiosis without evidence of parabiosis intoxication or mutual rejection. Parabiosis permits exchange of blood and extracellular fluid between partners, and by joining R with S animals we were able to study humoral aspects of the pathogenesis of hypertension. Most striking was the observation that on 8% NaCl the S animal survived and developed only moderate hypertension, while the R co-twin developed an unprecedented hypertension of the same magnitude as the S partner [2].

We may not have the definitive explanation for these findings but subsequent studies have revealed that in part, at least, the response is caused by a hypertensinogenic humoral factor produced in S rat kidney [8, 10].

A knowledge of the nature of parabiotic exchange was necessary for a proper interpretation of the observations. In particular, in experiments that involved complete nephrectomy of one partner, the parabiosis junction not only served as a channel for transfer of humoral agents but it became the lifeline on which the anephric partner depended for its existence. Under those circumstances, preparations of two R rats (in our jargon called R–R parabionts) were more viable than those involving at least one S partner (R–S or S–S parabionts). Two possible explanations were either that S rats produced an agent which was toxic under anephric conditions, or that the S rats provided a poorer exchange and consequently clearance of waste products from the nephrectomized partner. A corollary to the latter explanation was that the exchange even in R–R parabionts was marginal for conditions of survival, and that a small deterioration was sufficient to tip the scales. Serial BUN measurements favored the latter hypothesis. We therefore decided to measure the rates of exchange in the different preparations. This paper outlines the method developed for this purpose and reports the most relevant observations.

MATERIAL

R and S rats bred in our laboratory were used. These rats were developed from the same

* This work was supported primarily by the U.S. Atomic Energy Commission; partial support was received from the USPHS (HE 13408-01) and a grant-in-aid of the American Heart Association (AHA 70-772) supported by the Dutchess County (N.Y.) Heart Association.
** Medical Department, Brookhaven National Laboratory, Upton, New York U.S.A.

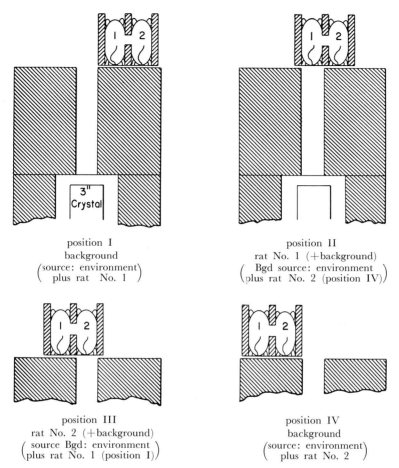

position I
background
$\left(\begin{array}{c}\text{source: environment}\\ \text{plus rat No. 1}\end{array}\right)$

position II
rat No. 1 (+background)
$\left(\begin{array}{c}\text{Bgd source: environment}\\ \text{plus rat No. 2 (position IV)}\end{array}\right)$

position III
rat No. 2 (+background)
$\left(\begin{array}{c}\text{source Bgd: environment}\\ \text{plus rat No. 1 (position I)}\end{array}\right)$

position IV
background
$\left(\begin{array}{c}\text{source: environment}\\ \text{plus rat No. 2}\end{array}\right)$

Fig. 1 Schematic drawing of whole body counter for rats in parabiosis. The tower
was built of lead bricks, the carrier of 1/2-inch lead plate.
Overall dimensions:
Collimator: 14" w × 16" d × 10" h
Opening: 2" w × 8" d × 10" h
Carrier: 5 1/2" w × 12" d × 4 1/2" h
The walls of the carrier could be adjusted, and it had a mechanism for reproducible
positioning.

original colony of Sprague-Dawley rats by selective breeding for the genetic traits of
resistance (R) and sensitivity (S), respectively, to development of salt hypertension [1].

The exchange studies were done on 10-week-old rats of both sexes. At the age of 4
weeks they had been joined in parabiosis, and one partner had been uninephrectomized.
They were scheduled to have a second nephrectomy 2 weeks after the experiments described here were completed. 39 pairs were examined: 13 R–R, 14 R–S, and 12 S–S preparations. ^{24}Na was chosen as the tracer; it was easily obtainable as a carrier-free ^{24}Na$_2$CO$_3$
and its physical half-life of 15.0 hrs. was long enough to permit counting for 24 hrs. yet
short enough for the isotope to be self-destructing in the two weeks before we intended
further procedures. It had high-energy gamma emissions. We built a "whole-body counter"
(Fig. 1) which could efficiently count doses less than 0.1μCi^{24}Na injected into a rat.

In the studies to be described, 10–20 μCi^{24}Na was injected into one rat via a polyethylene
catheter inserted into a tail vein and brought up to the root of the tail. Counting was

started at once as a series of 1 minute counts in the positions shown in Fig. 1. The count sequence was I–II–III–IV–IV–III–II–I and took 8–10 minutes to complete. Time was recorded when counting started, and 5 minutes were added to this value when decay curves were constructed, using the average for each position to calculate activity.

Calculation of exchange rates:

We chose a two-compartment closed system as the model for calculations. This model has been thoroughly analyzed and leads to a simple computation of the desired parameters. The model and its relevant equations are presented by ROBERTSON [12]. The application to the present problem is discussed here.

Nomenclature:

S_i = Amount of substance (labelled plus non-labelled) in ith compartment. (Here, i will take the values 1 and 2, only.)

x_i = Specific activity of radio-active label in S_i

$x_{i,o}$ = x_i at time zero

x_E = x_i at equilibrium ("infinite" time)

r_{ij} = Rate of flow of substance (labelled plus unlabelled) into ith compartment from jth compartment

t = elapsed time in minutes

In our calculations we considered two compartments, S_1 and S_2. We assumed a steady state $r_{1,2} = r_{2,1} = r$

The appropriate equations are

$$x_i = x_E + (x_{i,o} - x_E) \; \text{Exp} \; (-(r/S_1 + r/S_2)t) \tag{1}$$

or, in logarithmic form

$$\text{Log}|(x_i - x_E)| = \text{Log}|(x_{i,o} - x_E)| - (r/S_1 + r/S_2)t \tag{2}$$

We did not calculate absolute values for r but the ratios r/S_1 and r/S_2. We arbitrarily set $x_E = 1$, and the total dose injected equal to 100%. In order to compensate for decay and excretion we recalculated all values in terms of per cent of total activity present. The equilibrium distribution served as a measure of S_1 and S_2, and x_i at any time would be

$$x_1 = \frac{\text{percent of total activity in rat } i}{\text{percent of total activity in rat } i \text{ at equilibrium}}$$

Table 1 gives an example of the computation.

A least squares fit of EQUATION [2], or a manual fit of a curve to the data as plotted on a semilogarithmic paper gave the slope $(r/S_1 + r/S_2)$ which in turn permitted the calculation of r/S_1 and r/S_2.

The model assumes instantaneous, perfect mixing of label in each compartment. This is obviously not the case in parabionts. Sodium is distributed in intravascular and extravascular spaces, and in the latter space there are necessarily gradients before equilibrium is established. What we assume is that exchange rates between these spaces are orders of magnitude larger than the exchange rate between partners, so that for the purpose of interest here, we can treat each rat as a single homogeneous compartment. It is the one most precarious assumption of the whole computation. The activity is initially confined to the blood stream. During this phase the values of the distribution spaces (S_1 and S_2) are smaller, and the exponential constant $(r/S_1 + r/S_2)$ may be larger than after an equilibration in the whole extracellular space has been effected. When the vascular anastomosis is good, this initial phase will contribute significantly to the exchange curve and the equation will need two or more exponential terms to describe the curve properly. To extract and interpret information from such curves is not an exact science, but involves educated guesses. Whenever it was evident that a single exponential equation was inade-

Table 1 Example of a computation of specific activity. "Positions" refer to Fig. 1. For further details, see text.

Time:	50 min.	1500 min.
A. Actual counts, average		
Position I	244 cpm	178 cpm
" II	4929 "	2985 "
" III	12766 "	2282 "
" IV	304 "	159 "
B. Background corrections		
Rat ♯ 1 (Pos. II – Pos. IV)	4625 cpm	2826 cpm
Rat ♯ 2 (Pos. III – Pos. I)	12522 "	2104 "
Total	17147 "	4930 "
C. Normalization of data (per cent of total)		
Rat ♯ 1	27%	57.3%
Rat ♯ 2	73 "	42.7 "
Total	100 "	100 "
D. Specific activity (x_i)		
Rat ♯ 1 (x_1)	.47 (=27/57.3)	1.00
Rat ♯ 2 (x_2)	1.71 (=73/42.7)	1.00

quate, we took the position that the late exponent reflected the exchange rates relative to total extracellular sodium.

The model assumes a steady state, *i.e.*, r (=$r_{1,2}$=$r_{2,1}$) is the same in both directions. We have no reason to doubt this assumption. It is unlikely, but conceivable that one rat does all the drinking, the other all the excretion, of fluid resulting in a net flux in one direction. Even so, it would at worst amount to 1–2% of the total flux. We have measured intakes and output; as long as both animals have at least one kidney the assumption is valid for present purposes.

Specific activity at equilibrium (x_E) is assumed to be the same in both partners.   We have measured specific activity in plasma samples one day after injection and found no significant differences.

In short, we believe the method to be adequate for the purpose, and the computations to be acceptable. They must be viewed in light of the implicit assumptions in order to avoid unwarranted conclusions. In particular, if the curves are irregular and/or do not go through the theoretical intercepts with the y axis (as computed from the expression ($x_{i, o}$ $-x_E$)) the potential for error is great. In the present study most of the curves were acceptable from that point of view.

RESULTS

Exchange rates varied by a factor of 10 from the best to the poorest; and there was a considerable overlapping of results between the groups. The mean exchange rate for R-R parabionts, 0.46% of total extracellular fluid of one partner per minute, was significantly higher than that of the other two combinations (R-S and S-S). Their average was 0.29% of ECF per minute; (P<0.1).

We also found a significant rank correlation between exchange rate and survival time after complete nephrectomy. Except for extreme values, prediction of individual cases

Table 2

A. Rate of exchange of ECF between parabiotic partners, expressed as fraction of ECF/min. Average and standard deviation.

B. Per cent survivors 4 weeks after complete nephrectomy of one partner.

		A			B	
		Exchange rates			4 week survival after complete nephrectomy. (240 pairs)	
Parabiont combination	No. of pairs	r/Si				
		mean	s.d.			
		min^{-1}			%	Combination
R-R	13	.0046*	.0024		61	R-R
R-S	14	.0029	.0016		40	R-S
S-S	12	.0029	.0009		23	S-S

*R-R is significantly different from R-S and S-S (p<.01)

was erratic but at comparable levels of exchange we could not observe a systematic difference between R-R, R-S, and S-S preparations.

The observations are summed up in Table 2.

DISCUSSION

The study was prompted by a specific problem, the mortality of nephrectomized parabionts and the apparent systematic difference between strains. Before we discuss it in those terms, it is worthwhile to take a broader look at the physiology of the parabiosis junction.

Early workers were puzzled by the fact that sex hormones were ineffectively transmitted compared to pituitary hormones. The concept of a "parabiotic barrier" emerged [3]. Hill [5, 6], who was the first to measure the rate of plasma exchange in parabiotic rats, demonstrated that this barrier was dynamic, not anatomical or physiological, in nature. There was no filtering effect based on particle size—at least up to the size of blood cells—and there was no selectivity on other basis residing at the site of the union. The relevant factors were rate of exchange in relation to rate of metabolic disposal in each partner. Grollman and Rule [4] and Huff, Trautman and Van Dyke [7] confirmed the values reported by Hill and stressed the important consequences of his conclusions.

Ledingham [11] was faced with the same problem as we were: Survival of nephrectomized parabionts. His estimates of plasma exchange rates confirmed those of Hill, and varied by a factor of 2 from good to poor. He concluded that..."the impression was gained that when the anastomosis was poor the nephrectomized member did not live long".

The clearance concept takes on a special aspect in this situation. Since the junction is non-selective, a clearance for any given substance is proportional to the concentration gradient between partners and to the exchange rate, and inversely proportional to the concentration in the nephrectomized rat.

$$\text{Clearance} = (C_2 - C_1)r/C_2 = r(1 - C_1/C_2) \qquad (3)$$

(C_1 and C_2 are concentrations in plasma of rats 1 and 2, respectively)

This equation and a knowledge of the range of r enabled us to establish reasonable conditions for metabolic studies without costly trial and error. Thus we estimated that, even at best, a diet with 8% NaCl would create a sodium gradient of minimum 13 mEq/L, unless the nephrectomized partner cut down on his intake, and got some of his nutrients from the blood of his co-twin. Consequently, we had to reduce the level of intake considerably for the study of sodium metabolism after nephrectomy.

Our exchange rates referred to "sodium space", not to plasma as did most of the available data in the literature. Other variables, which we did not test, may therefore be significant. To all intents and purposes, red blood cells (RBC) are not part of the sodium space. Since RBC carry urea and other substances, the ratio of vascular to extravascular transport at any level of sodium exchange is a factor of importance. A more complete test should involve labeling of both sodium and RBC. We did one such study. Tagged cells were obtained from a donor that had incorporated ^{59}Fe *in vivo*. In each partner the exchange per minute amounted to 0.65 per cent of the total blood volume and 0.25 per cent of sodium space. We estimated that 30 per cent of sodium exchange in this pair was carried by plasma.

HILL [6] emphasized the day-to-day variation which he claimed to be as great as the variation between pairs. He therefore thought that all the observed variance was random, and not related to different efficiency of the anastomosis. To our knowledge, no one has tried to confirm or refute this statement. His mean values agree remarkably well with those obtained with today's superior instrumentation. The same may not be true for the variance. He could measure one point on the exponential curve, only, and the variance of his method may have been too large to permit the detection of variance in his preparations.

We must conclude from our study that the vascularization of the parabiosis junction was less efficient when at least one S rat was part of the preparation. The reason for this is not presently known. It is a fact that S rats have a more vulnerable vascularization of *kidneys* in that branching pads at the site of small arterioles easily proliferate and may occlude the lumen [9]. Similar problems may exist in the vascular network of the parabiosis junction.

We were satisfied that this systematic difference, and the uncontrolled variables discussed above, sufficed to explain the observations on survival of nephrectomized parabionts. Although we had not ruled out a toxic influence from the S rat we did not have to postulate one in order to explain our observations.

SUMMARY

Rats of the Brookhaven strain were united in parabiosis and the rate of exchange of extracellular fluid between partners was measured 6 weeks after the union, when the rats were 10 weeks old.

When the pairs consisted of two R rats, (from the colony resistant to experimental hypertension), the exchange was more efficient than in pairs involving at least one S rat (from the colony sensitive to experimental hypertension).

The method for measuring exchange rate is presented. Some consequences of the findings are discussed.

REFERENCES

1. DAHL, L. K., HEINE, M. and TASSINARI, L. (1962): J Exp Med, **115**, 1173.
2. DAHL, L. K., KNUDSEN, K. D., HEINE, M. and LEITL, G. (1967): J Exp Med, **126**, 687.
3. FINERTY, JOHN C. (1952): Physiol Rev, **32**, 277.
4. GROLLMAN, A. and RULE, C. (1943): Am J Physiol, **138**, 587.
5. HILL, R. T. (1931): Proc Soc Exp Biol Med, **28**, 295.
6. HILL, R. T. (1932): J Exp Zool, **63**, 203.

7. HUFF, R. L., TRAUTMAN, R. and VAN DYKE, D. C. (1950): Am J Physiol, **161**, 56.
8. IWAI, J., KNUDSEN, K. D., DAHL, L. K., HEINE, M. and LEITL, G. (1969): J Exp Med, **129**, 507.
9. JAFFÉ, D., SUTHERLAND, L. E., BARKER, D. M. and DAHL, L. K. (1970): Arch Pathol, **90**, 1.
10. KNUDSEN, K. D., IWAI, J., HEINE, M., LEITL, G. and Dahl, L. K. (1969): J Exp Med, **130**, 1353.
11. LEDINGHAM, J. M. (1951): Clin Sci, **10**, 423.
12. ROBERTSON, J. S. (1962): *In* "Handbook of Physiology" Section 2: Circulation, (W. F. HAMILTON and P. DOW, eds.) Vol. 1, p. 617, American Physiological Society, Washington, D. C.

RENIN INHIBITOR IN THE HYPERTENSION-PRONE RAT*

J. IWAI**, K. D. KNUDSEN** and L. K. DAHL**

By selective inbreeding, two strains of rats were evolved with opposite genetic propensities for hypertension (HT) from high salt intake as well as other common renal manipulations used to induce experimental HT [2, 3]. We have been looking for inherent differences between these two strains of rats that will account for the disparity in blood pressure response. In previous experiments we reported that rats from the strain with a genetic predisposition to HT (the Sensitive or S strain) produced a humoral factor which was transmittable in parabiosis and induced HT in rats genetically resistant (the Resistant or R strain) to this condition [4].

We surmised that the factor was identical both in salt hypertension and in renal

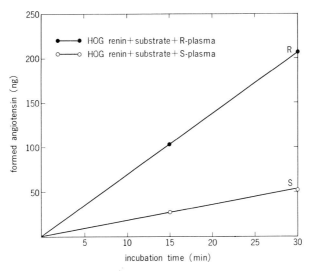

Fig. 1 The velocity of reaction between hog renin and rat renin substrate in the presence of plasma from intact R and S rats.

hypertension and have evidence that it is produced by the kidneys of hypertension-prone rats [4, 5, 7, 8]. We have explored to renin angiotensin system in our two strains of rats and have studied its possible relationship to the hypertensinogenic factor encounted in hypertension-prone rats.

The two strains of rats were tested for the responses to injections of angiotensin-II and hog renin and the influence of their plasma on the reaction velocity between hog renin and rat substrate *in vitro*. Renin activity level was measured by the micromethod of BOUCHER et al. [1]; a detailed report on the method used here has been published [6]. The pressor response to angiotensin II (Hypertensin - Ciba) of intact S rats on low salt was significantly higher than that of comparable R rats. High salt intake increased the

* This work was supported primarily by the U.S. Atomic Energy Commission; partial support was received from the USPHS (HE 13408-01) and a grant-in-aid of the American Heart Association (AHA 70-772) supported by the Dutchess County (N.Y.) Heart Association.
** Medical Department Brookhaven National Laboratory, Upton, New York, U.S.A.

response of S rats but not of R rats. After bilateral nephrectomy, there were no significant differences in responses between R and S rats ($p > 0.05$). In contrast to the results with angiotensin II, the pressor response to renin of intact S rats on low salt was significantly lower than that of R rats. These results have led us to suspect the existence of a block in the series of reactions from renin to the production of angiotensin II. Therefore, we have measured the reaction velocity between hog renin, (0.01 units) and rat substrate (150 mg) in the presence of plasma from R and S rats. Plasma from intact S rats inhibited hog renin activity *in vitro*, whereas plasma from intact R rats showed no inhibition (Fig. 1). Plasma from bilaterally nephrectomized rats from either strain showed no inhibition.

The lower pressor response of S rats to renin might be explained by assuming that the S rats had a lower activity of converting enzyme than R rats, but in the system which we used *in vitro* experiments, only the inactive angiotensin I was generated and only S rats were used for bioassay.

The reaction velocity between renin and substrate was inhibited by plasma from intact S rats. This inhibition was not due to less amounts of substrate, since this was present in excess *in vitro*.

The disappearance of the inhibition after bilateral nephrectomy suggested that the agent responsible for the inhibition was produced by the kidney of S rats.

These results suggest that there is an agent controlling the renin activity in the plasma and kidney of these hypertension-prone rats. We further speculate that this agent may be identical with a hypertensinogenic factor.

REFERENCES

1. BOUCHER, R., MENARD, J. and GENEST, J. (1967): Can J Physiol Pharmacol, **45**, 881.
2. DAHL, L. K., HEINE, M. and TASSINARI, L. (1962): J Exp Med, **115**, 1173.
3. DAHL, L. K., HEINE, M. and TASSINARI, L. (1962): Nature, **194**, 480.
4. DAHL, L. K., KNUDSEN, K. D., HEINE, M. and LEITL, G. (1967): J Exp Med, **126**, 687.
5. DAHL, L. K., KNUDSEN, K. D. and IWAI, J. (1969): Circ Res, **24-25**, Suppl. I, 21.
6. IWAI, J., KNUDSEN, K. D. and DAHL, L. K. (1970): J Exp Med, **131**, 543.
7. IWAI, J., KNUDSEN, K. D., DAHL, L. K., HEINE, M. and LEITL, G. (1969): J Exp Med, **129**, 507.
8. KNUDSEN, K. D., IWAI, J., HEINE, M., LEITL, G. and DAHL, L. K. (1969): J Exp Med, **130**, 1353.

SPONTANEOUS HYPERTENSION AND ERYTHROCYTOSIS IN RATS

S. SEN*, G. C. HOFFMAN*, N. T. STOWE*,
R. R. SMEBY* and F. M. BUMPUS*

OKAMOTO and AOKI [4, 5] bred a strain of rats which spontaneously developed hypertension when they reached about 150 g body wt. During our studies with these animals, we found that red blood cell counts rise concomitantly and in direct proportion to the blood pressure. The present study reports our findings concerning the nature and cause of this erythrocytosis and its relationship to hypertension.

METHODS AND MATERIALS

The SH rats used in this study were either bred at Cleveland Clinic Foundation or obtained from Purina Laboratory. Normal Wistar rats or Sprague-Dawley strain rats served as controls. Blood was collected for all studies either from the tail artery or from the orbital sinus, using 15% K_3 salt of EDTA as anticoagulant. Blood pressure was measured everyday using a tailcuff [2]. Blood counts and red cell indices were determined on a Model S Coulter particle counter.

RESULTS

Hematological characteristic of normotensive, spontaneously hypertensive and renal hypertensive rat blood samples are summarized in Table 1. A significant increase in erythrocyte counts was observed in SH rats when compared to normotensive rats and renal hypertensive rats. The SH rats were divided into 4 weight groups as follows: Pre-hypertensive (130–150 g), early hypertensive (180–200 g), established hypertensive (200–250 g), and older, established hypertensive (250–300 g). The results show that during the pre-hypertensive stage the RBC counts remain normal but with the onset of hyper-

Table 1 Hematological characteristics of normotensive, spontaneously hypertensive and renal hypertensive rats.

	Normal rats	Spontaneously hypertensive rats				Renal hypertensive rats
Weight, grams	200–300	130–150	180–200	200–250	250–300	200–300
B.P., mm Hg	110–120	110–130	180	200	200	210
Number	25	10	25	25	25	8
RBC $\times 10^6$ / mm^3	6.8 (0.1)	6.4 (0.2)	8.1 (0.1)	8.7 (0.1)	10.0 (0.1)	6.8 (0.1)
WBC $\times 10^6$ / mm^3	9.2 (0.3)	8.4 (0.5)	9.3 (0.3)	8.4 (0.4)	10.6 (0.5)	10.5 (0.6)
Hemoglobin, g/100 ml	14.7 (0.2)	13.5 (0.2)	14.8 (0.1)	15.7 (0.2)	16.6 (0.1)	13.3 (0.7)
Hematocrit, %	37.6 (0.6)	36.5 (0.5)	37.6 (0.1)	40.8 (0.3)	44.1 (0.4)	39.8 (0.5)
Mean cell volume, μ^3	54.2 (0.6)	55.5 (0.6)	47.0 (0.2)	45.8 (0.1)	45.4 (0.1)	53.5 (0.6)

Mean, with standard error of the mean in parenthesis.

* Research Division, Cleveland Clinic Foundation, Cleveland, Ohio, U.S.A.

Table 2 Plasma volume in normotensive and spontaneously hypertensive rats.

	Normotensive rats				Spontaneously hypertensive rats		
	ml		ml/kg		ml		ml/kg
Mean	8.76	Mean	39.18	Mean	8.96	Mean	39.08
SE	0.13	SE	0.46	SE	0.25	SE	0.88
	N=15				N=15		

Table 3 Incorporation of ^{59}Fe into erythrocytes of spontaenously hypertensive and normo-tensive rats (Results expressed as % of incorporation in 24 hrs.).

Rat No.	Normotensive		Spontaneously hypertensive	
Total 5	Mean	8.8	Mean	41
	SE	0.77	SE	2.16

tension, the RBC counts increase significantly while the WBC counts remain more or less constant for all groups.

The hemoglobin concentration and hematocrit readings were elevated in the older, established SH group of rats (250–300 g) while all other were the same as normotensive controls. The mean red cell volume (MCV) in hypertensive SH rats was lower than that in normotensive SH rats, renal hypertensive rats and normal controls. Hence, the hematocrit and hemoglobin content of the blood measured in SH rats were only slightly higher than normal controls.

When plasma volume (PV) was measured in SH and normal rats as ^{131}I distribution space, no significant differences were observed. The mean PV normal rats was 8.76, whereas in SH rats it was 8.96 (Table 2). This observation suggested that the increase in erythrocyte counts was an absolute increase.

Incorporation of ^{59}Fe into red cells of SH and normal rats, shown in Table 3, was

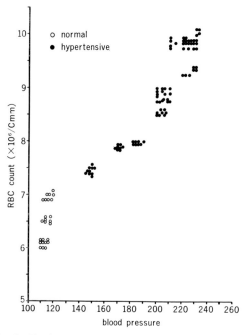

Fig. 1 Erythrocyte counts and blood pressure in SH rats.

measured as the percentage of ^{59}Fe reappearing in circulation 24 hrs after intravenous injection. The result shows a four-fold increase in Fe turnover. This observation also suggested increased red cell production. The reticulocyte counts are slightly higher than normal rats and bone marrow in SH rats showed erythroid hyperplasia. But histological study on spleen did not show any significant difference.

The observed increase in erythrocyte counts paralleled an increase in body weight. The body weight and RBC counts were followed in a group of normal and SH rats, which were born on the same day. A direct correlation between body wt and RBC counts was found in SH rats as they grew from 70–240 g, whereas in normal they remained same.

The erythrocytosis in SH rats was also accompanied by an increase in blood pressure. A significant linear relationship was observed between erythrocyte counts and blood pressure (Fig. 1).

Table 4 Effect of antihypertensive drug (α-methyldopa) on blood pressure and erythrocyte counts on spontaneously hypertensive and normotensive rats.

	Normotensive			Spontaneously hypertensive		
	A Before	B During	C After	A Before	B During	C After
Blood pressure (mm Hg)	110±10	100±10	100±5	200±10	145±15	200±10
RBC×10⁶/mm³ Erythrocyte counts (×10⁶/mm³)	6.3±0.2	6.5±0.3	6.5±0.3	10.3±0.1	6.18±0.1	8.9±0.2
Plasma volume, ml	9.3±0.2	8.5±0.4		9.5±0.5	7.9±0.6	

Results expressed as mean ± S.E.M. of 8 rats

A: Control data before drug treatment.

B: Data obtained after 18 days of drug treatment.

C: Data obtained 14 days after discontinuation of drug.

Table 5 Plasma erythropoietin titre in normotensive and spontaneously hypertensive rats (Results expressed as IRP units* /ml).

Assay material	wt	ESF units/ml (IRP)
Saline	—	None
SH - Rat plasma	150–160 gm	0.27 units
SH - Rat plasma	180 gm	0.15 units
SH - Rat plasma	250–270 gm	0.17 units
Normotensive - Rat plasma	200–250 gm	Not detectable

* International Reference Preparation.

When a group of SH rats was treated with α-methyldopa (200 mg/kg I.P.) for 18 days the RBC counts were significantly reduced, while the blood pressure was reduced from 200 mm Hg to 145 mm Hg (Table 4). No such change in RBC counts or blood pressure was observed in normotensive rats. Fourteen days after the treatment was stopped, the RBC counts rose along with the blood pressure. Plasma volumes were not altered by this treatment.

Measurement of plasma erythropoietin of SH and normal rats indicates that it is elevated in prehypertensive animals. The plasma erythropoietin apparently falls with the establishment of hypertension but it remains higher than that of normal rats (Table 5).

DISCUSSION

These studies show that the strain of Wistar rats which spontaneously develop hypertension also develop an erythrocytosis. Plasma volume measurements indicate that the erythrocytosis is absolute. The erythroid hyperplasia in the bone marrow and the four-fold increase in iron turnover are further evidence of increased red cell production. The red cells that are produced during this phase have a significantly smaller MCV than the cells produced before the development of erythrocytosis. As a result the blood hemoglobin content and hematocrit reading increase at a slower rate and this may in part account for the fact that the erythrocytosis has not been previously reported. The survival of these small red cells is normal.

Erythropoietin is apparently the immediate stimulus to the increased red cell production. Plasma levels of the hormone are highest at the onset of the erythrocytosis but remain very high even when the red cell count is $10 \times 10^6/mm^3$. The direct correlation between the blood pressure and the erythrocytosis suggests a causal relationship. Not only does the red cell count increase as the blood pressure rises, but also the red cell count decreases when the blood pressure is lowered by antihypertensive drugs. Furthermore, when the drug treatment is discontinued, the blood pressure and the red cell count increase again. We have no evidence as to the source of erythropoietin in these SH rats. However, different investigators have suggested the kidney is a major source of erythropoietin [1, 3]. It has also been suggested that renal hypoxia may be the stimulus to its production. Analysis of blood gases showed no change in oxygen tension in the arterial blood as the red cell count increased. One could postulate that hypertension reduces the renal blood flow or alters its intrarenal distribution in such a way that oxygen supply to the erythro-poietin-producing cells is reduced.

AOKI (1963) has shown that adrenalectomy reduces the blood pressure in the SH rats. We have studied 4 adrenalectomized SH rats and the red cell count decreased from a mean of $10 \times 10^6/mm^3$ to $6.5 \times 10^6/mm^3$ in 14 days and the blood pressure decreased from 200 mm Hg to 150 mm Hg. Although plasma volumes were not measured, these preliminary studies suggest that the adrenal gland may be involved in the production of hypertension and secondarily in the production of erythropoiesis.

Whatever the ultimate cause of the erythrocytosis and the hypertension is proved to be, the SH rats provide a readily available model for the study of spontaneous erythro-cytosis due to increased erythropoietin production.

AKNOWLEDGEMENTS

We thank Dr. J. W. FISHER, Dept. of Pharmacology, Tulane University, New Orleans for the erythroipoietin assays.

We are grateful to Miss Betty ROOT, B.A., Miss Judy RANKIN, M.T., ASCP, Mrs. Rita BLOCK and Miss Essie FOSTER for their expert technical assistance.

N.T.S. is a recipient of a National Kidney Foundation Research Fellowship Grant. This work was supported in part by a NHLI Grant HE-6835 and a grant from John A. Hartford Foundation.

REFERENCES

1. FISHER, J. W. and LANGSTON, J. W. (1968): Ann N Y Acad Sci, **149**, 75.
2. FRIEDMAN, M. and FREED, S. C. (1949): Proc Soc Exp Biol Med, **70**, 670.
3. JACOBSON, L. O., GOLDWASSER, E., FRIED, W. and PLZAK, L. (1957): Nature, **179**, 633.
4. OKAMOTO, K. (1962): Nippon Naibunpi Gakkai Zasshi, **38**, 782.
5. OKAMOTO, K. and AOKI, K. (1963): Jap Circ J, **27**, 282.

Chapter VIII

ESSENTIAL HYPERTENSION AND SPONTANEOUS HYPERTENSION

MODIFICATION OF HYPERTENSION BY ANTIHYPERTENSIVE DRUG TREATMENT IN SPONTANEOUSLY HYPERTENSIVE RATS

E. D. FREIS*

The SH rat presents an experimental model which in many ways resembles essential hypertension in man. One of the great advantages of this model is that the entire life history of the disease is compressed into a period of less than two years. Clinically, in the treatment of patients with essential hypertension, we as well as others have observed, that following prolonged reduction of blood pressure, the hypertension may regress to a much milder form or occasionally remit entirely for long periods. However, we have not been able to determine in man whether control of the blood pressure prior to the appearance of the hypertension could alter the progression of the disease. This question is approachabl, however, in the SH rat and we decided, therefore, to study the question as to whether hypertension could be modified or prevented by antihypertensive drug treatment before the establishment of a definitely elevated blood pressure.

Prior investigations by IWAKI, ISHIKO, KUDO and IRIKURA [2] in 1967 indicated that many antihypertensive agents were effective orally in reducing the blood pressure of SHR. NAGAOKA, KIKUCHI and ARAMAKI [4] found that hydralazine, reserpine guanethidine and alpha methyldopa were effective antihypertensive agents in SHR.

In preliminary experiments we found that a combination of reserpine, hydralazine and chlorothiazide given in slightly larger doses than those used clinically, effectively lowered the blood pressure of young SHR, and that this reduction could be maintained indifinitely without apparent toxicity to the animals.

METHODS

The design of the experiment was as follows: the experiment was begun when the SHR's were 3 months of age because at this time their blood pressures were still normal (as measured during recovery from ether anesthesia) and the rats had become large enough to allow us to measure the blood pressure easily by the tail method. The rats were randomly divided into a treated and a control group. The treated group received the combination of reserpine, hydralazine and chlorothiazide added to the drinking water while the control litter mates received only tap water without drugs. The concentrations of drugs in the drinking water were as follows: for the males, reserpine 1.4 mg, hydrala-

* Veterans Administration Hospital and Department of Medicine, Georgetown University School of Medicine, Washington, D.C., U.S.A.

zine 80 mg and chlorothiazide 1000 mg per liter of water and for the females, half of the concentrations used for the males. In occasional rats these doses were insufficient. In such cases the concentration of chlorothiazide was doubled.

Drug treatment was continued for 6 months or until the rats were 9 months of age and then was abruptly withdrawn. We then continued to observe both groups of animals for an additional 4 months after the drugs were withdrawn or until they were 13 months of age at which time they were sacrificed.

Blood pressure was measured in a warm room by the tail cuff method during recovery from light ether anesthesia beginning at the first sign of twitching of the fore whiskers or movement of the eyes and continuing until the time the animal was fully awake. A Statham P23dB strain guage was used to record cuff pressure while the arterial pulsations in the tail were detected by a mercury-in-rubber tubing resistance guage (Whitney) which encircled the tail just distal to the cuff [3]. Recordings were made on a 2-channel Hewlett-Packard direct writing oscillograph. The average of 3 recordings of blood pressure taken at approximately 1 minute intervals was taken as the systolic blood pressure of the rat.

RESULTS

The mean changes and standard errors in blood pressure in the two groups of rats over the 6 month period of drug treatment are shown in Fig. 1. The controls are indicated by the broken lines and the treated by the solid lines. There were 17 animals in each group.

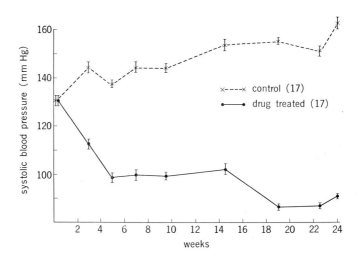

Fig. 1 Average systolic blood pressure of control (broken lines) and antihypertensive drug treated (solid lines) SHRs beginning when the rats were 3 months of age and continuing until they were 9 months old.

It is evident that the blood pressures are significantly different in the control and treated animals. The blood pressures of both treated and control rats at 3 months of age started from the same point, that is, at about 130 mm Hg. These average levels of blood pressure are considerably lower than those recorded by other workers but is should be recalled that the readings were taken just before the animals awakened from ether anesthesia rather than in the unanesthetized rat. It should be noted that in the treated group the blood pressure was lower at 4 weeks than at 2 weeks but this may have been due to manipulation of doses of the antihypertensive drugs which occurred during this period. However,

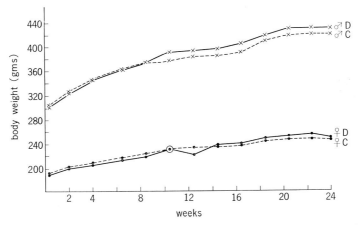

Fig. 2 Average body weights of control (broken lines) and antihypertensive drug treated (solid lines) SHRs during the 6 month period depicted in Fig. 1. Rats are further subdivided by sex. Note that the body weights of the drug treated animals kept pace with that of the controls.

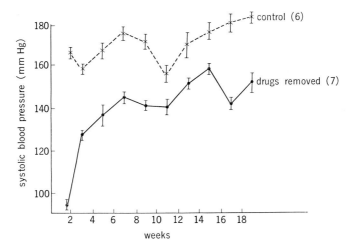

Fig. 3 Average systolic blood pressure of control (broken lines) and antihypertensive drug treated (solid lines) SHRs beginning at the time when drugs were abruptly withdrawn (9 months of age) and continuing for 4 months until the rats were 13 months old.

there was a further fall in blood pressure between 15 and 19 weeks when the doses were not changed. Just prior to discontinuing treatment, when the animals were 9 months of age, the systolic blood pressure averaged 92 mm Hg in the treated group which contrasted markedly with the controls whose systolic blood pressure averaged 159 mm Hg.

In contrast to the marked differences in blood pressure the two groups of animals appeared to be identical in their rate of growth, general health and activity. The average changes in body weight over the 6 month period are shown in Fig. 2. The upper solid line indicates the treated males and the broken line the control males. The treated and control females are shown below. As expected the males are heavier and gained weight more rapidly, but the important point to note is that there is no difference between the control and treated groups.

It is interesting to compare these rats with a prior group of SHR who were given 1%

salt to drink instead of tap water [1]. This high salt intake group, which began excess salt somewhat earlier at 2 months of age, exhibited a rapid acceleration of their blood pressure so that at less than 15 weeks of such treatment their average systolic blood pressure taken during recovery from anesthesia had risen to 195 mm Hg, and some had developed manifestations of malignant hypertension.

Fig. 3 shows the systolic blood pressure over a 4 month period in the control and treated groups beginning at the time of drug withdrawal when the rats were 9 months of age and continuing for another 4 months without further treatment. Following drug withdrawal the blood pressure rose steeply over the succeeding week from 92 to approximately 130 mm Hg. After this initial steep rise, however, the systolic blood pressure rose more gradually paralleling the rate of rise seen in the controls. The blood pressure of the SHR's who had been treated, therefore appeared to have been modified as it always remained significantly below that of the controls. By the fourth month following withdrawal of drugs when the animals were 13 months of age the systolic of 6 control rats averaged 185 mm Hg as compared to 150 mm Hg in 7 of the treated animals. Thus far, the remaining drug treated animals have not been followed for more than two months following discontinuation of drugs but over this period of time the blood pressure of the drug treated animals has behaved similarly to the smaller group described above.

Measurements of body weight indicated that the pre-treated animals gained more weight than the controls. At approximately one year of age some of the controls developed respiratory infections which were successfully treated with antibiotics.

The animals were sacrificed at 13 months of age. The tissues of the hypertensive control animals showed hypertensive changes which were not seen in any of the treated rats. The typical nodular changes seen in the mesenteric arteries of rats with severe or long standing hypertension were seen only in the control rats. The hearts of the control animals weighed more than that of the treated and the heart weight-body weight ratio was increased in the controls as compared to the treated rats. In addition, the myocardium of the control but not the treated animals exhibited microinfarcts with necrosis of muscle cells, fibrosis and an infiltrate of inflammatory cells.

The kidneys of 3 control animals showed extensive changes consistent with hypertension. There was fibrous hyperplasia and fibrinoid necrosis of the glomeruli, intimal hyperplasia of arterioles with areas of fibrinoid necrosis and proteinacious material in the tubules. These various hypertensive changes are similar to those previously reported by OKAMOTO [5].

In 5 control and 6 treated rats plasma volume changes with Evans Blue and extracellular fluid volume changes with thiocyanate were determined immediately before and one week after withdrawal of treatment. Plasma volume increased by an average of 12% in the animals in whom treatment was withdrawn as opposed to 6% in the controls. Thiocyanate space increased 2% in the treated animals and fell 7% in the controls following withdrawal of drugs. In hypertensive man the withdrawal of thiazide diuretics is associated with a significant increase in plasma and extracellular fluid volumes [6]. These volume changes in the rat, however, were not significant. Neither were there significant changes in serum sodium or potassium concentrations following withdrawal of the antihypertensive drugs. More animals will need to be studied to determine whether the increase in blood pressure is associated with significant increases in extracellular volumes or electrolyte shifts.

DISCUSSION

The present results support the contention that antihypertensive treatment did more than suppress the developing hypertension; it actually modified it. If drug treatment had been suppressive only, the blood pressure of the treated animals would have risen to the level of the control litter mates following withdrawal of treatment. On the contrary, the blood pressure failed to reach the level of the controls, and after an initial sharp elevation remained at a significantly lower level than the controls.

In the treated animals the process appeared to have been arrested for the 6 month period of treatment, and when treatment was stopped blood pressure rose quickly back to the level it had been when the SHR were 3 months of age, that is to 130 mm Hg *the level existing at the time that treatment was started*. Furthermore, over the subsequent 4 months the blood pressure rose to the *same* level of 150 mm Hg that the controls exhibited 4 months after the experimental period had begun. To state this crucial observation in another way when treatment was discontinued the experimental group of SHR, who were then 9 months of age, rose to the same level as they and the controls exhibited when they were 3 months of age; and when the experimental group were 13 months of age they exhibited the same level of blood pressure as the control SHR when they were 7 months of age. Thus, over the 6 months of treatment the progression of the hypertension appeared to have been entirely arrested. For the entire period of treatment the hypertensive process "stood still". When treatment was discontinued the hypertensive process resumed from the level where it had been arrested at the time antihypertensive treatment had been initiated.

These results indicate that the age of the animal, *per se*, is not the important determinant of the level of blood pressure in SHR. Rather, it appears to be the duration of the hypertension, which is uncontrolled, proceeds to higher and higher levels by gradual increments. This progressive process may be accelerated by excessive salt administration as we and others have shown or it may be completely arrested for the duration of antihypertensive drug administration.

The failure of the blood pressure to rise to the level of the controls cannot be ascribed to ill health or poor condition of the treated SHR. The treated animals gained more weight from 9 to 13 months of age, were less subject to respiratory illnesses and were as active or more active than the untreated controls who at one year of age began to suffer from the consequences of hypertensive cardiovascular-renal disease. Further, the treated animals showed none of the advanced pathological changes seen in the control group.

The hypertension of the SHR while genetically determined appears subject to considerable environmental influences. The hypertension can be accelerated by excessive salt ingestion or it can be arrested for the entire period of antihypertensive drug treatment. Thus, genetic and environmental factors appear to interact in determining the rate of development of hypertension in SHR. Furthermore, the biological processes associated with aging do not appear to play a role in the development of hypertension since, if progression is arrested for a long period of time (in the present case for 6 months-equivalent to 20 years in the life span of man) the process simply starts off again at the same level of blood pressure and at the same rate of progressive elevation as existed at the time the hypertensive process was originally arrested, even though the animals are now considerably older.

It seems unlikely that any of the antihypertensive drugs used in this experiment was a specific antagonist of the basic pathogenetic mechanism operative in SHR. And yet, the drugs appeared to act as if they affected the basic mechanism, since the hypertension was completely arrested during the period of treatment. This suggests that if treatment were begun even earlier and was continued throughout the life of the animal, such a continuously treated SHR would live as long or longer than a normal Wistar rat, and at death it would not exhibit any of the pathological stigmata seen in the untreated SHR. Such a result would be quite different from the effects of treatment of certain other chronic diseases, such as diabetes mellitus for example, where reduction of the blood sugar fails to halt the progress of the associated vascular disease.

It also seems evident that the treated SHR will provide a useful experimental tool in differentiating primary from secondary changes in the SHR. If a biochemical or other observed abnormality in the SHR is secondary to the hypertension it should not be found if the blood pressure is controlled at low levels beginning at an early age of the animal. However, if the observed abnormality is the primary congenital cause of the hypertension it should remain present even when the blood pressure is reduced.

Finally, it seems possible that very early treatment of the SHR beginning with the treatment of the parents before breeding and continuing for the first 6 months of life of the offspring may prevent the development of the hypertension in SHR. This intriguing possibility will be the subject of our future investigations in the SHR.

SUMMARY AND CONCLUSIONS

The blood pressure of SHRs was controlled at low levels using antihypertensive drugs for a 6 month period beginning at a time when the animals were 3 months of age. Treatment was then withdrawn and the animals were observed for an additional 4 months, or until they were 13 months of age. Antihypertensive drug treatment arrested the progression of the hypertension for the duration of the treatment period. Following withdrawal of the drugs the blood pressure did not rise to the level of the controls of similar age but rather returned to the pretreatment level and then progressed at the same rate as the controls exhibited when the latter were 3 months of age.

These results indicate that, (1) although the tendency toward hypertension is an inherited characteristic, the degree of hypertension which becomes manifest depends also on environmental factors. The hypertension can be arrested by chemotherapeutic interventions and it can be aggravated by an excessive salt intake (2). The hypertension in the SHR appears to be a progressive time-dependent process but is independent of any of the biological processes associated with aging, *per se* (3). The present technique for arresting the hypertension should prove useful in differentiating abnormalities which are secondary to hypertension itself from other observed abnormalities including those that are associated with the primary pathogenetic process.

ACKNOWLEDGEMENTS

The author wishes to acknowledge the assistance of Mary MATTHEWS, M.D. who reviewed the pathological findings. The technical assistance provided by Miss Jean BARSANTI and Mr. Dennis RAGAN also is gratefully acknowledged.

REFERENCES

1. BARSANTI, J. A., PILLSBURY, H. R. C., III and FREIS, E. D. (1971): Proc Soc Exp Biol Med, **136**, 565.

2. Iwaki, R., Ishiko, J., Kudo, Y. and Irikura, T. (1967): Nippon Taishitsugaku Zasshi,
    30, 170.
3. Maitsrello, I. and Matscher, R. (1969): J Appl Physiol, **26**, 188.
4. Nagaoka, A., Kikuchi, D. and Aramaki, Y. (1967): Nippon Taishitsugaku Zasshi, **30**, 165.
5. Okamoto, K. (1969): *In* "International Review of Experimental Pathology" (G. W. Richter
    and M. A. Epstein eds.), Vol. 7, p. 227, Accademic Press, New York.
6. Wilson, I. M. and Freis, E. D. (1959): Circulation, **20**, 1028.

THE SPONTANEOUS HYPERTENSIVE RAT: AN EXPERIMENTAL ANALOGUE OF ESSENTIAL HYPERTENSION IN THE HUMAN BEING*

A. GROLLMAN**

I am deeply honored by the privilege of contributing this paper in honor of Professor KOZO OKAMOTO on the occasion of the First U.S.-Japanese Seminar on the Spontaneously Hypertensive Rat (SHR). Professor OKAMOTO's contribution to the elucidation of the nature and pathogenesis of essential and chronic hypertension by his development of the SHR is inestimable. Although future studies may demonstrate certain secondary differences between the SHR and other forms of chronic experimental hypertension, the available data indicate that the SHR represents the analogue of the human disorder designated euphemistically as "essential" hypertension. The usefulness of the SHR as a model for experimental studies requires no elaboration. Its introduction has also served to establish essential hypertension as a true clinical entity and to dispel the many current theories as to its pathogenesis which have confused and retarded progress in the elucidation and management of this common clinical disorder.

That the kidney plays a role in the pathogenesis of most forms of hypertension is now well-established although the mechanism of its action is still disputed, particularly as regards the nature and role of various pressor and other humoral agents in its pathogenesis. There is overwhelming evidence that the rise in blood pressure in essential hypertension and in most forms of chronic hypertensive disease observed clinically or induced experimentally in laboratory animals, is not mediated by a demonstrable circulating pressor substance. The available data also indicate that renin and angiotensin are not the mediators of surgically remediable hypertension in the human although a high renin level is often but not invariably found in patients suffering from surgically remediable hypertension [12].

The presently reported studies are concerned with a comparison of the hypertension of the SHR with that induced in rats and other laboratory animals by a variety of procedures. These experimental studies and the available data on the human have been used as a basis for a theory regarding the pathogenesis and rational treatment of the various forms of hypertensive cardiovascular disease as observed in man [7, 8, 9].

EXPERIMENTAL STUDIES

The SHR derived from the original colony of Professor OKAMOTO [15] has been found to react similarly to animals rendered hypertensive by the application of a figure-of-eight ligature to the kidney [4], infarction of one kidney with contralateral nephrectomy [10], subjecting weanling rats to a choline or potassium-free diet, unilateral [6] or bilateral nephrectomy [8], and "teratogenically" induced hypertension by subjecting rats during a critical period of pregnancy to varying procedures [9]. Previous studies have indicated that these procedures induce a condition which resembles that encountered in the human disorder [7, 8, 9].

* Unpublished experiments included in the present report were performed with the aid of a Grant (71-1113) from the American Heart Association.
** Laboratory for Experimental Medicine, Department of Pathology, University of Texas Southwestern Medical School, Dallas, Texas, U.S.A.

In many studies of hypertension, confusion has resulted from the failure to differentiate an initial acute phase of experimental hypertension and its clinical analogue, surgically remediable hypertension in the human, from chronic hypertension in the experimental animal and essential and other forms of chronic hypertensive cardiovascular disease in man. The former is mediated by the elaboration of the kidney of a newly described pressor agent (nephrotensin); the latter has been attributed to the loss of a normal function of the kidney concerned in the maintenance of the normotensive state [9]. In all of the above-mentioned forms of chronic hypertension and in the SHR no pressor agent is demonstrable in the circulating plasma in contrast to the acute hypertension of the immediate postoperative period induced by drastic restriction of the blood flow through the kidney or infarction of one or both kidneys [10]. The latter procedures when applied to the young SHR with only a moderately increased blood pressure result in an exacerbation of the hypertension and the appearance of a pressor agent in the circulating plasma.

There is substantial evidence supporting the view that acute experimental and surgically remediable hypertension in the human are mediated by a circulating renal pressor-agent [10, 13]. Although immunoassay procedures indicate that this pressor agent may be angiotensin I [2], there is substantial evidence to indicate that this is not the case. It may be emphasized here that immunologic specificity is not absolute and it is necessary to examine any given system for possible interference.

The response of vascular smooth muscle has been used as a bioassay procedure for differentiating the pressor agent formed by the kidney in acute experimental and surgically remediable hypertension. The response of the SHR has been found to be similar to that of the rat rendered chronically hypertensive by other procedures.

Effect of Unilateral Nephrectomy

Elevations in blood pressure alone represent simply a hemodynamic variation which may be secondary to a number of conditions. The wide variation in basal blood pressure generally accepted as normal may actually represent varying degrees of hypertension. That this is actually the case may be inferred from the effect of unilateral nephrectomy on the blood pressure.

As shown in Fig. 1, unilateral nephrectomy results in no appreciable elevation of blood pressure in animals with pressures in the lower range of normal. The contralateral kidney under these conditions undergoes hypertrophy and compensates apparently for any deficiency of renal function induced by removal of the kidney. As the basal blood pressure increases, unilateral nephrectomy induces an increasingly greater rise in blood pressure. Removal of one kidney in the SHR, the blood pressure of which is only moderately elevated, also results in the development of hypertension at an accelerated pace as shown in the uppermost curve of Fig. 1. The SHR thus responds to unilateral nephrectomy as does the human being with pyelonephritis [14] or the rat with lesions of the kidney which are of a degree not sufficient of themselves to induce hypertension.

The above-described experiments on the effect of unilateral nephrectomy on the normotensive and on the SHR suggest that the laboratory rat *(Mus norvegicus)* like the human being has an inheritable congenital tendency to develop hypertensive disease. In most animal colonies used in the laboratory this congenital defect results in hypertension in less than 1 per cent of the animals but the elevation in blood pressure may be accentuated by age, infection, unilateral nephrectomy, application of a clip to one kidney, a high salt intake, and other procedures having an adverse effect on the renal function concerned in maintaining the normotensive state [3, 5, 9]. This congenital tendency has been taken advantage of by selective breeding to produce the SHR [15].

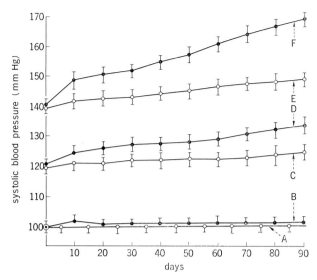

Fig. 1 The effect of unilateral nephrectomy on the arterial blood pressure of the rat.

Curves B, D and F (●—●) represent the effect of right nephrectomy; curves A, C and E (○—○), the effect of a sham operation (controls). Operations were performed at day 0. Rats of curves E and F were from a spontaneously hypertensive colony; those of curves A, B, C and D were from an inbred strain reared in the laboratory. Each point of the curves represents the average of readings on 10 animals ± S.E. (standard error), represented by the vertical lines.

Effects of Bilateral Nephrectomy

Removal of both kidneys in the frog, opossum, rat, dog, and man results in an elevation in blood pressure [6, 9, 15]. The removal of the sole remaining kidney of an hypertensive animal results in a decline in blood pressure only when the animal becomes moribund. Bilateral nephrectomy of the SHR as shown by AoKI [1] and confirmed in this laboratory intensifies the hypertension. This elevation of blood pressure, as in the case of normotensive animals, is not dependent on overexpansion of the extracellular fluid induced by the parenteral administration of fluids but as might be anticipated is not manifested in moribund individuals.

Effect of Renal Extracts

It has been suggested that essential hypertension is a disorder attributable to a deficiency of renal function [6, 9]. Strong support for this concept is the fact that extracts may be prepared from renal cortical tissue which fed to the chronically (but not to the acute surgically remediable) hypertensive animal results in a decline in blood pressure to normotensive levels. The availability of synthetic depressor agents acting on the nervous system and the small yields and instability of active material obtainable from kidneys have militated against the use of such renal extracts in the treatment of hypertension. The fact that such extracts are effective when administered orally in small amounts and the nature of the hypotensive response to their ingestion speak for their physiologic role and potential therapeutic usefulness [9].

The SHR as shown in Fig. 2 responds to the administration orally of renal extract to a degree comparable to that of animals rendered chronically hypertensive by other procedures and of the human being suffering from essential hypertension.

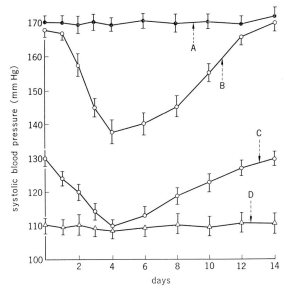

Fig. 2   The effect of the administration of renal extract orally to spontaneously hypertensive (Curves B and C) and normotensive (Curve D) rats.
Curve A represents results on untreated SHR controls. Each of the treated animals received an extract derived from 2 pounds of fresh pork kidneys admixed with its usual food on Day 0 and was consumed by Day 2. Each point represents the average of readings on 10 animals ± S.E. (standard error), represented by the vertical lines.

DISCUSSION

The presently available data indicate that the hypertension of the SHR is comparable to that of other forms of experimentally induced chronic hypertension and represents an analogue of essential hypertension of the human being. The laboratory rat like the human being apparently suffers from a congenital heritable defect. In the rat this tendency results in most individuals in no or only a modest rise in blood pressure. By selective breeding a strain with the more intense form of the disorder may be developed [15]. Most animals apparently have been freed of the disorder in its more intense manifestation through survival of the "fittest" but by inbreeding of the residual congenital defect, strains of hypertensive rats, mice, rabbits and possibly other animals can be developed, comparable to the spontaneously occurring human disease.

Although many forms of experimental hypertension conform closely to that of essential hypertension, the SHR provides the closest analogy to the disease as it occurs in the human being and is of great practical importance since it necessitates no dietary, surgical or other manipulation of the kidney for its induction. The clinical course and pathological findings on the SHR are similar to those observed in the human being. As in essential hypertension of the human being, the blood pressure is relatively normal in the young SHR, increases with age, and terminates in heart failure, cerebrovascular accident, renal insufficiency, or the malignant phase of the disease. The elevation in blood pressure is not mediated by a circulating pressor agent. Only in its "malignant" phase and in the acute hypertension which follows drastic restriction of the renal artery or infarction of the kidney does a pressor agent appear in the circulating blood.

Pathologically, the principal hallmarks of hypertension, namely, cardiac hypertrophy and arteriolar sclerosis, in the SHR are comparable to other forms of chronic experimental and clinical hypertension. The observed changes in the endocrine organs of the SHR and its response to hormones [1], are in accord with earlier observations on experimentally induced hypertension and the general concept that the endocrine organs exert a permissive rather than a direct action in maintaining the elevated blood pressure. Endocrine disturbances may, of course, elevate the blood pressure indirectly particularly through their action on salt and water metabolism and the volume of the body fluid compartments but there is no evidence to indicate that they induce classical hypertensive cardiovascular disease.

REFERECES

1. AOKI, K. (1964): Jap Heart J, **5**, 57.
2. CAREY, R. M., SCHWEIKERT, J. R. and LIDDLE, G. W. (1971): Endocrinology, **88**, A-115.
3. DAHL, L. K., HEINE, M. and TASSINARI, L. (1964): Circulation, **29**, Suppl. II, 11.
4. GROLLMAN, A. (1944): Proc Soc Exp Biol Med, **67**, 102.
5. GROLLMAN, A. (1946): J Am Dietetic Assoc, **22**, 864.
6. GROLLMAN, A. (1946): Special Publications, New York Academy of Sciences, **3**, 99.
7. GROLLMAN, A. (1959): Perspect Biol Med, **2**, 208.
8. GROLLMAN, A. (1969): Cardiovasc Clin, **1**, 1.
9. GROLLMAN, A. (1969): Clin Pharmacol Ther, **10**, 755.
10. GROLLMAN, A. (1970): Proc Soc Exp Biol Med, **134**, 1120.
11. GROLLMAN, A. (1970): Am J Physiol, **218**, 80.
12. GROLLMAN, A. and EBIHARA, A. (1968): Texas Rep Biol Med, **26**, 313.
13. MCPHAUL, J. J., Jr., MCINTOSH, D. A., WILLIAMS, L. F., GRITTI, E. J., MALETTE, W. G. and GROLLMAN, A. (1965): Arch Int Med, **115**, 644.
14. MJOLNEROD, O. K. and PRYDZ, H. (1959): Tydschr Nor Laegeforen, **79**, 826.
15. OKAMOTO, K. and AOKI, K. (1963): Jap Circ J, **27**, 282.

A COMPARISON OF THE FUNDUS FINDING BETWEEN ESSENTIAL HYPERTENSION IN HUMAN BEINGS AND SPONTANEOUSLY HYPERTENSIVE RATS

K. IRINODA*, S. MATSUYAMA* and S. TAKAHASHI*

Ophthalmoscopic findings give much information in the study of hypertensive diseases, and a considerable amount of study has been made of fundus changes in essential hypertension, but still many problems remain to be solved [2, 3, 4, 5]. One of the reasons is that in human beings it is very difficult to follow up exactly the fundus changes as well as other clinical data, all through the course of the disease. So the authors decided to compare the changes of retinal vessels in human beings suffering from essential hypertension with those of spontaneously hypertensive rats. This study was undertaken because according to previous studies spontaneously hypertensive rats are thought to be suitable for the experimental study of essential hypertension, as found in human beings.

As the detail of the fundus findings in SHR have already been reported in the other session of this symposium by Dr. TAKAHASHI, one of the authors, from the histological and ophthalmoscopic point of view, here we would like to present the results of the comparative study concerning ophthalmoscopic changes in the retinal arterioles, because the most important and interesting of the many eyeground changes is that of the retinal arterioles themselves.

CLINICAL OBSERVATION

Materials and Method

The systemic blood pressure and the fundi of 45 patients suffering from essential hypertension were examined repeatedly and followed up. The age of the patients at the first examination and the duration of the observation are shown in Table 1.

The fundus examination was carried out by the use of an ordinary ophthalmoscope

Table 1 Age of the patients at the first observation and duration of the observation.

Duration of the observation (yr$_0$) \ Age at the 1st observation	10–19	20–29	30–39	40–49	50–59	60–69	70–79	Total
2	1				3	1		5
3	1				8			9
4				1		3		4
5			3	2	4	2		11
6				2	3	3	1	9
7			1	1	2	1		5
8								0
9		1			1			2
Total	2	1	4	6	21	10	1	45

* Department of Ophthalmology, Hirosaki University School of Medicine, Hirosaki, Japan

and color fundus photographs. Thus the ophthalmoscopic changes of the fundus, especially the changes of the retinal arterioles such as narrowing, tortuosity and increase of the reflex from the wall were checked and compared in each step of the hypertension. Some of them were studied also by fluorescein fundus angiography.

Results

The results are summarized in Table 2.

In essential hypertension, the retinal arterioles showed some narrowing with or without caliber-irregularities. In younger patients suffering from essential hypertension, the narrowing of the retinal arterioles was in the earlier stages of the disease not always stable or progressive but reversible and varied in caliber; however, in most cases, the arterioles came to reveal sclerotic changes in the long run.

Table 2 Change of the ophthalmoscopic findings during the observation.

Change of the ophthalmoscopic findings* during the observation	Age at the first observation 10 – 19	20 – 29	30 – 39	40 – 49	50 – 59	60 – 69	70 – 79	Total
H. I＝H. I			1					1 ＝
→S. I				1		1		2 +
H. II→H. I			1					1 −
→S. I	2		3	1	1			7 +
S. I＝S. I					8	6	1	15 ＝
→S. II				2	4	1		7 +
→H. R. (a)						1		1 +
S. II＝S. II					5	2		7 ＝
→H. R. (a)					1			1 +
H. R. (b)→S. I				1				1 ?
→S. II					1			1 ?
→H. R. (a)				1				1 ?
	2	1	5	5	21	10	1	

＝......stationary; 23   −......improved; 1
+......progressive: 18   ? ......undetermined: 3
* classified by the author's classification [7].

In the advanced stages of essential hypertension, the retinal arterioles revealed sclerotic changes such as reflex-increase, crossing phenomena and narrowing with caliber-irregularities in most cases. However, in older patients with essential hypertension, the progression in the narrowing of the arterioles was very slight or very slow. Twenty-two out of thirty-two patients over fifty years of age did not reveal any progression in the fundus changes.

The following case is an example of essential hypertension which occurred in a younger patient.

The patient is a forty-eight year-old female. She has suffered from essential hypertension for 11 years, and was under our observation for seven years. Her blood pressure fluctuated between 210/110 and 110/70 mm Hg. The measurement of the caliber of the retinal arterioles showed narrowing with temporal fluctuation of the caliber. This finding suggested to us the presence of functional narrowing of the retinal arterioles.

When the patient came to our clinic on Dec. 11, 1969, the most evident ophthalmoscopic findings were diffuse narrowing accompanied by straightening and caliber variations (segmental narrowing). Reflex-increase and crossing phenomena were observed, too. Arteriolar sclerosis of the retina associated with hypertonus was the diagnosis we made. Then a vasodepressor test was carried out. Apresoline (20 mg/1 ml) was administered intramuscularly. The blood pressure was 210/130 mm Hg before the injection and 180/90 mm Hg 60 minutes after the injection. Disappearance of the segmental narrowing and slight dilatation of the arterioles were recognized. The findings were recorded by ordinary fundus photography and fluorescein fundus photography.

From the results of this experiment, the narrowing of the retinal arteriole found in this case was considered to be functional and hypertonic.

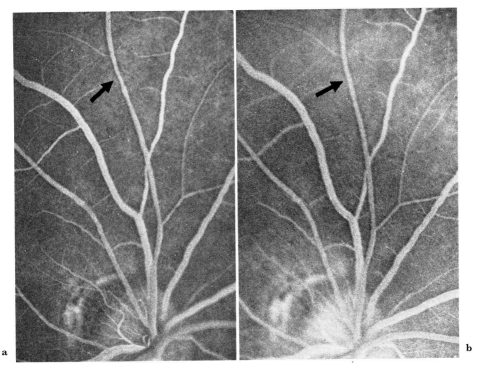

Fig. 1 A fourty-eight year-old female. Essential hypertension. Fluorescein angiography shows a real and functional narrowing of a retinal arteriole.
a. Focal narrowing (arrow) is marked before the injection of Apresoline.
b. The narrowing disappeared 60 minutes after the injection of Apresoline (arrow).

OBSERVATIONS IN REGARD TO SHR

Materials and Methods

Eighty-one spontaneously hypertensive rats were examined. The filial generations examined were between the 13th and the 16th.

Fundus examinations were performed once every week and recorded on color film by a hand fundus camera. Systolic blood pressures were measured on the tail artery every week by the plethysmographic method.

The reaction of the retinal arterioles of SHR to vasodepressive drugs was examined to ascertain whether the ophthalmoscopically observed narrowing of the arterioles of the retina was functional or organic.

Results (Table 3)

The rats spontaneously developed elevation of blood pressure within 9 to 10 weeks after birth in most cases, and by the sixteenth week in all cases.

Table 3 Ophthalmoscopic changes in the retinal arterioles in Spontaneously Hypertensive Rats.

Filial generation and number of rats examined	Onset of hypertension; Weeks after birth		Ophthalmoscopic changes				Systolic arterial blood pressure (mmHg)	
				caliber irregularities			At min. level of each rats	At max. level of each rats
			Narrowing	Rosary-like dilatation	Caliber irregularity (Mixed type)	Indentation		
F13 6			5	1			177.5 (170–180)	193.3 (180–200)
F14 21	9	16	21	6	4	11	177.4 (160–190)	203.6 (180–230)
F15 30	6	9	30	11	3	16	180.3 (170–200)	211.1 (190–244)
F16 24	7	13	24	14	6	14	180.4 (160–200)	212.7 (175–250)

As the blood pressure rose, straightening and diffuse narrowing of the retinal arterioles appeared first, and then caliber-irregularities followed, and sometime later, indentation of the arterioles appeared in some rats. Various types of caliber-irregularities were found; namely, (1) caliber-irregularities in a narrow sense, (2) aneurysm-like dilatation and (3) rosary-like dilatation. The term from the onset of high blood pressure to the appearance of the aneurysm-like changes was 7 to 11 weeks in F14, 3 to 11 weeks in F15 and 2 to 7 weeks in F16. The blood pressures of the rats at the time of the sppearance of these changes were in most cases between 170 and 200 mm Hg in systole.

Table 3 shows the ophthalmoscopic changes of retinal arterioles in SHR. Narrowing and caliber-irregularities were found in almost all cases.

The retinal arterioles showed straightening in the early stage of hypertension in most cases, though some exceptional rats showed tortuosity of the retinal arterioles with the onset of hypertension.

Reflex-increase and arterio-venous crossing phenomena were not found in SHR. But dilatation and tortuosity of the retinal venules were observed in some rats after a long of duration of hypertension.

The results of the examination of the reactivity of the retinal arterioles to vasodepressors is summarized in the Table 4.

The injection of a vasodepressor or ether inhalation caused lowering of blood pressure, dilatation of retinal arterioles, disappearance of caliber-irregularities including aneurysm-like dilatation and irregular tortuosity of the vessels.

The constricted arterioles of SHR were more responsive to Apresoline (1-hydrazino-phthalazine hydrochloride) than to Serpasil (reserpine), Methobromine (hexamethyl-1,6-bistrimethyl ammonium bromide), Priscol (2-benzyl-imidazoline hydrochloride) and Kallikrein.

Table 4   Reaction of retinal arterioles of SHR to vasodepressive drugs.

Drugs	Doses and methods of administration	Number of rats examined	Vasodilatative effect	Hypotensive effect
Apresoline	20 gm/kg, subcutaneously	4	++	++
Serpasil	1 mg/kg, subcutaneously	4	+	+
Methobromine	25 mg/kg, subcutaneously	4	+	+
Priscol	10 mg/kg, subcutaneously	4	+	+
Kallikrein	10 U./kg, intramuscular	4	±	+
Ether	Inhalation	4	++	++

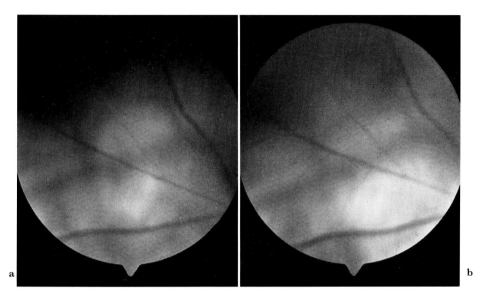

Fig. 2   Functional narrowing of the retinal arteriole in SHR.
a.   Caliber-irregularities of the retinal arteriole before the injection of Apresoline.
b.   Dilatation of the same arteriole after the injection of Apresoline.

COMMENT AND CONCLUSION

According to the reports of many investigators hypertension in SHR is considered to be analogous to and an ideal model of essential hypertension in man, from the stand point of its spontaneous occurrence [1] and its histopathology.

Hypertension in SHR is considered as belonging to the juvenile type of hypertension. Therefore, the observation of the arteriolar changes in the retina in SHR may contribute very much to an interpretation of the initial changes in the retina in human hypertensive patients.

The authors found that a diffuse narrowing of the retinal arterioles is an initial sign which is common to essential hypertension in man and in SHR. But the diffuse narrowing of the arterioles appeared more clearly in SHR than in human beings suffering from essential hypertension.

The narrowing of the retinal arterioles in patients suffering from essential hypertension is now an indisputable fact. This narrowing of the retinal arterioles is classified into two types; one is functional or hypertonic, and the other is organic or sclerotic.

However, there has been some discussion as to the existence of the two types of narrowing. There is no investigator who doubts the existence of organic or sclerotic narrowing of the retinal arterioles because it has been morphologically proved by histological methods. On the other hand, there are a few investigators who doubt the presence of the functional or hypertonic narrowing of the retinal arterioles [2, 4].

From our investigation of essential hypertension in man and hypertension in SHR, we found that the narrowing of the retinal arterioles play an important role in the onset of hypertension, and that the narrowing is functional or hypertonic, at least in the earlier stage of hypertension.

In the advanced stage of essential hypertension, as we observed is in older human patients, sclerotic changes such as reflex-increase, crossing phenomena and organic narrowing or attenuation of the arterioles were found, however such changes were not found in SHR.

Secondly, in regard to caliber irregularity of the retinal arterioles, the change was found in human beings as well as in SHR. Caliber-irregularity was observed both in younger and in older human patients.

In the younger patients, caliber-irregularity appeared mostly in the form of segmental narrowing with a smooth contour of the arteriolar wall, and this is thought to be a kind of hypertonic narrowing. In the older patients, on the other hand, it appeared in the form of indentation with an irregular and uneven contour of the arteriolar wall, and this type of caliber-irregularity is considered to be an organic and sclerotic change.

In SHR, caliber-irregularity occurred following diffuse narrowing and straightening after some duration of hypertension. Moreover, the caliber-irregularities found in SHR are more remarkable than those found in human patients. The formation of rosary-like or aneurysm-like caliber-irregularities in SHR is an interesting change compared with the aneurysm formation in mesenteric arteries of SHR. However, according to a histological study by one of the authors, TAKAHASHI [6], the change in caliber of arterioles in the retina was not organic but functional.

Thirdly, concerning the changes in the course of the retinal arterioles, SHR revealed straightening accompanied by narrowing from the beginning of the hypertension and did not reveal marked tortuosity except in some rats.

This differs from findings in essential hypertension in man and in other type of experimental hypertension using rats [6]. For instance, in DCA hypertensive rats, tortuosity of the retinal arterioles appears in accordance with diffuse narrowing, and tortuous retinal arteries in the main tributaries with narrowing of the peripheral branches are recognized very often in younger patients of essential hypertension.

In younger human hypertensive patients in man, straightening of the retinal arterioles is observed very often in association with the appearance of diffuse or focal narrowing and tortuosity of arterioles is also observed.

Tortuous retinal arterioles, are observed in association with some dilatation in main tributaries and narrowing and straightening in the peripheral small arterioles in the case of human being. Older patients with hypertension of longer duration sometimes reveal tortuous arterioles with an increase of reflex, and older patients in whom hypertension occurred after they were fifty never reveal tortuosity.

Results show that, in the early stages, functional constriction of arterioles occurred in the retina both in human beings with essential hypertension and in spontaneously hypertensive rats. In the later stages, human retinal arterioles revealed sclerotic changes but the retinal arterioles of the rats revealed no sclerotic changes.

Further investigation of these changes is being continued.

REFERENCES

1. OKAMOTO, K., AOKI, K., NOSAKA, S. and FUKUSHIMA, M. (1964): Jap Circ J, **28**, 943.
2. IKUI, H., TOMINAGA, Y. and KIMURA, K. (1964): Acta Soc Ophthalmol Jap, **68**, 899.
3. IRINODA, K., MATSUYAMA, S. and TAKAHASHI, S. (1970): "Proceeding of the XXI International Congress of Ophthalmology", International Congress Series. No. 222 Ophthalmology, p. 912, Excerpta Medica, Amsterdam.
4. McMICHAEL, J. and DOLLERY, C. T. (1963): Transact Ophthalmol Soc U K, 83, 51.
5. TAKAHASHI, S. and MATSUYAMA, S. (1967): Acta Soc Ophthalmol Jap, **71**, 1615.
6. TAKAHASHI, S. and WATANABE, J. (1969): Acta Soc Ophtalmol Jap, **73**, 1429.
7. IRINODA, K. (1970): Colour Atlas and Criteria of Fundus Changes in Hypertension, p. 132, Igaku Shoin Ltd., Tokyo.

CHARACTERISTICS OF THE NEW ZEALAND STRAIN OF GENETICALLY HYPERTENSIVE RATS CONSIDERED IN RELATION TO ESSENTIAL HYPERTENSION

F. H. SMIRK*

During the last few years the mean blood pressure of the rats of our New Zealand hypertensive rat colony [13] has been in the region of 170 mm Hg and there is now no difficulty in assembling a group of rats selected for blood pressures of 190 mm Hg or more. Male rats have a mean blood pressure of 8 mm Hg above the females. It has been shown by successful reciprocal skin grafts that subline A is a pure strain.

PHELAN [10] has traced the effect of selection for high blood pressure in the New Zealand strain since 1955. The rate of increase of the blood pressure up till 1970 has been approximately 2 mm Hg per generation.

In man the extent to which genetic and environmental factors are responsible for the high blood pressure of essential hypertension has been much debated. Observations on our rat colony are relevant to the human situation in that they show that, by selective breeding, it has been possible to establish a colony of rats with frank spontaneous hypertension which, so far as we can tell, is due solely or almost solely to genetic factors.

We were delighted when OKAMOTO and AOKI [9] also developed a spontaneously hypertensive rat colony. But note, by the F3 generation they achieved blood pressures of 177 mm Hg. This contrasts remarkably with our breeding experience with the New Zealand colony. Our first attempt failed. We started again in 1955 and it took fifteen years, including as many as twenty seven generations of inbreeding, to obtain the present high blood pressure levels.

Such differences in the breeding, and others to be mentioned later make it likely that there are at least two distinctive genetic types of spontaneous hypertension in rats, the Japanese and New Zealand strains, both leading to pathological changes such as cardiac hypertrophy, polyarteritis nodosa, advanced renal damage and occasionally to medial necrosis of arterioles.

Also we have the important salt-sensitive and salt-insensitive rat strains developed and investigated by DAHL et al. [2]; the former developing severe hypertension when 8 percent or less of salt is present in the food. This constitutes an experimental demonstration of the interaction of genetic and environmental factors, both of which appear to be concerned in the pathogenesis of essential hypertension.

Evidence reported by PHELAN [10] makes it probable that an additive polygenic inheritance without strongly dominant characters is responsible for blood pressure elevation in our genetically hypertensive rats.

JONES and DOWD of our group have shown that a difference between the blood pressures of our New Zealand strain of spontaneously hypertensive rats and controls is present already at the second post natal day.

If one may compare the life spans of man and rat; at 7 weeks of age, that is one forteenth of a rat life span, our spontaneously hypertensive rats have risen almost to the top

* Wellcome Medical Research Institute, Department of Medicine, Medical School, Dunedin, New Zealand.

level of their mean systolic blood pressures. This time is roughly equivalent to 5 years in man, namely, to one fourteenth of a 70 year life span.

The Japanese strain of rats also have considerable blood pressure increase present at an early age. We may say therefore, that in these strains of rats the hypertension is not to be regarded as a geriatric phenomenon.

In the course of an investigation in man I made a study of about 519 first dgree relatives of substantial hypertensives and of about 290 controls, thought to be representative of the general population. The rise in the blood pressure with age was greater in our first degree relatives than in controls.

This suggests that the rise of blood pressure with age in man is influenced to an important degree by genetic factors as it is in rats with spontaneous genetic hypertension. In man, however, the rise up to frank hypertensive levels occurs at a later stage in the life span.

As in man an important part of the blood pressure elevation in genetically hypertensive rats of the New Zealand and Japanese strains is neurogenically-maintained [6]. The term neurogenically-maintained is used so as to avoid the assumption that there is necesarily an increase in the discharge down sympathetic nerves. An increased response of the cardiovascular system to an unchanged amount of sympathetic nervous discharge could also explain an increased drop of blood pressure or of peripheral resistance after the administration of hexamethonium [3].

Table 1   Pressure baselines of isolated perfused mesenteric arteries from genetic hypertensive (GH) and control normotensive (C) rats.

		Baseline perfusion pressures (mm Hg)	
		GH	C
1.	Blood perfusion no drugs	40.1 ± 2.2	32.4 ± 1.2
2.	Saline perfusion no drugs	27.4 ± 0.9	23.2 ± 0.9
3.	Saline perfusion $+50$ $\mu g/ml$ sodium nitroprusside	26.3 ± 0.9	21.4 ± 0.9
4.	Saline perfusion $+50$ $\mu g/ml$ sodium nitroprusside intestine removed	18.1 ± 1.1	13.7 ± 0.6

(The perfusion rate was 1 ml/min for blood and 2 ml/min for physiological saline. Differences between GH and C rats are significant $p < 0.005$ or 0.001)

When our rats had only modest increases of their blood pressure large doses of hexamethonium brought the blood pressure down to almost the same level as it did in normotensive controls. Since 1961 the blood pressure within the colony has increased considerably and now the hexamethonium floor pressure is higher in rats from the genetic hypertensive colony than it is in the controls, so that the present situation is that there is not only a neurogenically-maintained but also a not neurogenically-maintained factor in the blood pressure elevation.

McGregor and Smirk (1968) [7] showed that perfusions at constant rate of mesenteric blood vessels from our genetic hypertensive and control rats show a significantly higher baseline perfusion pressure with the blood vessels of genetic hypertensives than with controls. This statement applies when the vessels are perfused with blood and when perfused with physiological saline. When sodium nitroprusside (50 $\mu g/ml$) is added to the saline, thus preventing contractile activity of the vascular muscle, the perfusion pressure baseline was 26.3 ± 0.9 mmHg in the genetic hypertensives and 21.4 ± 0.9 mmHg in the controls.

In part the increased baseline peripheral resistance may be due to hypertrophy of blood vessels, this having been suggested as a factor in hypertension by the present speaker (1949) [14], but it may also involve non-contractile elements.

Such findings in the perfused blood vessels of New Zealand rats and by FOLKOW et al. in the Japanese rats with spontaneous hypertension are in agreement with the demonstrations by FOLKOW [4] in essential hypertension patients that, even with full dilatation of forearm blood vessels, there was an increase of the peripheral resistance above the normal.

We now have good evidence that the blood pressure elevation in young rats of our New Zealand strain of spontaneous hypertensives is *not* a Goldblatt-type of hypertension. There is also eividence that essential hypertension in its early stages is not a Goldblatt hypertension. Later it is possible that a Goldblatt-type of hypertension is added on [14] in both genetic hypertensive rats and essential hypertension.

In our New Zealand strain of young genetic hypertensive rats SMIRK and PHELAN [15] showed that the major blood vessels of the kidney do not appear to differ from those of control rats, and up to about six weeks of age they found no change in the renal parenchyma by light microscopy. This corresponds with the findings at an early stage of essential hypertension in man.

McKENZIE and PHELAN [8] showed that in genetic hypertensive rats aged 120 days the plasma renin was less than that in control rats and at aged 90 and at 120 days the renal renin was significantly less in genetic hypertensive than in control rats. HOLLENBERG et al. [5] found that in their patients with uncomplicated essential hypertension the rate of renin secretion was extremely low, being unmeasurable in 3 our of 7 patients. With increasingly advanced renal vascular changes in intra-renal arteries the renal secretion rate of renin increased from 1.1 ± 0.5 in the absence of vascular damage to 5.3 ± 1.1 up to 13.5 ± 1.7 nanograms of angiotensin per ml. of plasma per 3 hours incubation with the increasing grades of vascular injury.

With increasing renal vascular damage there was a corresponding increase in the renin activity in the arterial plasma (nanograms per ml. plasma per 3 hours incubation).

PHELAN and WONG [11] showed that the changes in water and electrolyte composition of the aorta in rats with chronic *renal* hypertension resemble those described by other workers namely, increase in the percentage of water, of sodium and of potassium whereas the aortas removed from our rats with *genetic* hypertension closely approximate in composition to aortas from normotensive control rats. This suggests that we are not dealing with any kind of esoteric change of the Goldblatt-type which might be presumed to be possible even in the absence of the narrowing of the renal blood vessels.

Cross-transfusion experiments, LAVERTY and SMIRK [6], in which an isolated rat hind limb was perfused alternately at constant rate by blood either from a control or from a genetic hypertensive rat, each for periods of 1 hour, revealed no evidence of any circulating pressor substance in the blood of the genetic hypertensives, whereas in acute renal hypertension pressor activity was readily detected.

PHELAN [12] showed that in genetic hypertensive and renal hypertensive rats matched for similar levels of the blood pressure the hexamethonium floor blood pressure—the not neurogenically-maintained part of the blood pressure is significantly greater in the renal than in the genetic hypertensive rats and the neurogenically-maintained part is significantly less in the renal than in the genetic hypertensive.

He also showed that there was a highly significant difference in the responses of genetic and renal hypertensive rats to vasopressin, the larger responses being encountered in the renal hypertensives. Furthermore in Goldblatt hypertension, the norepinephrine content of the brain does not differ from controls; whereas, in our genetic hypertensive rats, there are highly significant increases of norepinephrine in the forebrain and cerebellum and of dopamine in the caudate nucleus.

However, there are some similarities between genetic and renal hypertensive rats. An increased response above the normal of perfused blood vessels is found in both renal and genetic hypertensive rat blood vessels.

It occurs in response to several pressor drugs: epinephrine, norepinephrine, angiotensin, pitressin and 5 hydroxytryptamine.

Several observations in man show that forearm blood vessels are also more reactive to pressor agents in hypertensives than in controls.

Increase in the reactivity of the vascular bed could be an important factor in the development of hypertension by increasing the response to other pressor agents.

Finally, our colleague CLARK [1] has shown that in our genetic hypertensive colony treated by immunosympathectomy the rise of blood pressure with age is greatly reduced, so that the adult blood pressure only rose to 142 mm Hg, whereas untreated litter mates developed blood pressures of 192 mm Hg.

Furthermore, after immunosympathectomy the hexamethonium floor of genetic hypertensive rats was reduced to fully normal levels.

It seems that if you greatly reduce the rise of blood pressure with age by immunosympathectomy you also prevent the increase in the *not* neurogenically-maintained part of the blood pressure.

In other words—it looks as if the neurogenically—maintained part of the blood pressure is primary and the not neurogenically-maintained part is, at least to some extent, secondary.

ACKNOWLEDGEMENTS

This work has been supported by the U.S. Public Health Service Grant HE 10942 from the National Heart and Lung Institute and the Medical Research Council of New Zealand. Thanks are due to Mrs. J. TOMLIN for much secretarial help.

REFERENCES

1. CLARK, D. W. J. (1971): Circ Res, **28**, 330.
2. DAHL, L. K., HEINE, M. and TASSINARI, L. (1962): Nature (London), **194**, 480.
3. DOYLE, A. E. and SMIRK, F. H. (1955): Circulation, **12**, 543.
4. FOLKOW, B. (1956): *In* "Hypotensive Drugs". (M. HARINGTON, ed.) 163, Pergamon Press, London.
5. HOLLENBERG, N. K., EPSTEIN, M., BASCH, R. I., COUCH, N. P., HICKLER, R. B. and MERRILL, J. P. (1969): Am J. Med, **47**, 855.
6. LAVERTY, R. and SMIRK, F. H. (1961): Circ Res, **9**, 455.
7. McGREGOR, D. D. and SMIRK, F. H. (1968): Am J Physiol, **214**, 1429.
8. McKENZIE, J. K. and PHELAN, E. L. (1969): Proc Univ Otago Med Sch, **47**, No. 1, 23.
9. OKAMOTO, K. and AOKI, K. (1963): Jap Circ J, **27**, 282.
10. PHELAN, E. L. (1970): Circ Res, **26** and **27**, Suppl II, 55.
11. PHELAN, E. L. and WONG, L. C. K. (1968): Clin Sci, **35**, 487.
12. PHELAN, E. L. (1966): Am Heart J, **71**, 50.
13. SMIRK, F. H. and HALL, W. H. (1958): Nature (London, **182**, 727.
14. SMIRK, F. H. (1949): Br Med J, **1**, 791.
15. SMIRK, F. H. and PHELAN, E. L. (1965): J Pathol Bacteriol, **89**, 57.

A MOLECULAR BIOLOGIST LOOKS
AT HYPERTENSION

S. UDENFRIEND*

Although investigators have discovered many systems which can elevate the blood pressure, it has long been apparent that no one of these systems is, in itself, the primary cause of the hypertension. The development and widespread distribution of the spontaneous hypertensive rat will, in my mind, prove to be one of the most important advances in this field. In any area of investigation it is not possible for basic scientists to participate significantly until models are available. The concensus of the participants at the symposium is that Professor OKAMOTO and his colleagues have finally come up with an acceptable animal model of essential hypertension.

In the few years that the spontaneous hypertensive rat has been available a number of questions about hypertension have been answered. These were discussed by the earlier participants of the symposium. First, sympathetic nervous activity is not elevated in these animals and is in fact diminished. The same is true of the renin-angiotension system. These findings, which are similar to those observed in patients with essential hypertension, have now been verified in many laboratories. Even if one questions, whether these rats are a correct model of essential hypertension, studies with them have proven conclusively that when the pressure is continuously elevated, sympathetic activity and the renin-angiotension system are depressed. Both changes appear to represent compensatory actions. As such, they provide the biologist with another group of regulatory actions whose mechanisms must be explored.

These compensatory changes are observed in the early stages of hypertension in the spontaneously hypertensive rat. Subsequently, with increasing age and increasing pressure, other changes are observed which also parallel those seen in patients with essential hypertension. There are changes in the heart, in the kidney and in blood vessels. The simple but elegant studies of Freis reported in this Symposium show that a regimen of antihypertensive drugs not only prevents the onset of the above pathologic changes in the spontaneously hypertensive rat but in many other ways maintains the animals in better health. If the same findings can be obtained by lowering blood pressure with a variety of agents, which act by different mechanisms, then we can infer that the continued elevation in blood pressure, in itself, triggers changes which lead to the pathologic lesions. With the spontaneously hypertensive rat it should be possible to dissect these changes and determine the mechanisms involved in each of the pathologies. Thus, it has recently been shown by Ross and BORNSTEIN [1] that the smooth muscle cells of the blood vessels, in the absence of fibroblasts, produce collagen and other fibers. They have further shown that mechanical damage to the blood vessels leads first to a migration of smooth muscle cells towards the lumen of the vessel which is followed by the formation of collagen and other fibers. Finally, there is a depostion of platelets and cholesterol onto the fibers. Thus, we have models for arteriosclerosis and atherosclerosis which are analogous to fibrosis; the response to injury observed in other tissues. The biosynthesis of collagen should become a subject for investigation by those interested in cardiovascular disease. It remains to be seen whether an elevation in blood pressure can in itself produce the damage which initiates the "fibrosis" of the blood vessels. It may well be that as the blood pressure increases above certain values each pulse produces some damage. If this is so, then it provides a rationale for early initiation of antihypertensive therapy.

* Roche Institute of Molecular Biology, Nutley, New Jersey, U.S.A.

The spontaneously hypertensive rat has already set off investigations in many laboratories around the world. Specialized experts in each area of biology, genetics, endocrinology, neurobiology, pharmacology, etc, are becoming more and more interested in studying this animal model. With time we will learn the reason for the hypertension in the experimental animals. I have no doubt that we will also have learned a lot about essential hypertension in man.

REFERENCE

1. Ross, R. and Bornstein, P. (1971): Sci Am, **224**, 44.

INDEX

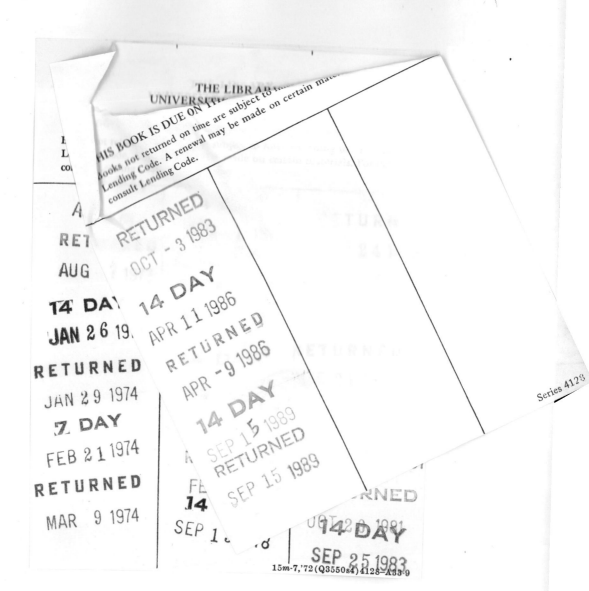